Celiac
Disease

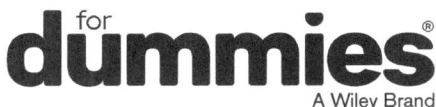

for
dummies®
A Wiley Brand

Celiac Disease

2nd Edition

by Benjamin Lebwohl, MD, MS
Anne Roland Lee, EdD, RD, LD
FOREWORD BY Peter H.R. Green, MD

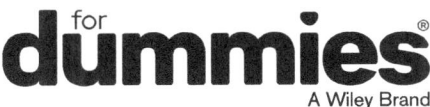

Celiac Disease For Dummies®, 2nd Edition

Published by: **John Wiley & Sons, Inc.,** 111 River Street, Hoboken, NJ 07030-5774, www.wiley.com

Contents at a Glance

Table of Contents

PART 4: THE LONG-TERM: LIVING AND THRIVING WITH CELIAC DISEASE

Foreword

I n 2001, when I founded the Celiac Disease Center at Columbia University, the conventional wisdom was that celiac disease was a rare childhood condition that was readily diagnosed. The subsequent years brought great awareness to the public regarding celiac disease and its manifold symptoms. It can be diagnosed at any age and can go undiagnosed for many years.

Since 2010, when the first edition of *Celiac Disease For Dummies* was published, we have learned more about how common the condition is, how it can affect multiple organ systems, and how to best treat it with a gluten-free diet that strikes a balance between taking key precautions while also maintaining a good quality of life. There has also been an explosion of interest in nondietary therapies — that is, medications — which are in clinical trials. These developments, and more, are covered in this updated edition.

I have known and worked with Ben Lebwohl and Anne Lee for decades. Ben first came to work with me as an aspiring medical student, when I was developing a celiac patient database for research purposes in the late 1990s. Anne's expertise in nutrition was a key part of our center's services from the very beginning. Both are valued partners in our mission to advance care and discovery for those living with celiac disease.

Peter H.R. Green, MD

Phyllis and Ivan Seidenberg Professor of Medicine

Celiac Disease Center at Columbia University

Introduction

When the first edition of *Celiac Disease For Dummies* came out, celiac disease was finally recognized as a common condition worthy of the public's attention. Up until that point, few had ever heard of celiac disease, and, when it was a subject of discussion, the conversation was typically rife with misconceptions, misapprehensions, and misinformation. Compounding this unfortunate scenario was the fact that celiac disease was little taught in medical schools, and, outside of select healthcare disciplines, was off the medical radar.

In more recent years, diagnosis rates of celiac disease have increased, and there's greater awareness of the gluten-free diet than ever before. Still, even with improved recognition, getting diagnosed with celiac disease often involves a long period of symptoms and a road that includes more than a few detours. After a diagnosis, having celiac disease requires constant treatment and vigilance. It's a lifelong condition. So if you think that being dealt a celiac disease diagnosis is patently and profoundly unfair, we won't disagree because you're right; it *is* unfair.

But here's the thing: Although having celiac disease is no piece of cake, the wonderful thing — the *absolutely . . . wonderful . . . thing* — is that you can be entirely healthy with your celiac disease. You can live a full, active, long, and productive life with your celiac disease. You can explore the ocean depths or climb the Himalayas. You can work on the city subway or have a top-floor office in the nearest skyscraper. And, as for celiac disease not being a piece of cake, well, actually you can have a piece of cake . . . so long as it doesn't contain a protein called gluten. As we look at in detail in this book, avoiding gluten is the key to successfully living with celiac disease.

About This Book

We've written this book for people living with celiac disease, and in case you think this phrase is ambiguous, this is by intention because if *one* member of a family has celiac disease, *everyone* in the family is very much living with celiac disease.

Which is all to say that we hope *Celiac Disease For Dummies* is helpful whether you're the one who has celiac disease or you're reading this book because someone you care about — a child, another family member, or another loved one — has the condition.

Throughout this book, when we discuss celiac disease as causing one or another problem, we're typically talking about untreated or insufficiently treated celiac disease. Celiac disease that is properly treated (by, as you will discover, meticulously following a diet free of gluten) typically causes . . . nothing! Also, whenever we use the term *active celiac disease*, we are again referring to celiac disease that is untreated or insufficiently treated, in which case there is still active inflammation in the small intestine.

We hope you find this book helpful, interesting, informative, and even entertaining.

Foolish Assumptions

We have written this book based on the assumption that whatever your knowledge of celiac disease, you want to learn more. Period. If you know nothing about celiac disease you will find this book allows you to readily discover the basics, and if you're already acquainted with the condition, you'll discover additional details to meet your needs.

YOUR HEALTHCARE TEAM

This book is cowritten by Ben and Anne. We work together as a gastroenterologist and dietitian at the Celiac Disease Center at Columbia University in New York City. As you will see throughout this book, the treatment and monitoring of celiac disease requires the expertise of both specialists, with complementary roles.

On the subject of dietitians, throughout this book, we discuss the terribly important role of *registered* dietitians in assisting people living with celiac disease to take charge of their condition by healthy, gluten-free eating. *Registered* dietitians have passed stringent academic requirements and are part of an officially certified healthcare profession. Because it gets awfully repetitious to add the word *registered* before each use of the word *dietitian*, whenever we use the word *dietitian*, we are specifically (*and only*) referring to *registered* dietitians. Similarly, when we use the word *nutritionist*, we are once again using this term interchangeably with *registered dietitian*.

Icons Used in This Book

There exist political, intellectual, social, and goodness knows how many other icons in society. Well, we don't discuss those here! No, the icons we mention here are those that serve as little flags or identifiers — bookmarks if you will — that let you know what information you're going to find in the paragraph that follows.

EXAMPLE

This icon signifies that we're sharing a story about a patient. These stories have been specifically selected because they contain elements that you may well relate to. (The names and other identifiers have been changed to maintain confidentiality.)

TECHNICAL STUFF

This icon indicates we're providing information of a technical nature. You may find this interesting to read, but it isn't fundamental to your understanding of celiac disease.

REMEMBER

When you see this icon, it means the information is essential and you would be well served to pay special attention.

TIP

This icon indicates that we're sharing a practical piece of information that will arm you with a time-saving or grief-avoiding measure.

WARNING

This icon means we're discussing critical issues and that immediate or imminent harm could come to you if the information is overlooked or not heeded.

Beyond the Book

Our online Cheat Sheet contains a quick reference that lists key pieces of information related to the diagnosis and treatment of celiac disease. This includes information on common symptoms, the blood tests used to test for celiac disease, and the basics of the gluten-free diet. You will be able to find the online Cheat Sheet by going to www.dummies.com and searching for **Celiac Disease for Dummies**.

We've also provided meal plans with both vegetarian and vegan options, which are available at www.dummies.com/go/celiacdiseasefd2e.

Where to Go from Here

Celiac Disease For Dummies is written in modular format, which is basically a fancy way of saying that this book is structured so that you can open it to whatever topic interests you at a particular time rather than having it to read it from front to back. Having said that, if you have no familiarity with celiac disease, you may find that reading it in just that way works best for you.

Not sure where to start? Well, recognizing there isn't a bad place to begin your journey of discovery, if you've just been diagnosed and are finding the whole notion of having celiac disease overwhelming, have a look at Chapter 1 to discover the emotional impact of being told you have celiac disease. Alternatively, you may want to flip to Chapter 2 and delve right into a description of the symptoms of celiac disease. Or you may want to get a bird's-eye view and start by reading the Part of Tens chapters. Sure, some of it won't make sense until you've read other parts of the book, but you may still find it the most interesting section of all to read.

1

What Is Celiac Disease, and Why Does It Matter?

Chapter **1**

Finding Out You Have Celiac Disease

When you first find out that you or your loved one has celiac disease, you may be shocked. No one likes to hear bad news, and, as so often happens in this type of situation, you may recall little other than the words *celiac disease* from the conversation you have with your doctor that day.

Over the next few days and weeks, your mind may race nonstop as you mull over your new diagnosis and try to come to grips with it. Or, if the diagnosis is brand new to you, perhaps you are right now in the process of trying to deal with the news.

Celiac Disease For Dummies provides you not just with the facts about celiac disease, but the tools to help you master it. In this chapter, our goal is to help you understand and come to terms with your diagnosis.

Getting to Know Celiac Disease

Celiac disease, also known as celiac sprue, non-tropical sprue, and gluten-sensitive enteropathy, is a condition in which consuming *gluten* — a protein found in wheat, rye, barley, and some other grains — leads, in susceptible people, to damage to the lining of the small intestine, resulting in the inability to properly absorb nutrients into the body. This can lead to many different symptoms, including fatigue, malaise (feeling generally poorly), bloating, and diarrhea. Left untreated or insufficiently treated, celiac disease can lead to damage to other organs. If properly treated, celiac disease typically leads to . . . nothing!

TECHNICAL
STUFF

In your travels, you may see the word *celiac* spelled as *coeliac*. Both terms refer to the same condition. *Celiac* is the spelling far more commonly used in North America and, hence, the spelling we use throughout this book. Incidentally, the term *celiac* (or *coeliac*) comes from the Greek word *Koila*, which refers to the abdomen.

Doctors have known about celiac disease for a long time. Articles describing individuals suffering from diarrhea (most likely due to what we now call celiac disease) first appeared over two thousand years ago. It was, however, Dr. Samuel Gee who, in London, England in 1887, first described the condition in detail and even presciently observed that successful therapy was to be found in changing a patient's diet, although he did not point to gluten as the culprit. That came later (see the "Discovering celiac disease" later in this chapter).

Knowing How Having Celiac Disease Feels

It could well be that you were diagnosed with celiac disease after having been unwell for quite some time. If so, then when you read this section's heading ("Knowing How Having Celiac Disease Feels"), you may have said to yourself, "Hey, I can tell you how it feels. It feels crummy. I had belly pain and I had indigestion and I had . . ." Yup, those things sure can happen. But so too can many other symptoms or, on the other side of the spectrum, few or even no symptoms at all.

In Chapter 2, we look at the whole panoply of symptoms a person with celiac disease can experience. Some of these may lead you to nod your head in recognition (such as the symptoms we just mentioned), and some may take you by surprise (such as discovering the link between celiac disease and conditions as varied as skin rash and infertility).

Dealing with the Diagnosis of Celiac Disease

Some diseases are easy to diagnose. Tell a doctor you have spells where you see flashing lights followed by a throbbing headache, and, dollars to donuts, the doctor will quickly inform you that you may be suffering from migraine headaches.

Diagnosing celiac disease is often not that simple. It involves an interview and examination by a physician and necessitates investigations typically including blood tests and *always* having a fiberoptic scope passed through your mouth, down your esophagus, through your stomach, and into your small intestine where a biopsy is then taken. Okay, we admit, that may not sound particularly pleasant, but as you see in Chapter 3, it ain't so bad at all.

The journey to a diagnosis of celiac disease can take a number of different paths. In Chapter 4, we discuss the different types of celiac disease based on symptoms (or lack thereof). Perhaps you're already aware (and if you're not, you soon will be because it's a recurring theme in this book) of the key role that a nutrient called *gluten* plays in triggering celiac disease. As we discuss in Chapter 5, however, although gluten *triggers* the condition, that's not quite the same as saying it *causes* the condition.

By way of analogy, if ever you were working on your computer and you routinely pressed a key only to suddenly have your computer crash, you could appropriately say that pressing the key *triggered* the crash, but an underlying operating system glitch *caused* the problem in the first place.

What, then, causes celiac disease? The quick answer is we don't know. The more complicated answer is a combination of having a susceptibility to the condition by virtue of your genetic make-up in conjunction with some as yet unknown environmental factor. Chapter 5 contains the full story on the cause, as best we understand it.

Unless people are ill with some sort of gastrointestinal (GI) ailment, they understandably generally think little, if at all, about the incredibly complex processes involved in extracting the good from the food they eat and ridding their bodies of the stuff they don't need. That makes sense. When celiac disease enters your life (either directly or by virtue of a family member now being affected by it), however, having some familiarity with your GI system proves beneficial. Chapter 5 explains how your GI system works when you're healthy and how it malfunctions when you have celiac disease.

DISCOVERING CELIAC DISEASE

The first definitive report of celiac disease was made by Dr. Samuel Gee in London, England in 1887 in his seminal study "On the Coeliac Affection." Dr. Gee astutely observed that "if the patient can be cured at all, it must be by means of diet."

He experimented with various diets and noted that "A child, who was fed upon a quart of the best Dutch mussels daily, throve wonderfully, but relapsed when the season for mussels was over." It is, perhaps no surprise to any parent that Dr. Gee also reported, "Next season (the child) could not be prevailed upon to take them."

By 1950, the link between celiac disease and wheat was finally established. In that year, Dr. Willem-Karel Dicke, a Dutch pediatrician, reported that children with symptoms of celiac disease got better when wheat was removed from their diet.

Dicke was suspicious that wheat was the culprit for decades, but this theory only gained traction during World War II. In 1943, wheat products were in short supply in Holland due to a Nazi blockade. During that time, previously unwell children, now deprived of wheat-based products, had relief from their symptoms with them only to return upon the reintroduction of wheat into their diet after the end of the war.

With his theory validated by these tragic circumstances, Dicke went on to publish his findings regarding gluten as the culprit, and the gluten-free diet as the treatment.

Some people have no symptoms, gastrointestinal or otherwise But even they may end up diagnosed with celiac disease. In Chapter 6, we look at who should be *screened* (tested) for celiac disease and how the screening should be done.

As we mentioned earlier in this chapter, if left untreated or insufficiently treated, celiac disease can not only make you feel unwell, but it can lead to serious damage to your body (including causing complications like osteoporosis, anemia, and more).

In Chapter 7, we take a detailed look at these potential complications and how to avoid them. In Chapter 8, we look at the many ailments that are not directly caused by celiac disease but are *associated* with it. We describe the kinds of symptoms these ailments cause and the symptoms to which you should pay the most heed.

For many people, the most feared complication of celiac disease is cancer. Thankfully, celiac disease seldom leads to this, but it can. In Chapter 9, we make you aware of the types of cancer that are linked to celiac disease and, most important, early warning signs for which you should keep a close watch.

Treating Celiac Disease

Celiac disease can make you feel unwell. It can be a hassle to live with. It can cause complications, including damage to your body. *Oh joy.* So now the good news: *You* have ultimate power over this condition. Even better, this power is derived not from taking a truckload of pills — or, indeed, any pills at all; no, this power is derived from you modifying your diet to eliminate any and all gluten.

Modifying your diet to eliminate gluten intake, however, isn't simple and requires lots of work and, like they say about the price of freedom, eternal vigilance. In Chapter 10, we look in detail at what constitutes a gluten-free diet and provide all sorts of tips to help you make the necessary changes to the way you eat and how you eat. And, speaking of vigilance, we also look at hidden sources of gluten for which you should be on the lookout.

When it comes to celiac disease, gluten is the most important nutrient that affects the health of your GI system, but it's not the only one. As you see in Chapter 11, celiac disease can lead to low iron levels and difficulty digesting certain milk products (a condition called *lactose intolerance*).

Sometimes, despite carefully following a gluten-free diet, a person continues to feel unwell. Could it be that gluten is sneaking its way into your diet? Or could it be, perhaps, that you don't have celiac disease (doctors do make mistakes, including mistaken diagnoses) or that you have an additional ailment that's causing your symptoms. In Chapter 12 we explore these possibilities.

Living and Thriving with Celiac Disease

Perhaps it's been some time since you were diagnosed with celiac disease and you're nicely on track with your gluten-free existence. What then? Do you need to be monitored for celiac disease-related health issues? If so, how should the monitoring be done? Chapter 13 describes the ongoing care of celiac disease and ways that you can continue to empower yourself.

Although people living with celiac disease share many similar challenges, differences exist for some people based on age, living condition (home or in a college dorm for instance), and special circumstances such as attempting to conceive, or being pregnant. Chapter 14 covers living — and thriving — with celiac disease in these situations.

Better ways of managing celiac disease may emerge in the future. Indeed, there may come a time when you may not need to follow a gluten-free diet. In Chapter 15, we explore these and other possible options for dealing with celiac disease that may come about someday.

Handling the News

From the time you were first told you (or your loved one) had celiac disease until the time you picked up and started reading this book, you probably have experienced many different feelings and conflicting emotions.

If you were feeling poorly — especially if this had been going on for a long time — with typical symptoms of celiac disease (we discuss these in Chapter 2), you likely felt relief that the cause of your troubles was identified and that treatment would make you feel better. At the same time, you may have been understandably upset that you had been saddled with a diagnosis for which there is no cure. All these feelings are perfectly normal.

In this section, we look at a few of the different types of feelings that people experience after being diagnosed with celiac disease.

Experiencing denial

Your first reaction upon being told that you had celiac disease may have been surprise; indeed, you may have been stunned. And it could be that, as the impact of being told you had this life-changing disease sunk in, you doubted it could be the case.

"Me? Celiac disease? No way," you may have said to yourself or others.

You may have then looked up information online and found that your symptoms didn't match all of those listed on some sites; this may have provided additional justification to your feelings of denial.

But you still weren't feeling as well as you should or your lab tests showed you were deficient in certain nutrients, or your bone density was low (as seen with osteoporosis), or you had some other feature of celiac disease which, try as you might, wasn't going to disappear. Eventually, you likely came — perhaps grudgingly — to accept that you had the condition. Or perhaps as you read this book, you have only recently been diagnosed and you still can't believe it. Either way, these feelings are perfectly natural.

Being angry

If you felt angry after you were told you had celiac disease, rest assured, this is normal and perfectly understandable. You've got enough going on in your life without being told there is another issue you have to contend with.

Having celiac disease isn't like having a strep throat or bladder infection that will quickly go away after a few days of antibiotics; if you have celiac disease today, you will have it tomorrow and next week and next month and next year, too. And who wants that? Nobody.

It's also perfectly understandable to be angered by the "work" of having celiac disease. All of a sudden, you need to spend far greater effort when shopping and cooking, not to mention the additional expense of buying food that's gluten-free. Also, in addition to the usual considerations regarding fat content, calories, sodium, and so forth, you now also need to scrutinize everything you eat to ensure that it doesn't have gluten.

The diagnosis of celiac disease may not be what led to anger. You may be angry that the diagnosis wasn't made earlier. Many people go months or even years, feeling unwell all the time, before their celiac disease is discovered. During this time, other, incorrect diagnoses may have been made or people may have been told that their problem was "all in your head" or "due to nerves." No wonder a person in this situation feels frustrated or angry.

Another source of anger arises when a person with a delayed diagnosis reflects on the lost opportunity to have prevented complications from celiac disease (such as, for example, osteoporosis).

By the way, we are not casting stones here. Celiac disease is a condition that can both mimic and masquerade as many other diseases and a delayed or missed diagnosis is not uncommon; indeed, many an excellent physician has overlooked this diagnosis.

Regardless of the source of your anger, feeling angry isn't useful. Eventually, anger has to be left behind so that you can get on with your life and get back to and maintain a state of good health.

Feeling sad and taking time to mourn

Feeling sad upon hearing bad news is perfectly understandable and normal. A diagnosis of celiac disease is experienced by some as a loss, who mourn the ending of the "before times" when they didn't have to think about gluten when traveling or eating in restaurants. You may find, however, that if you've been feeling unwell (especially if it's been for quite some time), your sadness will be mixed with relief now that treatment will get you feeling better in short order. You should realize, however, that even after your celiac disease symptoms are controlled, you may at times feel sad that you have celiac disease. With time, that too will pass.

Taking the next step

Regardless of what feelings you experience after finding out you have celiac disease, none of them have gotten your symptoms to go away or your blood tests to normalize, and now you're ready to take the bull by the horns and deal with your diagnosis. As you learn the ins and outs of living a gluten-free existence, don't get mad at yourself if, from time to time, some of your old angst shows up. That is normal and will pass.

When you're feeling down or frustrated or simply upset at having celiac disease, you may find the following coping strategies helpful:

>> **Be a positive thinker.** Focus on how much better you will feel once you're following a gluten-free diet or, if you're already on treatment, how much better you already feel. Unlike so many other diseases, you have the power to control things without requiring medication.

>> **Know that you're not alone.** Recognize that there are healthcare professionals — most importantly, dietitians — who are there to help you learn what you need to know. You're not on your own!

>> **Involve your family.** As you learn about living gluten-free, you can share your newfound knowledge about nutrition with your partner and your children. You will find that you are — or will shortly become — a true nutrition resource! Also, involving your family allows them to provide you with the support and encouragement you may need and want from time to time.

>> **Seek out a celiac disease community.** Find a support group, either one that meets in your community or online. We discuss online support groups in the next section.

Finding Information and Support on the Internet

We certainly hope that you will find this book a helpful tool to assist you in your quest to find out more about your celiac disease, but we also recognize that a vast amount of additional information is available online.

Some of the information you find online is good, and some is, to put it charitably, not quite as good (or downright awful to be quite frank). In this section, we look at how you can use the web to find more information about celiac disease and how you can seek out Internet support groups to lend you a hand when you need it.

Knowing whether an Internet site is reputable

Okay, sure, sometimes it's obvious when an Internet site is not to be trusted, like if you were to come across a site called `www.wesellusedcarsandwealsocure celiacdisease.com`. But most of the time, it's not nearly so easy to tell whether you've reached a cutting edge, state-of-the-art site, or one that is far less reputable.

A website that is credible and provides reliable information and advice (recognizing that, of course, none of these criteria guarantees the site will be sound) generally does the following:

» **Reports facts objectively:** The site provides information in an even-handed way and avoids sensationalism.

» **Relies on science:** The site doesn't rely on testimonials to the exclusion of science. An unusual or unique treatment that appeared to help a person with celiac disease isn't proof that it worked; perhaps the person got better for an unrelated reason.

» **Uses ads responsibly:** The site doesn't have advertising or, if it does, the ads, like the site, are not over-the-top declarations encouraging you to buy "instant cure" miracle-type products.

» **Aims primarily to inform, not to sell:** If the site is run by a scientific organization, hospital, healthcare clinic, or recognized expert on celiac disease, the site is likely very reputable. If the site is owned and run by a company that is marketing a product, question whether the information on the site is appropriately dispassionate and even-handed. Such company-owned sites may be perfectly reasonable and good sources of information; it's just necessary to question it, that's all.

» **Identifies its author:** The author or authors of the site are identified and, ideally, the site provides background information regarding important details such as their professional qualifications and academic affiliations (if any).

TIP

Google the names of a site's authors. You may discover an author has written hundreds of scientific articles, which is good, or you may discover that they've just lost their medical license because of incompetence — which is, well, bad.

>> **Uses verifiable facts:** Information on the site is referenced or at least supported by verifiable facts rather than just being "stream of consciousness" opinion. Also, if the site quotes scientific studies, check to see whether they were published in obscure-sounding journals; they may be obscure for good reason. (Although, of course, some excellent scientific journals have unusual names.)

>> **Does *not* engage in conspiracy thinking:** If the site talks about conspiracies among the medical community or "big business" or government or some other organization said to be participant in some Machiavellian scheme to "hide the cure" to celiac disease, then you should take a pass on the site.

In Appendix D, we list some helpful and reputable organizations with extensive online resources.

Finding an online celiac disease support group

An Internet-based support group (which, depending on the specific nature of the group, may also be referred to as a discussion group, discussion forum, or chat group) is a place where people affected by a condition, either directly because they have it or indirectly because a loved one has it, can exchange thoughts, ideas, facts, and suggestions. These may be freestanding or may be a group within a social media platform such as Facebook.

Support groups are designed to provide support. That is, however, just the tip of the iceberg. Indeed, support groups provide myriad other functions above and beyond this. They can also have their downsides, however. In the sections that follow, we look at these issues.

Understanding how an online support group can help you

An online support group can help you by providing the following:

>> **Other people's stories:** If you don't know other people with celiac disease and as a result are feeling isolated, reading other peoples' stories about how they have been affected by celiac disease can help you realize that you're not the only person out there battling the condition.

>> **Patient-provided tips:** You can find many tips that others with celiac disease have posted regarding helpful shopping, cooking, and other "living with celiac disease" topics. For example, a person may have discovered a great place to

buy gluten-free foods (either online or at a bricks-and-mortar store) and may be keen to share this information.

>> **Opportunities to share your story:** You may find it cathartic or stress-relieving to share with others your own trials and tribulations with celiac disease.

>> **Encouragement:** Support groups are designed to provide support! Having a bad day? Feeling fed-up with living gluten-free? Let the group know, and you'll likely find members quickly commiserate and encourage you to keep up your efforts.

>> **Opportunities to help others:** You can gain satisfaction by helping others if you share your own how-to tips with the cybercommunity.

>> **Success stories:** If celiac disease is new to you, you may find it reassuring to read postings from people who have successfully lived with celiac disease for many years.

>> **Substitute for a "real" support group:** Local, "real" (as opposed to online) support groups are less common than they were 20 years ago and may not be available nearby. Online forums allow you to still participate in group discussion and to do so at times that are convenient for you.

>> **Multi-language support:** You may be able to find discussion groups that converse in the language in which you are most comfortable.

>> **Resource to take to your doctor:** If you're having symptoms of one sort or another, you may find postings describing similar issues and what was eventually found to be their cause. You could then ask your healthcare provider if your symptoms, too, might be attributable to this.

Recognizing the downsides of online support groups

Like the web in general, online support groups have both upsides (see the immediately preceding section) and downsides. Here are some of these downsides and what you can do to avoid these pitfalls:

>> **Question your sources.** Anyone can post to a discussion forum. *Anyone.* You could be reading a posting that has been written by a well-informed, knowledgeable, well-meaning individual who has something important to share . . . or you could be reading a posting by someone who is ill-informed and is sharing nothing more than misinformation.

>> **Avoid endless complainers.** Some people participate in a support group for no other reason than because they've got an axe to grind. Although

sometimes reading about someone else's complaints can be helpful in its own way, to read complaint after complaint after complaint can get to be a real downer.

>> **Scrutinize sales pitches.** Online support groups may contain postings by people whose main goal is to try to sell you something, whether or not the product is of proven value or benefit.

>> **Turn away sites dominated by a few individuals.** Online support groups may have posting after posting after posting by a single or small group of individuals who dominate, take over, and hijack discussions.

>> **Leave mean-spirited groups.** Support group postings sometimes degenerate into nothing more than name calling, insults, and other derogatory rants. Not a pretty sight (or site!).

TIP

Look for support groups that are moderated; that is, they have someone (typically a well-meaning, reasonable, and knowledgeable person) who supervises the postings and removes those that fall below or outside an appropriate minimum standard.

Looking at "Real" (Non-Virtual) Support Groups

Regardless of whether you elect to participate in an online support group, we recommend you consider joining a local, non-virtual-world group. By participating in such a group, you can do the following:

>> **Get to know real people.** You get to meet in the flesh other people living with celiac disease. Getting to know snippets of someone's life by reading postings online is one thing; spending time with a "real" person is quite another.

>> **Expand your conversations.** Spending time with others allows you to have expanded conversations not constrained by the limitations of interacting exclusively online. Online postings are, by their very nature, typically a few sentences long and necessarily limited in scope.

>> **Meet people who know your locale.** Local people live locally! The great benefit of meeting local people is that your neighbors likely know the best places in your community to buy gluten-free foods, the most knowledgeable and helpful dietitians and doctors, and so much more.

>> **Mobilize the group to work together.** There is strength in numbers. The group can order food items in bulk to minimize shipping charges and can then divide up the goods among the people that ordered the product; that way, you (and the others) can help avoid storing large amounts of a product that you may use only occasionally. The power of a group can also be helpful in persuading a local health food or specialty food store to stock their shop with gluten-free products that the group identifies as tasty and worth having available locally.

>> **Participate in organized activities.** Participating in such group activities allows you to learn the "gluten-free" ropes of shopping, cooking, and eating out while making new friends and acquaintances. Local support groups often organize helpful events such as

- Cooking demonstrations
- Food tastings
- Restaurant outings
- Seasonal parties

>> **Attend presentations.** Support groups often invite speakers to talk with the group. A speaker may be a celiac disease specialist, dermatologist (skin specialist), dietitian, or a nurse who specializes in celiac disease.

>> **Join a well-managed support group.** People participating in a real support group are less likely to dominate and take over conversations than what you find on some online forums.

>> **Get real, live human support.** Sometimes, in moments when you're feeling down, a real hug can feel a heck of a lot better than another hour staring at a screen.

TIP

Here are a few ways you can find a local support group:

>> **Ask your healthcare provider.** Ask your dietitian or celiac disease specialist.

>> **Look up the listings.** If you live in the United States, have a look at the state-by-state listings on the National Celiac Association website: `https://nationalceliac.org/celiac-disease-support-groups`. You can also find a directory of Gluten Intolerance Group local support groups at `https://gluten.org/community/support-groups`. Other suggestions are listed in Appendix D.

IN THIS CHAPTER

» Exploring gastrointestinal symptoms of celiac disease

» Finding out how celiac disease can lead to weight loss

» Looking at skin rashes

» Assessing mood, thinking, and neurological symptoms

» Evaluating endocrine (hormonal) problems

» Discovering symptoms caused by musculoskeletal conditions and other organs

Chapter **2**

Examining Symptoms of Celiac Disease

When we speak to groups of people with celiac disease, we are struck by the fact that the label — celiac disease — is often the only thing that the roomful of people has in common. All people with celiac disease have their individual stories, journeys with celiac disease and, in the case of symptoms, personal ways in which the condition has affected them.

As you read through this chapter, you may recognize symptoms you've been experiencing. In that case, take heart; if you've not yet begun your gluten-free diet or if you've only very recently started it, once you're on track with your new diet, you will likely find your symptoms soon start to ease. In other words, throughout this chapter when we say that celiac disease causes this or that symptom, we are — unless we specifically state otherwise — invariably talking about *untreated* or *insufficiently treated* celiac disease.

Many people with celiac disease recognize just how bad and just how long they've been feeling unwell only *after* they've been diagnosed and treated and their symptoms have started to ease. That is, their symptoms had been present for so long, they had simply become "part of the wallpaper." (Sort of like after your car has had a tune up and you only then notice a conspicuous absence of a longstanding rattle has suddenly disappeared.)

Some of our patients tell us this makes them feel guilty — as if they did something wrong by ignoring their symptoms. They feel badly that if they had mentioned their symptoms to their doctor earlier, they would have been diagnosed — and therefore, felt better — sooner.

If you feel this way, we hope your guilt quickly falls by the wayside. First, perhaps you're just stoic. Second, it's perfectly reasonable that you might have attributed such everyday symptoms as stomach upset or abdominal cramps that *everyone* (whether one has celiac disease or not) gets from time to time to something else. Third, guilt isn't going to make you feel any better, so there's no point in dwelling on the past.

Symptoms 101: Looking at the Big Picture

Because celiac disease can be such a many-headed hydra, it's important to recognize that there isn't one set of symptoms that reliably points to a diagnosis of celiac disease. Though "classical" symptoms refer to diarrhea and weight loss, this is more of an historical reference. Today, the substantial majority of people with celiac disease have what is called the "nonclassical" form of the disease. We discuss the classification of celiac disease in detail in Chapter 4, but with regard to symptoms, here are the key attributes of these types:

>> **Classical celiac disease** is associated with gastrointestinal symptoms such as abdominal bloating and discomfort, diarrhea, and weight loss.

>> **Non-classical celiac disease** may have gastrointestinal (GI) symptoms such as bloating or constipation. However, it also may not have any GI symptoms and instead have symptoms due to complications from celiac disease being the predominant features.

>> **Silent celiac disease** does not cause symptoms.

As this list indicates, it is only the classical and nonclassical forms of celiac disease that cause symptoms.

Gut Feelings: Gastrointestinal Symptoms

If you've been experiencing gastrointestinal symptoms, but, out of embarrassment, have been hesitant to see your doctor about them, you're certainly not alone. Indeed, lots of people find themselves in this same boat. Doctors, however, are *never* embarrassed discussing GI symptoms, and your doctor's comfort with this will soon put you at ease, too. (In fact, GI specialists have been known to say, "It may be poop to you, but it's bread and butter to me!" Well, actually, they word it somewhat less, ahem, tastefully, but we've edited the saying for this family-oriented book.)

EXAMPLE

Jerry was a 25-year-old man who hadn't been feeling well for quite some time. He was feeling constantly bloated, and he was spending lots of the time in the bathroom with diarrhea. He had put off seeing a doctor, initially because he had hoped things would clear up on their own and, when they didn't, because he thought he'd be embarrassed talking about his bowel habits. As it turned out, it took less than 30 seconds for him to realize he'd had no reason to fear; the discussion with his family doctor was no more embarrassing than had they been talking about the weather. Jerry's physician astutely concluded that Jerry's symptoms were not to be passed off and referred Jerry to a gastroenterologist for further investigation. The gastroenterologist discovered Jerry was also having problems with excess burping, heartburn, and flatulence (*farting* in nonmedical speak). Testing included a blood test for tissue transglutaminase, which was elevated. Jerry underwent an endoscopy and small intestine biopsy (we discuss these procedures in Chapter 3), which confirmed the diagnosis. Jerry was placed on a gluten-free diet and within a short period of time, he felt like new.

The gut stops here: Diarrhea, celiac disease, and you

Diarrhea is the frequent passage of watery or semiformed stools. Pretty well everyone — whether they have celiac disease or not — gets diarrhea from time to time, often from relatively harmless (but decidedly unpleasant) conditions such as viral gastroenteritis ("stomach flu").

Loosely speaking: Diarrhea due to celiac disease

Diarrhea is the symptom of celiac disease that is best known to the world at large. It often comes as a surprise to most people — including many doctors — when they learn that more than 50 percent of people with celiac disease *have no diarrhea at all*; indeed, for some people living with celiac disease, the main bowel problem is that of constipation! Contrary to popular belief, diarrhea is no longer considered a hallmark of this disease.

Of those people with celiac disease who do get diarrhea, its nature can vary to a great extent — both between people and even for a given person. If you have diarrhea, it could be that you've noticed that you have some days where you feel that you're spending the entire day on the toilet and other days where you could be a hundred miles from the nearest bathroom and care not a whit (well, passing urine aside).

If you have not been diagnosed with celiac disease and you see your doctor to report that you are having alternating constipation and diarrhea, your doctor may not have celiac disease high up on their radar as a possible cause for your problem. Instead, they're more likely to consider irritable bowel syndrome (or IBS; which we discuss in Chapter 12). This is perfectly understandable because IBS is a very common cause of these kinds of symptoms. Nonetheless, it can't hurt for you to mention — especially if you're not responding sufficiently well to treatment for IBS and have never been tested for celiac disease — that you've read (here) that celiac disease can also cause these symptoms. Who knows; perhaps you will end up being responsible for figuring out your own diagnosis?

Celiac disease does *not* cause blood to appear in or on the stool. If you see blood with your stool, you should let your doctor know. It may be that there's nothing going on beyond some minor problems with hemorrhoids, but much more serious causes exist, including colon cancer. Blood in the stool is not a symptom to be ignored.

An absorbing discussion about malabsorption

Some people, especially those with the classical form of celiac disease, have severe, unremitting diarrhea. This can be evidence of *malabsorption*. Malabsorption is a condition in which one is unable to properly absorb nutrients from food. If you malabsorb fat, the fat you eat stays in your intestine and — it has to go somewhere — becomes part of your stool. Having stool that contains fat is called *steatorrhea*. If you have steatorrhea, your stools are liquidy. These fatty stools tend to stick to the toilet bowl, so you may find yourself needing to get a brush to scrape off the remnants of your trip to the bathroom, lest the next visitor get an eyeful. Other features of steatorrhea are that the stools are bulky and include oil droplets.

Eating when you're suffering from severe malabsorption is like filling your car's gas tank only to find the fuel gauge showing you're nearly empty because you have a hole in your tank. The gas goes in but gets drained out without being used; your food goes in but also does not get used, and the nutrients are instead passed out of your body with your stool.

Malabsorption isn't an all-or-none phenomenon. Some people with celiac disease — especially children with the classic form — have severe malabsorption and, as a result, lose a great deal of ingested nutrients from the body. This can result in loss of muscle mass, fat stores, fatigue, lethargy, and weight loss. In children, this can lead to an overall picture where development and growth has slowed (see the, "Failure to Thrive in Children" section later in this chapter). Much more commonly, however, malabsorption is selective, with only a limited variety and amount of nutrients (particularly iron) being lost from the body and with virtually no symptoms being present. This is seen in many people with the nonclassical form of celiac disease. Because of the frequent absence of symptoms, it's often only after a routine blood test done at an annual checkup or for some other, coincidental reason comes back abnormal that the diagnosis of celiac disease eventually gets made.

Treating diarrhea due to celiac disease

The mainstay of treating diarrhea (and other bowel complaints) due to celiac disease is to follow a gluten-free diet. Within a few weeks of getting on track with your diet, you will likely notice an improvement in your bowel troubles. It may, however, take months before things are back to normal. If your symptoms don't settle, then you and your healthcare providers will need to determine whether some other problem is going on. Considerations, which we discuss in detail in Chapter 12, include

>> Having some other, coexisting intestinal problem (such as irritable bowel syndrome)

>> Having a complication from your celiac disease (such as lactose intolerance)

>> An incorrect diagnosis of celiac disease

>> Ongoing, typically inadvertent, ingestion of gluten

Olfactory challenges: Sniffing out the importance of flatulence

One of our favorite pieces of trivia is the fact that the average adult farts 10 to 20 times per day. Although everyone (yup, *everyone* — even presidents, prime ministers, and princes, not that we know firsthand mind you) routinely passes gas, people with celiac disease can be particularly prone to flatulence.

When it comes to celiac disease, there is no classical or typical pattern of flatulence. Note that if you're passing more wind than the last Nor'easter, it's likely you have a problem with your gut (celiac disease or otherwise), but the absence of lots of flatus doesn't necessarily mean that all is well and, in particular, doesn't rule out the possibility you have celiac disease.

Flatus is caused by bacteria in the large intestine acting on undigested or incompletely digested food (specifically, carbohydrates) that's made its way down to the colon after not being absorbed into the body by the small intestine. As the large intestinal bacteria munch on the nutrients that have come their way, they produce gasses, including the infamous hydrogen sulfide that is the main cause of flatus' malodor.

TIP

If you have steatorrhea (see the preceding section), your gas may be particularly malodorous. This can be an important clue for your doctor, so share this — so to speak — with them, and don't feel embarrassed (see the preceding anecdote to find out why).

Abdominal symptoms: Belly pain, bloating, and beyond

As with flatus (see the preceding section), every person on the planet experiences abdominal symptoms of one sort of another from time to time. When it comes to celiac disease, however, abdominal symptoms are often much more of a problem. They may even be part and parcel of your existence.

TECHNICAL
STUFF

When we consider abdominal symptoms, in addition to well-known and commonly understood terms (like cramps), there are a few other, sometimes misconstrued terms worth looking at:

>> **Abdomen:** The part of your body between your chest and your pelvis. We mention this to differentiate it from your stomach which, of course, is the organ connecting your esophagus and (small) intestine.

For example, if you were to mention to a healthcare provider that you're having "stomach pain," how your words are interpreted may be very different than if you were to mention you're having "abdominal pain." Many people use these two terms interchangeably, and most healthcare providers recognize this. Nonetheless, to avoid confusion, it's best to just use the word "abdomen" unless you are very certain your symptom really is coming specifically from your stomach (which, by the way, is often exceptionally difficult to know).

>> **Bloating:** The symptom of feeling that your abdomen is overly full. Typically, if someone says they feel bloated, they're referring to a feeling of fullness as if they have too much gas in the intestine, but the term is also used by people to describe a similar feeling due to other causes, such as feeling overly full with food or feeling constipated.

>> **Abdominal distension:** The physical equivalent to the symptom of bloating. In other words, bloating is something that a doctor observes when they examine you. Having said that, the word *distension* is also often (and perfectly legitimately) used synonymously and interchangeably with the term *bloating*.

Bloating (and, therefore, abdominal distension) due to celiac disease is typically most bothersome after a meal but can also be present even if you haven't recently eaten. Although bloating is not a life-threatening symptom, it can be very unpleasant and can interfere with your everyday function. Marked and persistent abdominal distension used to be seen quite often in very young children affected by severe celiac disease, but thankfully this seldom happens nowadays because children with celiac disease are typically diagnosed (and treated) much earlier in the process than used to be the case.

Abdominal cramps are sharp, often piercing, pains that can be felt in a variety of places. They are typically fleeting, lasting from seconds to minutes. Cramps are usually caused by contractions of the intestine; as the contraction relaxes, the discomfort eases. Passing flatus sometimes also helps ease a cramp, which you probably know from personal experience.

ABDOMINAL SYMPTOMS AND THE MISDIAGNOSIS OF CELIAC DISEASE

Abdominal symptoms from celiac disease don't have features that are specific to this particular condition, which is part of the reason that celiac disease so often gets overlooked. Perhaps you had the experience, before your celiac disease was diagnosed, of telling your healthcare provider that you were having abdominal discomfort, bloating, and so on, and you were then misdiagnosed with some other ailment like, for example, irritable bowel syndrome (IBS). If so, you're in good company because this happens all the time. All we can say is that we hope that as both healthcare providers and healthcare recipients become more aware that celiac disease is so common, and how often celiac disease presents with nonclassical features (see Chapter 4 for a discussion of the different types of celiac disease), that they will have a heightened level of alertness to look out for this condition, and the condition will be more quickly diagnosed.

Reflux and heartburn

Reflux is a condition in which acid from within the stomach passes back up into the esophagus (as shown in Chapter 5, the esophagus is the swallowing tube that connects the mouth to the stomach) giving rise to a burning feeling behind the breastbone (sternum). Reflux is common in the general population and may be even more common in people with celiac disease. Eosinophilic esophagitis, an allergic condition that affects the esophagus, can cause heartburn as well as the sensation of food being stuck in the chest after it's been swallowed. It may be more common in people with celiac disease.

TECHNICAL STUFF

Reflux is the short form for *gastroesophageal reflux*. If someone has chronic problems with reflux, the condition is called *gastroesophageal reflux disease* (or GERD).

As we discuss in Chapter 5, the stomach produces acid, which helps to digest food. How much acid is in the stomach? Well, the stomach produces so much hydrochloric acid that stomach fluid is, brace for this fact, 1,000,000 times more acidic than water.

The stomach has special protective mechanisms so that all this acid doesn't normally damage the stomach lining. (When this mechanism fails, people are susceptible to stomach ulcers.) The esophagus, however, doesn't have these same protective features; as a result, it's susceptible to damage from acid. To protect the esophagus from being exposed to the stomach's acid, the part of the esophagus that attaches to the stomach has a valvelike feature (called the *lower esophageal sphincter*) that blocks the stomach acid from entering. When this valve is weak, acid travels up from the stomach into the esophagus and damages it, giving rise to the symptom of heartburn.

Most people, regardless of whether they have celiac disease, experience reflux and heartburn from time to time — particularly after a large meal or drinking more than their fair share of coffee. Heartburn is more likely to be a problem as a person enters middle age. Heartburn is also particularly common during pregnancy.

Nondrug therapy

If you have celiac disease, you may be more prone to reflux and, therefore, heartburn. The reflux (and heartburn) may be present both more often and more persistently. Following a gluten-free diet can help lessen your reflux but often is insufficient.

Here are some nondrug therapies that may help ease your symptoms:

>> Avoid ingesting — or, at the least, limit the consumption of — those things that trigger your symptoms, such as caffeine and spicy foods.

>> Avoid overeating — especially in the late evening before going to bed. (When you're lying down, you're especially prone to reflux because you don't have gravity helping to keep acid in the stomach and out of your esophagus.)

>> Avoid excessive liquid intake for a few hours before going to bed.

>> Try to lose weight if you are overweight. (Being overweight is a contributory factor leading to reflux.)

Drug therapy

Despite the measures we just discussed, many people still have problematic symptoms. In this case, a variety of medications are available to help you, including the following:

>> **Antacids:** Antacids —including Maalox, Mylanta, and many others — can be obtained without a prescription and are often an excellent treatment choice if you get heartburn just occasionally.

>> **H$_2$ blockers:** Many H$_2$ blockers are available over the counter and have various trade names, such as cimetidine (Tagamet) and famotidine (Pepcid and Zantac 360). These drugs can be used on an "as needed basis" to treat an episode of heartburn or, under a doctor's supervision, on a routine basis to prevent heartburn. Some of these can be obtained without a prescription.

>> **Proton pump inhibitors:** Proton pump inhibitors are especially potent at suppressing acid production from the stomach and have become very popular therapies. They go by a variety of names, including dexlansoprazole (Dexilant), esomeprazole (Nexium), lansoprazole (Prevacid), omeprazole (Prilosec and Zegerid), pantoprazole (Protonix), and rabeprazole (Aciphex). Some of these can be obtained without a prescription.

>> **Potassium competitive acid blockers:** This newest class of drugs — vonoprazan, or brand name Voquenza — is even more potent that proton pump inhibitors. It can be obtained only by prescription.

We recommend that if you get just occasional heartburn, you take an antacid or an H$_2$ blocker when you need to. If your problem occurs regularly, follow the nondrug preventative strategies in the preceding section. If, however, your heartburn is occurring frequently or is particularly bothersome for you, speak to your doctor about whether you might benefit from taking a proton pump inhibitor or potassium competitive acid blocker.

WARNING

Rarely, people with severe and intractable reflux that the recurring presence of stomach acid in your esophagus leads to scarring and, eventually, narrowing of the esophagus (a *stricture*). If this happens, you will have difficulty swallowing solid foods such as bread or steak because the food can get stuck in your esophagus. You typically experience this as a sudden pain behind the lower part of your sternum that comes on as you are eating. The pain eventually eases as the food finally passes through the obstruction. If you experience this symptom, be sure to mention it to your doctor so that they can determine if you have a stricture. Whether you have a stricture is typically determined by performing an endoscopy. An endoscopy can also determine whether you have eosinophilic esophagitis, which can cause difficulty swallowing and, sometimes, strictures (we discuss this procedure in Chapter 3).

Indigestion

Indigestion (*dyspepsia*) is a common gastrointestinal symptom of celiac disease. Though indigestion can be defined in many different ways, most commonly it refers to an aching, uncomfortably full, or burning discomfort which typically occurs after eating. The sensation is in the upper part of the abdomen (as opposed to GERD where the main symptom is a burning behind the breastbone).

Pretty well everyone, whether having celiac disease or not, experiences indigestion from time to time (think third helping of Thanksgiving turkey, or beer and pizza when out with friends). If you have celiac disease, however, you are more prone to indigestion, and it may occur without any obvious food overindulgence.

Many people with celiac disease have put up with years of bothersome indigestion only to have it nearly vanish within a few months of starting a gluten-free diet. Indeed, eliminating gluten from your diet will likely be the only therapy you require.

Weight Loss

Until the developments of recent years when much has been learned, it had been thought that celiac disease was primarily a childhood ailment, and it was almost always associated with weight loss. Although this is true of what is called *classical celiac disease*, it is, in fact, not true of the majority of people with celiac disease, most of whom have *non-classical celiac disease* (see Chapter 4 for a discussion on the classification of celiac disease) and do not experience weight loss. Having said all this, weight loss in adults with celiac disease can and does occur and, if it happens to you, it's important that you are aware of the possible causes.

When you lose weight due to celiac disease, you typically lose no more than a few pounds and have no cause for alarm. If, however, you are losing substantial amounts of weight, you should seek medical attention right away.

Looking at the issue of weight loss in four different settings is helpful. Weight loss can be caused by

>> Active celiac disease

>> Dietary changes once a person starts following a gluten-free diet

>> A coexisting condition

>> Complications from celiac disease

In the next few sections, we look at each of these scenarios.

Weight loss due to active celiac disease

Having active celiac disease — that is, ongoing damage to the small intestine — can lead to weight loss from two main causes:

>> **Loss of appetite:** Celiac disease can make you feel generally crummy, which means you may not have much of an appetite. That, in turn, will lead you to eat less. This reduced intake of calories will result in weight loss.

>> **Malabsorption:** As we discuss earlier in this chapter in the section, "An absorbing discussion about malabsorption," celiac disease damages the small intestine, which is the place that nutrients are absorbed into your body. If you have a reduced ability to absorb these nutrients *into* your body, they — and the calories they contain — are then lost *from* your body with your stool. This is called *malabsorption*. Lost calories causes lost weight.

Weight loss due to the gluten-free diet

People with celiac disease may find that they lose some weight once they start on a gluten-free diet. As we discuss in detail in Chapter 13, following a gluten-free diet entails giving up certain calorie-rich gluten-containing foods. As a result of ingesting fewer calories, you may find yourself losing weight after you've started your gluten-free diet.

Weight loss due to a coexisting condition

As we discuss in detail in Chapter 8, a number of different diseases are not caused by celiac disease but occur with greater frequency if you have celiac disease. Several of these can result in weight loss *unrelated* to your celiac disease.

If you have celiac disease, have gotten on track with your gluten-free diet, and are ingesting sufficient calories, but are still losing weight, then you and your doctor should consider the possibility you have one of these coexisting conditions:

>> **Addison's disease:** The adrenal glands are underfunctioning.

>> **Depression:** People who feel depressed often lose their appetite.

>> **Diabetes:** Having high blood glucose levels (as is a hallmark feature of diabetes) causes weight loss.

>> **Hyperthyroidism:** The thyroid is overfunctioning.

Weight loss due to a complication of celiac disease

As we discuss in Chapter 12, celiac disease can cause complications which, in turn, can cause weight loss. These are *not* common occurrences, but if other causes of weight loss have not been found, your healthcare professional should investigate further to see if one of them may be the cause. Here are the most important ones to be aware of:

>> **Pancreatic insufficiency:** This is a condition in which the pancreas is unable to make sufficient quantities of digestive enzymes; as a result, you get malabsorption.

>> **Small intestinal bacterial overgrowth (SIBO):** This is a condition in which there are excess numbers of bacteria in the small intestine; these excess bacteria consume some ingested dietary nutrients and also damage the small bowel; consequently, digestion is impaired, and malabsorption develops.

>> **Intestinal cancer:** Cancer of the small intestine, which we discuss in depth in Chapter 9, is a rare complication of celiac disease and is most likely to develop if you've had many years of severe, uncontrolled celiac disease.

TIP

Save yourself untold grief: Before you and your healthcare providers start an extensive search for one or more of the conditions we mention in the preceding list, make sure you have eliminated all gluten from your diet. What a shame it would be if you went through all sorts of tests to look for why you were unexpectedly losing weight if, in fact, the cause was nothing more than the fact that you were still (inadvertently) ingesting gluten.

Failure to Thrive in Children

As we discuss in detail in Chapter 14, although children with celiac disease can have symptoms (like abdominal discomfort and diarrhea) similar to adults' symptoms, youngsters may also have one unique group of symptoms, which are collectively called *failure to thrive*.

A child who is failing to thrive will have stopped growing and developing at the rate of his or her siblings or peers. The child may also be less energetic, less able to concentrate (and therefore, their schoolwork may suffer), and less socially engaged. These symptoms improve when your child is on track with a gluten-free diet . . . in which case, if they still don't feel like doing their homework, they'll have joined the ranks of many other healthy kids!

Nongastrointestinal Symptoms and Celiac Disease

When most people think "celiac disease" — when they think of it at all — they think "gut." And indeed, the gut is the root of the condition and the place where many people experience symptoms. Nonetheless, if you have celiac disease, you are at increased risk of other organs malfunctioning.

Your other organs may malfunction

>> **As a *direct result* or your celiac disease:** An example of this direct effect would be celiac disease damaging your intestine to result in impairing your ability to absorb vitamin D into your body. In turn, the vitamin deficiency may lead to osteoporosis.

>> *In association* **with celiac disease:** If you have blond hair, you are more likely to have blue eyes but, of course, your blond hair did not cause you to have blue eyes. This is an *association*, not cause and effect. In the same vein, celiac disease affecting the gut may be associated with other bodily ailments without directly causing them. Sometimes, this is because if you have one type of immune disorder (like celiac disease), you are at increased risk of having other immune disorders (like type 1 diabetes). More often, however, the reason for this association is either only partly known or is simply obscure.

In the following sections, we look at nongastrointestinal symptoms that you may experience if you have celiac disease. Depending on the symptom in question, it may be present as a direct result of your celiac disease or, alternatively, may be present because you have an associated condition. For a detailed discussion on the diseases we mention in this section, have a look at Chapters 7 and 8.

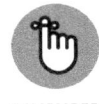

REMEMBER

As you read in this section of the many ailments that are associated with celiac disease, please do us — and, more importantly, *yourself* — a favor and bear in mind that most people with celiac disease *never* experience *any* of the problems we discuss here. Having said that, some people do, and thus, we feel it's important that you be aware of them.

TIP

With some important exceptions (such as the skin rash called *dermatitis herpetiformis,* which we discuss in a moment), each of the conditions we discuss in this section requires their own specific treatment. In other words, the gluten-free diet you need to follow to help control your celiac disease does not generally help you manage these other ailments.

Rash decisions

If you have celiac disease, you are at increased risk of having one of several different types of skin rash. We discuss these conditions in detail in Chapter 8. In this section, we note the visual changes associated with some of the skin diseases most commonly linked to celiac disease:

>> **Dermatitis herpetiformis:** If you develop small, intensely itchy, pinkish blisters on the elbows, knees, or buttocks (less often on the shoulders, scalp, face, and back), you may have dermatitis herpetiformis (DH). The link between DH and celiac disease is so strong that DH is sometimes referred to as "celiac disease of the skin." Both conditions are triggered by exposure to gluten, have the same antibodies present, and respond to the elimination of gluten from the diet.

>> **Psoriasis:** Should you have red, scaly sores affecting your skin — particularly the scalp, elbows, knees, and back, this may indicate you have psoriasis.

>> **Vitiligo:** If you develop patches of pale (to the point of being white) skin, you may have vitiligo.

Mulling over mood, thinking, and neurological issues

People with celiac disease are at increased risk of having certain mood, thinking, and neurological disorders. It is far from clear why this association exists, and it is always worth bearing in mind that an association isn't the same thing as cause and effect. These are the related conditions to be aware of (and which we discuss in detail in Chapter 8):

>> **Ataxia** is a condition in which the balance is affected, causing a person to walk unsteadily.

>> **Epilepsy** ("seizures") is a condition in which episodes of abnormal electrical discharge occur in the brain, leading to abnormal movements or behaviors that correspond to the particular area of the brain that's affected.

>> **Migraine headaches** are intense, typically throbbing headaches, which are often preceded by visual warning symptoms.

>> **Peripheral neuropathy** is a condition in which the nerves in the feet (far less often, the hands) are damaged, typically causing numbness.

>> **Attention-deficit/hyperactivity disorder (ADHD)** is a condition in which a person experiences challenges with paying attention, may be highly energetic or overly active, and often acts impulsively.

>> **Autism spectrum disorder** is a group of conditions that affect how a person communicates, learns, behaves, interacts with others, and experiences the world around them.

>> **Depression** and other psychiatric disorders that can affect a person's mood and state of emotional well-being.

Feeling fatigued

In the previous section, we list various mood, thinking, and neurological issues. But what if your problem is simply that you feel tired? Run down. Exhausted.

Worn out. Could this be due to your celiac disease? The quick answer is, well, there is no quick answer. In this section, we look at the possibilities.

You might imagine that, if you have chronic abdominal pain, are getting recurring bouts of diarrhea, and are malnourished because you're not sufficiently absorbing important nutrients into your body, that you'd feel tired. You bet! So yes, if you have these symptoms, it would likely be no surprise to you that fatigue is part and parcel of the process. Fortunately, soon after you start your gluten-free diet, these symptoms start to ease (though, if you're very malnourished, your tiredness may take longer to improve than the other symptoms we just mentioned).

Some people with celiac disease, however, feel fatigued even in the absence of gastrointestinal symptoms (and, as we discuss in detail in Chapter 4, most people with celiac disease have the nonclassical type in which GI symptoms are minimal or nonexistent). Although the cause may be unrelated and coincidental (literally thousands of different ailments can cause fatigue), there are a few celiac-related/-associated conditions that can lead to fatigue and, therefore, should be considered by you and your doctor:

>> **Anemia:** As we discuss in Chapter 7, there are several types of anemia that may occur if you have celiac disease. Of these, the most common one, which is also the one most likely to lead to tiredness, is *iron-deficiency anemia*. This is typically readily determined by performing a simple blood test.

>> **Depression:** Tiredness is a common symptom experienced by people who are depressed. It is, however, not the only symptom seen with depression; rather, it occurs in the context of a number of other features including difficulty sleeping and feeling helpless and hopeless. We discuss depression in detail in Chapter 8.

>> **Fibromyalgia:** Fibromyalgia is a musculoskeletal condition in which tiredness is a very common feature. We look in detail at fibromyalgia in Chapter 8.

>> **Thyroid disease:** The thyroid gland is a small hormone-secreting gland located in the front of the neck just above the breastbone (sternum). As we discuss in detail in Chapter 8, the thyroid helps regulate a great many different processes in the body. If the thyroid is underfunctioning (a condition called *hypothyroidism*), fatigue commonly results. What is far less widely known is that if the thyroid is overfunctioning (a condition called *hyperthyroidism*), fatigue is also very frequently experienced. If you have celiac disease and you have unexplained fatigue, be sure to ask your healthcare provider if your thyroid function has been checked. Your thyroid function is readily tested by performing a simple blood test. (The most commonly used test to screen for thyroid malfunction is called a TSH, which stands for *thyroid stimulating hormone*.)

If your celiac disease is well-controlled, yet you feel fatigued on an ongoing basis, you're doing yourself a disservice if you simply attribute your tiredness to your celiac disease. Instead, you should discuss your symptom with your doctor to determine what else might be causing it.

Hormonal (endocrine) problems

If you have celiac disease, you're at increased risk of certain hormonal (endocrine) conditions (which we discuss in detail in Chapter 8):

» **Addison's disease** is a disorder of the adrenal glands in which one loses weight and has low blood pressure and the skin darkens.

» **Type 1 diabetes** is a condition in which the body is unable to produce insulin. As a result, high blood glucose levels develop. Symptoms of elevated blood glucose include excess thirst, frequent urination, and weight loss.

» **Thyroid over-functioning (hyperthyroidism)** can cause weight loss, fatigue, tremor, palpitations, diarrhea, and other symptoms.

» **Thyroid under-functioning (hypothyroidism)** can cause weight gain, fatigue, dry skin, brittle hair, muscle aching, and other symptoms.

Musculoskeletal problems

If you have celiac disease, you may be at increased risk of the following musculo-skeletal disorders:

» **Rickets and osteoporosis** are conditions in which there is insufficient bone strength and mass. We discuss these ailments in detail in Chapter 7.

» **Rheumatologic problems** (we discuss these in detail in Chapter 8) including

- **Sjogren's syndrome** is a condition in which you have decreased ability to make saliva and tears.

- **SLE** ("lupus" or, more fully, *systemic lupus erythematosis*) is a disorder in which the joints and other body tissues become inflamed and painful.

- **Raynaud's phenomenon** is a condition in which blood flow to the fingers and toes is temporarily impaired upon exposure to cold temperatures leading to episodes of pallor of the digits.

- **Fibromyalgia** is a condition in which one experiences a variety of aches and pains but without evidence of inflammation in the body.

Cancer

Fortunately, cancer related to celiac disease (which we discuss in detail in Chapter 9) seldom occurs, but it can. Following are the most important types to be aware of:

>> **Enteropathy-associated T cell lymphoma** is a form of lymph cell cancer.

>> **Small intestine adenocarcinoma** is a form of cancer of the small intestine.

Gynecological and obstetrical problems

A variety of different, but related gynecological and obstetrical problems may occur if a woman has celiac disease, including

>> Irregular periods.

>> Infertility. We discuss infertility in detail in Chapter 7.

>> Miscarriages. We discuss pregnancy issues in detail in Chapter 14.

>> Early (premature) delivery.

Other problems

Of the remaining, important disorders associated with celiac disease, the key ones to be aware of are the following:

>> **Mouth ailments:** See Chapter 7 for more on mouth ailments, such as aphthous ulcers ("canker sores").

>> **Dental problems:** We discuss dental issues, such as loss of the tooth's protective enamel coating, in Chapter 7.

>> **Liver and bile duct disorders:** Liver disease can lead to jaundice, bleeding problems, and, potentially, many other problems. See Chapter 8 for a discussion on liver and bile duct disorders.

>> **IgA deficiency:** This is a congenital (meaning that one is born with it) inability to produce normal amounts of the IgA form of antibody. We discuss IgA deficiency in Chapter 8.

>> **Chromosome defects:** Turner syndrome and Down syndrome are conditions due to abnormalities in the chromosomes. (Chromosomes contain DNA, which is the genetic blueprint responsible for many of the traits of living organisms.) We discuss these conditions in Chapter 8.

Silent Celiac Disease

We can't leave this chapter about symptoms without pointing out that some people with celiac disease have no symptoms whatsoever!

As we discuss in Chapter 4, silent celiac disease can be uncovered due to laboratory abnormalities discovered during a routine physical, or it may be discovered in the context of a family history. The tremendous diversity of symptoms that people with celiac disease can experience means that some people reading this chapter can rightfully say, "None of the above," when reviewing the many symptoms of celiac disease.

Chapter **3**

Diagnosing Celiac Disease

C eliac disease affects about one percent of the North American population, and a significant portion of people with celiac disease either don't know they have it or, in some cases, are suspected to have it (and are treated for it) without first having objective confirmation of the diagnosis with appropriate testing. (As we discuss later in this chapter, we recommend against treating celiac disease unless the diagnosis is first proven.)

A key reason that so many people with celiac disease are undiagnosed is that, as we discuss in Chapter 2, the symptoms of celiac disease frequently occur with other, more common ailments and, common things being common, are attributed (by patients and doctors alike) to one or more of these other conditions. Fortunately, both healthcare providers and people in general are becoming more aware of celiac disease and, as a result, celiac disease is now being looked for more often.

In this chapter, we discuss what should be done once the suspicion first arises that you have celiac disease. In particular, we look at the tests that should be done to determine whether you have it.

Figuring Out Whether You Have Celiac Disease

To figure out whether you have celiac disease, your doctor typically follows four steps:

1. Learns about your symptoms.

   If you've been diagnosed with celiac disease, you probably recall having had symptoms of one sort or another that ultimately led you to see your doctor who then interviewed you to learn more about how you were feeling. "Taking a history" is always the first step that doctors follow in figuring out what may be the cause of a patient's symptoms.

2. Examines you.

   The second step in determining whether you have celiac disease is a physical examination in which the doctor measures your weight, looks at your skin, feels your abdomen, and looks for other physical abnormalities that can be seen with this ailment.

3. Orders blood tests.

   We hope that you notice that blood tests don't come up until this step. Medical tests are always complementary to the essential information that a doctor learns from talking to you and examining you.

4. Sends you for an endoscopy and small intestinal biopsy.

   In the great majority of cases, the diagnosis of celiac disease is certain only if you first have an endoscopy and small intestinal biopsy with the latter being interpreted by the pathologist as showing the appropriate features of the condition.

The rest of this chapter discusses each of these steps in detail.

Understanding the Importance of Symptoms

If the real estate world is all about "location, location, location," the world of medicine is all about "history, history, history." By medical history, we don't mean the balms and salves of ancient Rome, but rather, history in the sense of what a patient tells a doctor. Ninety percent of a diagnosis is based not on a physical examination or laboratory testing but on the story you relate when you meet with your physician. (That's why medical students are taught to pay great attention to listening to patients; in medical circles, this practice is called "taking a good history.")

A key part of the history is reviewing what symptoms you are experiencing. As we discuss in Chapter 2, some symptoms are considered classical of celiac disease. These include diarrhea, weight loss, abdominal discomfort, and really smelly gas and bowel movements (worse than other people's, if that's possible!), and, in children, failure to grow normally.

Your doctor doesn't need to be Sherlock Holmes to think of celiac disease when these are the symptoms; however, as we review in Chapter 2, many people with celiac disease instead have other, more subtle GI symptoms that point less obviously toward this condition as their cause. Other people who are eventually found to have celiac disease may have few or even no GI symptoms, but rather, have seemingly unrelated (to celiac disease) complaints like fatigue, depression, or muscle and joint aches and pains.

In the twentieth century, the classical form of celiac disease (see Chapter 4) was largely what led patients, families, friends, and doctors to think of celiac disease, but today, people increasingly recognize that these other, less obvious symptoms can be due to celiac disease. For this reason, doctors and other healthcare providers have to be alert to the possibility that a person's symptoms may be due to celiac disease.

TIP

If you are not yet diagnosed with celiac disease but are experiencing the symptoms we discuss here and in Chapter 2, ask your healthcare provider if these might be due to celiac disease. Who knows; you may be the one that first sets the wheels in motion leading to discovering your own as yet undiscovered diagnosis.

Knowing What to Expect from the Physical Examination

Although the history is a very important part of a medical visit, an examination of your body (a *physical examination*) can be helpful in the path to a diagnosis. Here are some of the things your doctor will check and explanations of what your doctor is trying to find:

» **Weight and height:** By knowing your weight and height, your doctor can calculate your body mass index (BMI), which indicates whether you are underweight, of normal weight, or overweight. Although BMI is an imperfect marker (see Chapter 13), it's one useful data point.

A normal BMI is between 18.5 and 24.9. Being underweight may be a sign that you aren't absorbing nutrients from your food properly as is often the case for people with celiac disease. (On the other hand, as we discuss in Chapter 2, many people with celiac disease aren't underweight or losing weight; in fact, you can have celiac disease and, like most North Americans, be overweight, even considerably so.) You can determine your own BMI by using an online tool such as the one available at https://cdc.gov/bmi/adult-calculator/index.html.

Measuring a child's height is especially important because being shorter than their peer group or not growing normally may be clues that the child also has a nutrient absorption problem like celiac disease.

>> **Blood pressure and heart rate:** Having low blood pressure and a rapid heartbeat can signify a number of different ailments, including dehydration (as you may experience if your celiac disease has resulted in profound diarrhea). A rapid heartbeat (without low blood pressure) can also be seen with celiac disease complications or associated conditions such as anemia (see Chapter 7) or hyperthyroidism (Chapter 8).

>> **Skin:** Celiac disease can be associated with a skin condition called *dermatitis herpetiformis* (see Chapter 8). Also, paleness may indicate you are anemic (Chapter 7).

>> **Mouth:** As we discuss in Chapter 7, celiac disease can be associated with oral health issues such as mouth ulcers.

>> **Abdomen:** Your doctor examines your abdomen to determine whether it causes you discomfort, your belly is soft or firm, or it is distended and to look for evidence of enlargement of your internal organs.

>> **Arms and legs:** Because celiac disease can affect the muscles and nerves in your extremities, your doctor will examine your arms and legs. Also, dermatitis herpetiformis (see the earlier bullet about skin abnormalities) can cause skin changes on your extremities.

>> **Rectal exam:** We saved this for the, ahem, end. A rectal exam is not done all the time but may be helpful if you are reporting symptoms such as blood in the stool or pain in the anal region during a bowel movement.

Getting Blood Tests

Although the history and physical examination are invaluable tools in figuring out whether you have celiac disease, in and of themselves they are usually not sufficient to establish a diagnosis, and you will need to have certain tests done. In most medical conditions, including celiac disease, the first tests to be done are blood tests.

You will be sent for blood tests for two main reasons:

» **To help determine if you may have celiac disease:** The two main types of blood tests that can help diagnose celiac disease are

- *Antibody tests* (also called *serologic tests* or *serology*): These are virtually always done.

- *Genetic tests:* These are not done routinely but are useful in certain circumstances, as described in the later section ("Genetic Testing").

» **To look for evidence of complications from or associated with celiac disease:** For example, blood tests may reveal that you are anemic, malnourished, dehydrated, or have evidence of liver injury. See Chapters 7 and 8 for more information on the complications from or associated with celiac disease.

In the remainder of this section, we look in detail at the various blood tests that are performed to help figure out whether you have celiac disease.

Antibody tests

TECHNICAL STUFF

Antibodies (abbreviated as Abs if plural, Ab if discussing just one) are special proteins called *immunoglobulins* (abbreviated as Ig) produced by certain white blood cells in our body. The body forms antibodies most commonly in response to — and to fight off — infections caused by germs like viruses and bacteria. (To discover more about the immune system, have a look at Chapter 5.)

Having antibodies to help us battle an infection is essential, but sometimes the immune system makes antibodies that are not only unhelpful but are actually harmful. Conditions in which the body makes antibodies that attack a person's own tissues are called *autoimmune* diseases. Rheumatoid arthritis is an example of an autoimmune disease. In this condition, antibodies attack the joints.

Celiac disease is also an autoimmune disease, but in addition to making antibodies against one's own tissues, people with celiac disease also make antibodies to *gluten*, a protein found in wheat and some other grains.

Medical scientists don't really know why celiac disease is associated with the various antibodies that are found with this condition, but knowing *if* they are present remains very helpful in making (or excluding) the diagnosis, as we look at next. In the next few sections, we look at the antibody tests that are used to diagnose celiac disease; following that discussion, we summarize how your healthcare provider can then use this information to help determine whether you may have celiac disease.

Tissue transglutaminase antibody

Tissue transglutaminase is a protein found in nearly all the body's tissues. If you have celiac disease, you form *tissues transglutaminase* (TTG) antibodies against this protein. (Two types of TTG antibody are formed: TTG IgA and TTG IgG. Most of the time, it's necessary to test only for TTG IgA; see the later section "The issue of IgA deficiency" for information on when TTG IgG test is recommended.)

The TTG IgA test is the single most important blood test you should have done if your doctor suspects you have celiac disease. As we discuss in Chapter 5, in celiac disease, gluten ingestion activates the immune system and leads to damage to the lining of the small intestine. Because TTG IgA is present in most people with celiac disease, doctors routinely look for TTG IgA if they suspect a patient has celiac disease.

REMEMBER

Even though TTG IgA is a particularly important test in diagnosing celiac disease, its presence does not guarantee you have celiac disease and does not preclude the need for a small intestinal biopsy. That is because there are situations where someone does not have celiac disease but nevertheless has an elevated TTG IgA, a situation known as a *false positive*.

In addition to helping doctors diagnose celiac disease, measuring your TTG IgA is also helpful in monitoring your condition. As we discuss in Chapter 13, as you remain on track with your gluten-free diet, your TTG IgA level will probably return to normal. If, on the other hand, it remains elevated, this may indicate that your gut is still being exposed to gluten, and your diet needs to be reviewed to determine how this is happening.

TIP

Different laboratories have different methods and, as a result, different normal ranges for many tests including TTG IgA levels. For this reason, to ensure apples are being compared to apples, if you need your TTG IgA test redone, it's best to go back to the same lab that did your earlier TTG IgA test.

Endomysial antibody

Endomysial antibody (EMA) is an antibody that, like TTG antibodies, targets the protein, tissue transglutaminase.

EMA testing used to be commonly performed, but because TTG antibody testing tells us similar information, is more readily available, and is less technically difficult (and therefore less expensive to perform), EMA studies are now ordered much less often.

DEAMIDATED GLIADIN PEPTIDE ANTIBODIES

Patients with active celiac disease often also have antibodies to a form of gliadin that has been modified by the tissue transglutaminase enzyme. This form of gliadin is referred to as *deamidated gliadin peptide* (DGP). The IgG form of this antibody can be helpful in people with IgA deficiency, as described in the later section "The issue of IgA deficiency." Both the IgA and IgG form of this antibody can be used to monitor adherence to the gluten-free diet, as described in Chapter 13.

One additional problem with the EMA test is that sometimes it can be normal *even in people who have celiac disease*; — a situation known as a *false negative* test result. As you can imagine, this can be very misleading because it could cause your celiac disease diagnosis to be overlooked. (Although the TTG IgA antibody test — covered in the preceding section — can also be falsely negative, this false result occurs less often.)

Gliadin antibody

As we discuss in Chapter 8, *gliadin* is the component of gluten that is the major trigger of celiac disease. Antibodies to gliadin are called *antigliadin antibodies* (AGA).

Because AGA testing is not nearly as accurate as the TTG antibody test in diagnosing celiac disease — it has both frequent false positive (meaning that the test is abnormal but the person being tested doesn't have celiac disease) and false negative results — the test is now seldom ordered.

The issue of IgA deficiency

People make five types of antibodies (immunoglobulins): IgA, IgD, IgE, IgG, and IgM. IgA is the major type of antibody made by the immune cells in the lining of the digestive tract. About 1 in 500 to 700 otherwise healthy people do not make IgA; this condition is known as *IgA deficiency*. As we discuss in Chapter 8, patients with IgA deficiency are at increased risk of infections of their respiratory and digestive tracts.

For some reason, patients with celiac disease are more likely to have IgA deficiency. This fact is important because if you are IgA deficient, some of the key tests that doctors order to figure out whether you have celiac disease (such as the tests we discuss in the previous few sections) may be normal even if you *do* have celiac disease. This is because if you do not have the ability to make IgA, you will make neither normal, healthy IgA antibodies (such as those to fight off infections of the respiratory and digestive tracts) nor the abnormal IgA antibodies (such as TTG antibodies) that are seen with celiac disease.

To get around the problem of diagnosing celiac disease when you have IgA deficiency, you can have a type of celiac disease antibody test other than the one typically used. These tests measure IgG antibodies instead of IgA. The two available IgG tests are DGP IgG and TTG IgG.

Though TTG IgG and DGP IgG can be useful when testing for celiac disease in people with IgA deficiency, they are more prone to be false positives. For this reason, they're not recommended to be used outside of this situation. Too often, physicians order a whole bunch of antibody tests and misinterpret an elevated TTG IgG or DGP IgG. In a person with a normal level of total IgA who has a negative TTG IgA level, an elevated TTG IgG or DGP IgG is very likely to be a false positive result. People with normal IgA levels and an elevated TTG IgG or DGP IgG are very unlikely to have celiac disease.

A stepwise approach to using antibody tests to help diagnose (or rule out) celiac disease

If your physician suspects that you have celiac disease, in the majority of cases, antibody tests will be ordered. In some instances, as discussed in the next section, genetic testing may also be requested. Because of its accuracy, the preferred antibody test is the TTG IgA antibody.

Looking specifically at your TTG IgA result:

>> **If your TTG IgA result comes back positive (that is, you *have* the TTG IgA antibody):** This result indicates a sufficiently strong probability of celiac disease that the next step is typically to proceed directly to a biopsy of your small intestine (as we discuss later in this chapter).

>> **If your TTG IgA result comes back negative (that is, you *do not* have the TTG IgA antibody):** Your doctor needs to ensure the negative result isn't because you have IgA deficiency and, therefore, will send you for an IgA level if this was not already checked. What happens next depends on whether your IgA level is normal or low:

  • *Normal:* IgA deficiency is excluded, your negative TTG IgA result is in keeping with a very low likelihood of celiac disease, and further testing for celiac disease is usually unnecessary *unless* your particular situation is so very suspicious for celiac disease that, despite these negative test results, you still require additional tests — such as an endoscopy and small intestine biopsy — to be as definitive as possible whether you do or do not have celiac disease. (An example of this situation might be a man or a postmenopausal woman who is iron deficient and for whom there is no evidence of bleeding.)

- *Undetectable:* You likely have IgA deficiency, and your negative TTG IgA result may be on this basis rather than the absence of celiac disease. Therefore, additional testing is required. If available, the next step is usually to measure your TTG IgG level or your DGP IgG level. If either of these are positive, the next step is typically to proceed with a small intestine biopsy. If this is *negative* then the probability of you having celiac disease is very low and further testing for celiac disease is typically unnecessary.

TIP

Some people have an IgA level that is lower than the normal range but is still detectable. TTG IgA is still considered a reliable test in the majority of people with low-but-detectable IgA levels. Still, some physicians will test for an IgG serology (TTG or DGP) to be sure.

Figure 3-1 is a schematic of the usual diagnostic steps your doctor performs when celiac disease is suspected. You will notice that the final common pathway make a diagnosis of celiac disease is almost always an endoscopy and small intestine biopsy. At present, as helpful as blood tests are, none exists that is sufficiently accurate, in and of themselves, to diagnose celiac disease.

CELIAC DISEASE SUSPECTED
- Clinical symptoms
- Abnormal blood tests
- Associated problems

ORDER ANTIBODY TESTS
- Tissue transglutaminase IgA (TTG IgA)
- Total IgA level

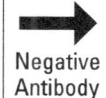

Negative Antibody Tests

Celiac disease unlikely: No further tests usually necessary

Positive Antibody Tests

ENDOSCOPY WITH INTESTINAL BIOPSY
- 4 to 6 specimens (minimum), including at least one from the duodenal bulb

FIGURE 3-1: Usual diagnostic steps to determine if you have celiac disease.

Can I skip the biopsy?

As shown in Figure 3-1, the road to a diagnosis of celiac disease runs through an endoscopy and intestinal biopsy. But as scientists have learned to interpret the fine points of antibody tests, there has been a call to skip the intestinal biopsy in some cases.

Why skip an intestinal biopsy? Well, the endoscopy can pose practical concerns (it typically involves taking a day off from work or school), and in some regions where specialists are scarce, it might take many weeks to get on the schedule for the procedure. Though the endoscopy with intestinal biopsy is extremely safe, there are rare circumstances that increase the risk of complications. For instance, people with hemophilia or other bleeding conditions have an increased risk of bleeding excessively after a biopsy.

In Europe, pediatricians have adopted a "biopsy-free" approach in children who meet certain criteria. They need to have a very highly elevated TTG IgA (greater than 10 times the normal limit), and a second abnormal antibody test drawn separately (which is, among other reasons, that the blood test result was not a laboratory mix-up). In those circumstances, families in Europe are being advised that their children can be considered to have celiac disease without an intestinal biopsy. This recommendation is based on the fact that antibody levels this high are very, very likely to mean that the child has celiac disease.

This approach has not caught on in the United States, and expert bodies have cautioned against skipping the biopsy, even in these cases. This hesitancy is mainly due to the fact that there is less certainty about the accuracy of the many different commercially available antibody tests used in the United States. Also, in adults, the false positive rate of these antibodies is higher than in children.

Still, there are situations where a patient may have a medical condition that poses increased safety concerns about having an endoscopy. Talk about this with your doctor. Although a biopsy is still recommended in the great majority of cases, the European pediatric approach is considered in select cases.

Genetic testing

As we discuss in Chapter 5, you need to have certain genes for celiac disease to develop. Because virtually all people with celiac disease have the HLA DQ2 or DQ8 genes, if tests show you do *not* have either of these genes, the likelihood that you will ever develop celiac disease is close to zero. In contrast, having one or even both of these genes does not mean you have or will later develop celiac disease. In fact, the great majority of people with these genes do not have celiac disease.

Medical scientists estimate that having the HLA DQ2 or DQ8 genes accounts for about half of the risk of getting celiac disease, which means many other factors exist that lead to celiac disease, as we discuss in Chapter 5. Scientists are working to discover other genes that are necessary for developing celiac disease. We discuss the work that scientists are doing in this field in Chapter 15.

HLA DQ2 and DQ8 genetic testing can be of value in several situations. Common to all of these situations is that the presence of these genes indicates a person may or may not have celiac disease, and the absence of these genes indicates a person almost certainly cannot have celiac disease.

Here are the situations in which genetic testing is of value:

» **If your doctor suspects you have celiac disease, but your other test results do not fit with the diagnosis.** For example, if your intestinal biopsy suggests celiac disease but your serology does not, or vice versa. In these situations, the fact that you have the HLA DQ2 and/or DQ8 genes means that despite the other test results, you still may have celiac disease. This may prompt a more concerted effort to find other evidence of celiac disease.

» **If you have started yourself on a gluten-free diet prior to a diagnosis of celiac disease having been made.** In this case, antibody and small intestinal biopsy results may be normal either because you have celiac disease and are successfully treating it or, on the other hand, because you didn't have celiac disease in the first place. We discuss this scenario further in the section, "Diagnosing celiac disease if you are already living gluten-free."

» **When a person within a family is discovered to have celiac disease, raising concerns that other family members may be at risk.** If these family members don't have the HLA DQ2 or DQ8 genes, they can be reassured they are highly unlikely to have or to later develop celiac disease. Doing such tests on undiagnosed — and asymptomatic — relatives is called *screening*. We discuss screening in detail in Chapter 6.

Other blood tests

In the preceding sections, we look at blood tests performed to help determine whether you might have celiac disease. In this section, we look at blood tests that your doctor will most likely order to see whether you have either complications from celiac disease or some other ailment associated with it. (We discuss these different conditions in detail in Chapters 7 and 8.)

These are other blood tests you may have:

>> **Hemoglobin level:** *Hemoglobin* is the molecule that carries oxygen in your blood stream. Your doctor will order your hemoglobin level to determine whether you are anemic.

>> **Electrolytes and other blood chemistry:** These tests are done to determine whether you are dehydrated or have low levels of body minerals such as potassium.

>> **Thyroid function:** Thyroid disease can occur with celiac disease and can also cause gastrointestinal symptoms.

>> **Liver tests:** Celiac disease can cause liver test abnormalities and may be associated with (autoimmune) liver and bile duct diseases.

>> **Nutritional tests:** Because celiac disease causes malabsorption, your doctor will most likely test your blood to look for evidence of deficiencies of vitamins and other nutrients.

Outside Looking In: How an Endoscopy Works

To determine whether you have celiac disease, your doctor must hear about your symptoms, examine you, and, almost always, order appropriate blood tests. At that point, if suspicion remains that you have celiac disease, you will need a simple and safe outpatient procedure called an endoscopy and small intestine biopsy. We discuss the endoscopy procedure in this section. (We discuss biopsies further in the next section; "Take a Little Piece: Small Intestinal Biopsy.")

You may be wondering, as some of our patients do, why a doctor wouldn't forego preliminary steps and go directly to an endoscopy and biopsy if a diagnosis of celiac disease is being considered. Although these procedures are the only definitive ones, and although they are straightforward and safe, they are still much more involved than a blood test, require a patient to give up time from work or other commitments, are much more expensive than a blood test, and do carry an element of risk — however slight. For these reasons and others, doctors seldom subject a patient to endoscopy and biopsy without first doing a preliminary evaluation to be certain that these procedures are truly necessary.

When you have an endoscopy, a specially trained physician places a narrow, flexible, fiberoptic tube (called an *endoscope*) into your body to look at one or another different parts of your gastrointestinal tract. Different endoscopes are used, depending on which part of your gut needs to be looked at. Figure 3-2 shows what a typical endoscope used to examine your small intestine looks like.

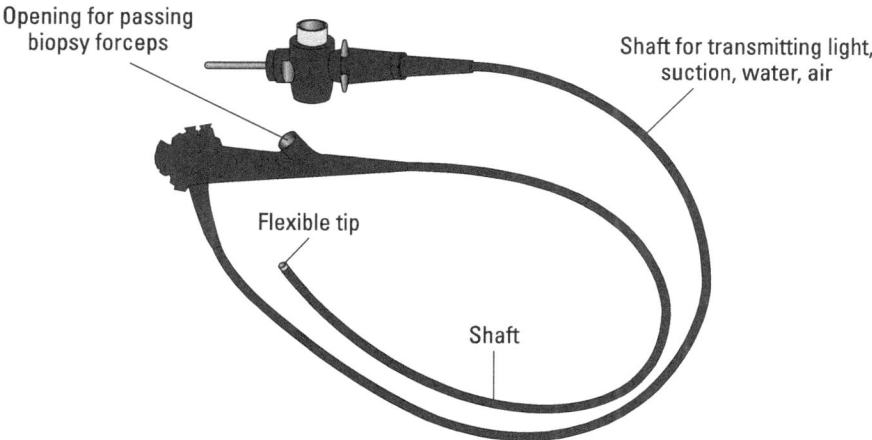

Opening for passing biopsy forceps

Shaft for transmitting light, suction, water, air

Flexible tip

Shaft

FIGURE 3-2: Typical endoscope used to examine the upper gastrointestinal tract.

TECHNICAL STUFF

Although *endoscopy* is a general term for this method of examining any part of your digestive tract, doctors typically reserve the term for those procedures done on the upper digestive tract (the esophagus, stomach, and duodenum), not the lower digestive tract. (When the lower part of the digestive tract — that is, the colon — is being examined, the procedure is called a *colonoscopy*.) Since the full name for endoscopy is *esophagogastroduodenoscopy* (EGD), you can see why it's easier to simply call it an endoscopy or an EGD.

Preparing for your endoscopy

Not much preparation is required prior to your endoscopy; however, there are a few helpful and important measures for you to follow:

>> **Plan to bring someone with you to your endoscopy appointment.** This serves two important functions because that person can

- *Accompany you home after the procedure:* This is especially important if you've received sedation because driving after being sedated is prohibited.

- *Provide an extra set of ears:* Bring someone to listen in when the doctor or nurse tells you the endoscopy results. Since you will have received sedation, you may be prone to forgetting what you were told. Far better to have that extra person with you at the time of your scope so that you don't have to later play telephone tag with your physician and, more importantly, so that you don't have to worry needlessly.

>> **Fast before the procedure.** You should not eat or drink for a number of hours prior to your test. (See the next section for the details on this requirement.)

>> **Check with your doctor about medicines.** Speak to your doctor to find out what, if any, changes to your usual medicines will need to be made. Here are some examples:

- *Diabetes medications:* Your doctor may need to change the dose, or you may not take them (or a portion of them) on the day of your procedure because you won't eat be eating fully that day.

- *Anti-obesity medications:* You may need to pause your medication before your procedure because it may affect the emptying rate of your stomach. (The stomach must not have any food in it for the procedure to be done safely.)

- *Anticoagulants ("blood-thinners") and anti-platelet medications:* Anticoagulants, including medicines such as warfarin (Coumadin), apixaban (Eliquis), and rivaroxaban (Xarelto), are typically not taken for two days prior to an endoscopy, and potent platelet-inhibiting drugs such as clopidogrel (Plavix) are typically not taken for about five days prior. Most endoscopy units do not require you to stop over-the-counter doses of aspirin (ASA) or anti-inflammatory drugs like ibuprofen or naproxen. Check with both the doctor who prescribes these medications for you and also the physician who will be doing the procedure to see what their recommendations are for you.

- *Medicine to be taken during the day of the procedure:* For those medicines that your doctor says you may continue to take the day of the procedure and that you customarily take first thing in the morning, ask the doctor who will be performing the endoscopy whether you can take them with a sip of water (even though you are fasting).

Undergoing the procedure

Physicians performing endoscopies are assisted by endoscopy nurses and technicians in an endoscopy unit of a hospital or a specialized endoscopy center. An endoscopy (and small intestinal biopsy) is a fast procedure; start to finish, it typically takes no more than 10 to 15 minutes or so (a bit longer if one includes the time that you rest after it's done). These are the steps involved with an endoscopy:

1. If you're having your endoscopy in the morning, you shouldn't eat or drink anything after midnight the night before the test (therefore, if your test is, say, at 8:00 a.m., you will have been fasting for eight hours). If your test is in the afternoon, your doctor will probably tell you that you can drink a small amount of clear liquids early that morning.

   Fasting is important because your stomach needs to be empty both to allow the doctor to see properly and also, so that you don't vomit (and, potentially, choke).

REMEMBER

2. You are brought into the endoscopy suite where you are asked to lie on your side on a special table. A small needle is placed in a vein (an "intravenous") in your arm.

3. To make swallowing the endoscope easier for you, the doctor or nurse may numb the back of your throat by either spraying it or by having you gargle with a local anesthetic medicine. To make it more comfortable for you to undergo the procedure, you will be given an intravenous injection of a small dose of sedative. Both the sedative and the spray will wear off within a few hours.

4. You are given a protective piece of plastic (a mouth guard) to place between your teeth. The scope is then inserted through the opening in the mouth guard into your mouth and passed down into your stomach and subsequently into your duodenum. The doctor examines the lining of your duodenum where, sometimes, highly characteristic changes (such as small notches and fissures) may be seen. Then, as we discuss in detail in the next section, the doctor uses long forceps to painlessly take biopsies of your duodenum.

5. The scope is withdrawn; within minutes, the sedation starts to wear off, and you awaken. The doctor (or nurse) discusses the findings with you and soon thereafter you're on your way home.

An endoscopy test is usually very well tolerated and you'll almost certainly be surprised when the doctor tells you the test is all done. Often, people don't know the test had even started!

Knowing what to expect after your endoscopy

As we mention in the preceding section, "Undergoing the procedure," you'll probably be surprised at how fast and easy the whole procedure goes. Here are a few things to be aware of after the endoscopy has been completed:

>> You may notice a bit of a sore throat. If you do, this fades over the course of a day or two.

>> You can return to normal eating and drinking within a few hours.

>> After sedation, you cannot drive, operate heavy machinery, or perform other such activities for the rest of the day. For that reason, it's necessary to have someone drive you home after your endoscopy.

Examining What the Doctor Looks for During Your Endoscopy

As the doctor performs your endoscopy, they will examine each part of your upper gastrointestinal tract. They'll look at the general health of the lining of the different organs and, in particular, will look for evidence of the abnormalities that can be seen with celiac disease. Equally important, the *endoscopist* (that is, the doctor performing your endoscopy), will look for abnormalities *unrelated* to celiac disease that could also explain any symptoms you've been having.

Exploring your esophagus

As we discuss in Chapter 5, the esophagus is the tube that connects the mouth to the stomach. The most important abnormalities that your doctor examines your esophagus for are evidence of inflammation related to gastroesophageal reflux andeosinophilic esophagitis. We discuss these conditions in Chapter 2.

Surveying your stomach

After examining your esophagus, the doctor will push the scope further down into your gastrointestinal tract to your stomach. The endoscopist will examine your stomach to look for ulcers, *gastritis* (stomach inflammation), and other abnormalities that may explain any symptoms — such as upper abdominal pain — that you may have been having.

Delving into your duodenum

After the endoscopist examines the stomach, they pass the scope through the small channel (the *pylorus*) that leads from the stomach into the duodenum and then, voila, the duodenum, the very first part of the small intestine, is reached. Although examining the other parts of your gastrointestinal tract is important, when it comes to celiac disease, the duodenum is where the action is.

Typically, the endoscope is advanced as far down the small intestine as possible. This can range from just beyond the first part of the duodenum (known as the *duodenal bulb*) to the first part of the jejunum. (The *jejunum* is the part of the small intestine just beyond the duodenum.)

Your doctor will carefully examine your duodenum for changes of celiac disease and will also take biopsies. (We discuss biopsies in the next section, "Taking a Little Piece: Small Intestinal Biopsy.") If an abnormal area is identified, the endoscopist will make a point of specifically biopsying this region.

The specific abnormalities in the duodenum that the doctor is looking for are

>> Scalloping or notching of the duodenal folds. Normally, the duodenum is smooth and free of scalloping or notching.

>> Fissuring or cracking of the mucosal lining between the folds.

>> Absence of the duodenal folds. This can happen in very severe celiac disease.

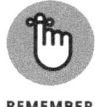

REMEMBER

A person can have celiac disease yet have a completely normal endoscopic appearance of the duodenum (or the entire upper gastrointestinal tract for that matter). Therefore, having an endoscopy is not sufficient to make (or rule out) a diagnosis of celiac disease. In all suspected cases, biopsies must be taken of the small intestine. It's only biopsy confirmation of celiac disease that establishes the diagnosis.

Taking a Little Piece: Small Intestinal Biopsy

As we mention in the preceding section, the diagnosis of celiac disease usually requires an intestinal biopsy. In a sense, everything else we discuss earlier in this chapter can be considered one long opening act and the small intestinal biopsy result the climax of your diagnostic journey.

As we discover in Chapter 5, the small intestine is more than 20 feet long, and virtually any part of it can be damaged by celiac disease. Fortunately, the part of the small intestine that's easiest to reach with an endoscope — the first part, called the duodenum — is abnormal if you have celiac disease; hence, it's ideally suited for obtaining a biopsy. A biopsy of the small intestine is performed at the same time as the endoscopy. After the doctor has passed the endoscope into your duodenum, a long forceps is inserted through a channel in the endoscope, allowing it to emerge into the intestine where the forceps can be opened and then closed, painlessly pinching off a tiny sample of the lining of the small intestine called the *mucosa*. The biopsy sample is very small — about the size of grain of rice.

It is important to take at least four to six biopsy samples of the duodenum, including at least one biopsy from the duodenal bulb. Taking fewer samples may miss affected areas of the intestine. (Sometimes celiac disease is "patchy," meaning that not every single area of a portion of the small intestine is equally affected.)

Interpreting a biopsy

To the naked eye, the biopsy sample that your doctor takes at the time of your endoscopy doesn't look particularly impressive; basically, it's a tiny fragment of pinkish tissue. But put that same biopsy under the microscope, and, if changes of celiac disease are present, whoa, is that ever a whole different story! As we describe in Chapter 5, a biopsy taken from someone with active celiac disease can show dramatic changes (well, okay, *dramatic* to the trained observer), resembling a microscopic war zone. However, because not everyone with celiac disease has this full-blown microscopic picture, the pathologist who looks at the biopsy will also look for milder forms of damage that are also consistent with the diagnosis of celiac disease.

REMEMBER

Of the microscopic changes seen on a small intestinal biopsy taken from someone with active celiac disease, the most important abnormalities are signs of inflammation, and shrinking (*atrophy*) of the finger-like projections (*villi*) that are key components in allowing absorption of nutrients into the body.

Knowing when the biopsy may potentially be wrong

Even though the small intestinal biopsy is considered the gold standard for making the diagnosis of celiac disease, there are some potential pitfalls:

>> A pathologist may misinterpret the biopsy findings and incorrectly attribute the observed abnormalities to some other condition even though, in fact, they are due to celiac disease.

>> A pathologist may overlook abnormalities altogether and report a specimen to be normal even though there are, in fact, features of celiac disease present.

Fortunately, in the great majority of cases, if you have a biopsy that has celiac disease findings present, the pathologist will find them and report them correctly. Also, as we mention previously in the section, "Take a Little Piece: Small Intestinal Biopsy," it's important that the doctor performing the endoscopy provide a sufficient number of biopsy samples to the pathologist.

If you have symptoms and physical examination findings and blood tests that all point toward celiac disease, but your biopsy report comes back stating otherwise, your doctor should consider having the biopsy slides reviewed again. A second opinion can't hurt. If the biopsies turn out to be truly normal, then genetic testing should be performed if it hasn't already been done. If these are positive for the HLA DQ2 and/or DQ8 genes, then additional testing to get biopsies from further down in the small intestine is sometimes recommended. We discuss this uncommon situation at the end of this chapter.

Having another small intestinal biopsy

If you have been diagnosed with celiac disease, gotten on track with a gluten-free diet, and had resolution of your symptoms and laboratory abnormalities (including antibody levels), then a second biopsy may or may not be recommended. Some celiac specialists recommend a repeat EGD and biopsy in *all* their patients two years after starting the gluten-free diet, but other specialists do not routinely recommend this course of action.

If you aren't responding to treatment the way you should (for example, you continue to have abdominal pain and diarrhea despite months of appropriate dietary therapy), then your doctor will probably recommend your endoscopy and small intestine biopsy be repeated. If the repeat procedure reveals ongoing abnormalities, you and your doctor will then need to do some digging and figure out why. Typically, the problem is that you are inadvertently still ingesting gluten. We discuss this situation further in Chapter 12.

EXPLORING OTHER DIAGNOSTIC TESTS

In your travels — especially of the online kind — you may come across other tests that bypass your doctor and are marketed directly to you. Here are some examples:

- **Home-based genetic testing:** This test involves swabbing your inner cheeks and then placing the swab into a container, which you mail to a laboratory. Weeks later, you will receive a result telling you whether you have a celiac disease-related gene. As mentioned earlier, the genetic test cannot tell you whether you have celiac disease. Its main value is that if it's negative for a celiac disease-related gene, it makes it highly unlikely that you have (or will ever develop) celiac disease.

- **Fecal and saliva tests for celiac disease antibodies:** These tests involve analyzing a stool or saliva specimen for the presence of celiac disease antibodies. These tests have not been very well studied or validated, so they neither replace standard testing nor should they be used routinely.

Diagnosing Celiac Disease When You Already Live Gluten-Free

More and more people are going on a gluten-free diet without having a confirmed diagnosis of celiac disease.

Sometimes, a gluten-free diet is started without any testing because a person believes that they're having symptoms that are so typical of celiac disease (see Chapter 2) that, in that person's opinion, the diagnosis seems overwhelmingly likely and doing tests seems unnecessary. Other times, a well-meaning doctor gets antibody tests that come back positive and instructs the patient to start a gluten-free diet without getting an intestinal biopsy.

With rare exceptions (see above, "Can I skip the biopsy?"), celiac disease specialists do not advocate starting a gluten-free diet without first having had a definitive, biopsy-proven diagnosis. Here's why:

- » **Risks treating wrong condition:** As we discuss in Chapter 11, other conditions can have similar symptoms to celiac disease, so you may end up treating the wrong disease with the wrong treatment.

- » **Potentially delays proper treatment:** Antibody results, although helpful in establishing a diagnosis of celiac disease, are still not as reliable as a small intestinal biopsy, so, once again, treating yourself without biopsy confirmation of celiac disease may end up delaying proper treatment for the condition that is actually present.

- » **Alters test results:** If you're on a gluten-free diet but aren't feeling better, it makes it more difficult to figure out if you do or do not actually have celiac disease. This is because antibody tests and biopsy specimens become less accurate once someone is on a gluten-free diet. We discuss this further in the next section, "Confirming a diagnosis of celiac disease when you live gluten-free."

- » **Causes unnecessary screening of relatives:** If you're the first person in your family to be diagnosed with celiac disease, you may have relatives that then want to be screened for the condition. Imagine the confusion and hassles to your relatives if they seek out screening tests for a condition which, as it turns out, they didn't need to be screened for because you, in fact, never had it to begin with.

Confirming a diagnosis of celiac disease when you live gluten-free

If you have *not* been biopsy-proven to have celiac disease but have been following a gluten-free diet, determining if you have celiac disease can be a challenge.

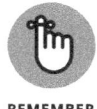

REMEMBER

The fact that your symptoms may have improved on a gluten-free diet should *not* be taken as proof that you have celiac disease. There may be many other reasons for the improvement. For example, people with irritable bowel syndrome (see Chapter 12) sometimes feel better on a gluten-free diet even if they don't have celiac disease.

If you have undiagnosed celiac disease and you've been on a gluten-free diet for less than a year and especially if you've not been meticulously gluten-free, then the odds are good that one or more of your antibody tests will still be abnormal, and a small intestinal biopsy may also be abnormal (thus confirming the diagnosis). Therefore, in this situation, your specialist will probably send you for these tests.

If, however, you've been living gluten-free for a year or more, your antibody tests and your small intestinal biopsy will most likely be normal. The challenge is to figure out if they're normal because you have celiac disease and it's under excellent control or, conversely, they're normal because you don't have the disease to begin with. To sort this out is a challenge, but the first step is to do genetic testing (see Chapter 6); only if you have the DQ2 or DQ8 genes would further tests, such as a gluten challenge (see the next section), be warranted.

EXAMPLE

Bianca, a 30-year-old nutritionist was evaluated for possible celiac disease. She had suffered from bloating and loose bowel movements for several years and, concerned that she had celiac disease, she had earlier placed herself on a gluten-free diet with subsequent improvement in her symptoms. Bianca's TTG IgA was normal but an HLA DQ2 and DQ8 test showed that Bianca did not have these genes. When Bianca returned to the doctor to discuss the results of her tests, she was told that she was very unlikely to have celiac disease. The doctor speculated that most likely the reason Bianca got better was that the gluten-free diet was helping an underlying irritable bowel syndrome, she could have non-celiac gluten sensitivity (see Chapter 5), or some other factor may have been responsible. Bianca gradually incorporated gluten back into her diet, and she continued to feel well thereafter.

The role of a gluten challenge

As we mention in the preceding section, if you're following a self-imposed gluten-free diet on speculation that you have celiac disease, and you then have a normal biopsy of the small intestine, this doesn't prove much. It could be that you have celiac disease and it has responded to your diet, or it could mean that you don't have celiac disease to begin with.

This conundrum can sometimes be resolved by having you perform a *gluten challenge*, meaning that you abandon your gluten-free diet and then, under your doctor's close supervision, see if you redevelop your previous symptoms or develop positive antibodies. If this happens, an endoscopy with small intestinal biopsy can then be performed. There are, however, some problems with the gluten challenge, including these:

>> **Becoming ill:** Some patients may become very ill soon after beginning the challenge, and they're unable to continue it long enough to see if evidence of celiac disease shows up in the blood test or biopsy results.

>> **Delayed onset of symptoms or antibodies:** Some patients, even if they have celiac disease, may not develop symptoms or antibodies for many weeks, in which case the diagnosis remains unclear.

Great variation exists among celiac specialists on how the challenge is conducted (amount of gluten, duration of challenge, timing of TTG IgA testing during the challenge, and timing of the endoscopy with intestinal biopsy). This depends on how long the patient has been gluten-free, the symptoms that occur during the gluten challenge, and other factors.

REMEMBER

If your doctor advises you to reintroduce gluten into your diet, be sure to do so only gradually. Consuming too much gluten too soon can potentially lead to marked gastrointestinal symptoms.

Questioning Your Diagnosis

No symptom, no physical examination finding, no blood test and, on rare occasion, not even a biopsy result can provide perfect accuracy in determining if someone has celiac disease. So, if no perfect way of diagnosing celiac disease exists, it could be that you have either been told you have it and you wonder whether you don't or, conversely, you might have been told you don't have it, yet you wonder if, in fact, you do. We look at these two issues in this section. We also examine the rare situation when everything points to celiac disease but the standard tests aren't enough to make the diagnosis.

Second-guessing celiac disease

If you've been diagnosed with celiac disease and are being treated with a gluten-free diet, yet you continue to feel unwell, you should consider it a red flag that perhaps something else is amiss. One possibility is that, despite your best efforts, you're inadvertently continuing to ingest gluten. (We discuss hidden sources of gluten in Chapter 12.) Another possibility is that the diagnosis is wrong, and you don't actually have celiac disease.

EXAMPLE

Bill was a 48-year-old veterinarian, who, after having had longstanding problems with heartburn, constipation, and bloating, was referred to a gastroenterologist. The gastroenterologist performed an EGD with small intestinal biopsy, which a pathologist concluded showed features of celiac disease. Bill was treated with a gluten-free diet, but despite dutifully following it, his symptoms didn't go away. Because of the lack of improvement, his gastroenterologist decided to treat Bill with a potent anti-inflammatory medication called prednisone. Alas, not only did this not help but Bill started to feel even worse. He sought a second opinion. The second gastroenterologist had Bill's biopsy slides reviewed by a pathologist with expertise in celiac disease, and lo and behold, the second pathologist's conclusion was that the specimens did not, in fact, show celiac disease but revealed changes typical of excess acidity (peptic duodenitis). The doctor took Bill off prednisone, had him start an anti-acid medication, and discontinued Bill's gluten-free diet. Within a few weeks, Bill's symptoms were almost gone, and he felt like a new person.

TIP

If you suspect that you do not have celiac disease, even though you've been diagnosed with the condition, speak to your doctor about your concerns. Your doctor can review the different factors that led to the diagnosis having been made, and the two of you can decide if further investigations or getting a second opinion (either from a gastroenterologist who has a special interest in celiac disease or by your doctor arranging to have your biopsy slides read by a different pathologist) is appropriate.

In some situations, your doctor may conclude that you don't have celiac disease, but you are unconvinced. In this situation, it's worth reviewing the results. For example, if you have an elevated TTG IgA but your intestinal biopsy was read as normal, it may be worthwhile to have your biopsy slides reviewed by a pathologist with specialized expertise in celiac disease because the diagnosis could be missed in the case of subtle biopsy findings.

Looking for suspected celiac disease when it can't be found

As we mention earlier in this chapter, on occasion, a person who has both clinical features (that is, symptoms and physical examination findings) and laboratory test abnormalities (including antibodies) strongly suggesting celiac disease nonetheless has a normal endoscopy and small intestine biopsy. This can be quite a conundrum. Does the person have celiac disease and it's being overlooked? Or, in fact, is celiac disease not present?

If you're in this situation, the next set of measures your celiac disease specialist can undertake to sort things out include the following:

>> Have another pathologist look at the small intestine biopsy slides to make sure some subtle signs of celiac disease were not overlooked.

>> Test your blood to see whether you have the HLA DQ2 or HLA DQ8 genes that place you at risk for celiac disease. If you have neither of these genes, then you are highly unlikely to have celiac disease.

If despite these measures, it is still unclear if you have celiac disease, depending on your symptoms, you may benefit from evaluation of the intestine further down — that is, in areas beyond the reach of a conventional endoscope. (The regular endoscope can only reach the duodenum and the very beginning of the jejunum.) This is done mainly to evaluate for other gastrointestinal conditions that can mimic celiac disease.

The following sections explain the ways your doctor can try to assess areas of your small intestine that cannot be reached with a regular endoscope.

Colonoscopy

The goal is to pass the scope beyond the colon and into the terminal ileum (this is the end part of the small intestine). This is called an *ileoscopy*. When the scope is in the terminal ileum, biopsies of this area can then be obtained. The ileum is the site where Crohn's disease most commonly affects the bowel. (Celiac disease can also affect the ileum but would be extremely unlikely to do so in the absence of abnormalities elsewhere in the small intestine.) While the endoscopist is performing the colonoscopy, they may take biopsies of the colon to look for microscopic colitis because, as we discuss in Chapter 7, this condition can sometimes mimic celiac disease and not infrequently occurs with celiac disease.

Capsule endoscopy

A *capsule endoscopy* (CE) is a procedure that allows video images to be taken of the intestine beyond the reach of an endoscope. During a CE procedure, you swallow an oversize "pill" that is a miniature video camera (see Figure 3-3). The pill takes high-resolution movies of the lining of the gut as it makes its merry way through the intestine, moved along not by a tiny propeller but by the bowel's natural contractions (something called *peristalsis*). As it journeys through your gut, the camera beams its video images to a specially designed recorder (attached to a belt) you wear for eight hours, at which time the recorder (and belt) are removed, and the captured images of the small intestine are downloaded onto a computer where a doctor analyzes them for evidence of signs of complications of celiac disease such as lumps, bumps, ulcers, and other abnormalities.

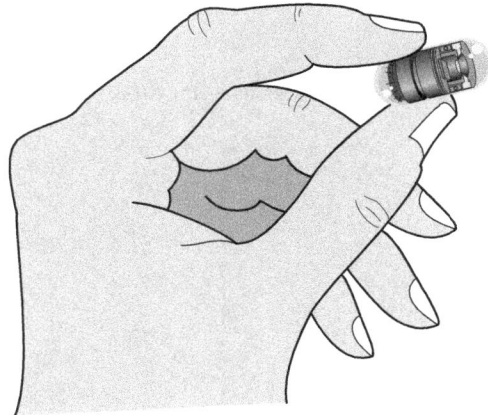

FIGURE 3-3:
Video capsule.

If you're wondering what happens to that high tech capsule, well, eventually, you pass it out of your body with your stool. Most people don't see it; it is mixed in with the stool and gets flushed down the toilet.

In addition to its role in monitoring celiac disease, capsule endoscopy can be used to help diagnose elusive cases. Specifically, there are occasional situations where a doctor strongly suspects a person has celiac disease, but a regular endoscopy and biopsies don't detect it. In this situation, it could be that celiac disease is indeed present but is only located further down the small intestine where a regular endoscope can't reach. In this situation, a capsule endoscopy can be performed, and if the images it captures are compatible with celiac disease in this more distant region of the small intestine, then a longer type of endoscope (a *push enteroscope* or a *double balloon enteroscope*) can be used to try to confirm the diagnosis by obtaining biopsies of this portion of the intestine. The following section has more details on this procedure.

Enteroscopy

Enteroscopy is the same as endoscopy but uses a long scope (an enteroscope) that, because of its length, can reach beyond where an endoscope is able. Because these techniques are time-consuming and require specific expertise, referral to a specialized center will often be needed to have such testing done.

If after all this, a diagnosis of celiac disease (or an alternative diagnosis) has *still* not been made, then further recommendations are made based on your individual clinical situation. Often, a trial of a gluten-free diet is undertaken to see whether this causes relief of symptoms. If you have an elevated TTG IgA and you're not feeling particularly unwell in the first place, your doctor may recommend you continue with your regular diet and have certain of your tests redone after 6 to 12 months to see whether they've become more definitive. (In particular, with the passage of time, if you have celiac disease, your small intestine biopsies will likely become more clearly abnormal.)

Fortunately, it is very rare that diagnosing celiac disease is as complicated as this!

IN THIS CHAPTER

» Looking at the types of celiac disease

» Exploring classical celiac disease

» Learning about non-classical celiac disease

» Discovering potential celiac disease

» Finding out about silent celiac disease

Chapter 4

Spotting the Chameleon: The Multiple Presentations of Celiac Disease

Although most people — including many healthcare professionals — think of celiac disease as being one condition, there are several different forms. In this way, celiac disease is like a chameleon, taking many forms. In this chapter, we look at these various forms of celiac disease, what they have in common, and how they differ. Most importantly, we discuss why this is relevant for you to know.

What's in a Name: The Different Types of Celiac Disease

In its *classical* — and best known — form, celiac disease is associated with abdominal cramping, diarrhea, and malnutrition. As you may expect, if there is a classical form, there is bound to be one or more other forms, including *non-classical* form, the *silent* form, and the *potential* form. It's now known that the majority of people with celiac disease do not have the classical variety but instead have one of these other types. Table 4-1 describes the key features of the different forms of celiac disease; you may find it helpful to refer to this table as you read the chapter.

TABLE 4-1   The Main Features of the Different Types of Celiac Disease

Type of Celiac Disease	Classical	Non-Classical	Silent	Potential
Typical Age of Onset	Childhood	Any age	Any age	Any age
Symptoms	Primarily gastrointestinal	Primarily non-gastrointestinal	None	None
Complications	Usually absent	Often present	None	None
Celiac Disease Antibodies	Present	Present	Present	Present
Small Intestine Biopsy	Abnormal	Abnormal	Abnormal	Normal
Treatment	Gluten-free diet Treatment of complications	Gluten-free diet Treatment of complications	Gluten-free diet	Uncertain

Looking at Classical Celiac Disease: The Textbook Form

For nearly two thousand years starting with the first mention of celiac disease by a doctor in ancient Greece, when people referred to celiac disease, they were discussing the classical form of this condition. Similarly, when celiac disease is discussed in the press or at the dinner table or at the office water cooler, it is often this variety of the condition that is described. The following sections discuss the symptoms, diagnosis, and treatment of this form of celiac disease.

Symptoms of classical celiac disease

Classical celiac disease can occur in adults but more typically begins in early childhood. It's characterized by symptoms that arise directly from damage to the small intestine. The affected person has abdominal bloating and discomfort and diarrhea. Also, because the damaged bowel becomes unable to properly absorb nutrients into the body (a condition called *malabsorption*), the individual with classical celiac disease starts to break down some of their tissues to provide nutrients to supply energy for the body's normal functioning. This leads to loss of muscle mass and weight.

In children, the malabsorption means there are insufficient nutrients present to allow for proper weight gain, growth, and physical maturation (a condition called *failure to thrive*). In particularly severe cases, a child's bones may not develop properly, leading to bowing of their legs (called *rickets*; see Chapter 7). We discuss celiac disease in childhood in detail in Chapter 14.

Diagnosing classical celiac disease

As with the other forms of celiac disease, a person with classical celiac disease has abnormal blood tests; most importantly, they typically have the presence of tissue transglutaminase IgA antibody (TTG IgA). We discuss this test in detail in Chapter 3.

TIP

The TTG IgA test will not be reliable if a person has a deficiency of the IgA antibody. Therefore, if you have the symptoms we discuss in this section yet after doing some blood tests, the doctor determines that celiac disease is not present, we recommend you ask the doctor whether the IgA level was tested. If it wasn't, it needs to be. We discuss the issue of IgA deficiency in detail in Chapter 3.

REMEMBER

Classical celiac disease cannot be diagnosed unless a small intestine biopsy is obtained and found to be abnormal. We discuss this test in detail in Chapter 3.

Treating classical celiac disease

The mainstay of treating classical celiac disease is following a gluten-free diet. Meticulously. Conscientiously. Strictly. Ah, we think you get the point. The speed with which a person responds depends, in part, on how long they've been unwell and how ill they are. In general, once treatment is underway, the person with classical celiac disease will soon start to improve with progressive resolution of the abdominal symptoms and diarrhea. If a child has had stunted growth and development, they may have a spurt and — depending on when the diagnosis was made and how severe the complication — may eventually catch up to their peer group in size and maturation.

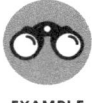

EXAMPLE

Lily was on the verge of tears when she brought Keisha, her four-year-old daughter, to see the pediatrician. Sick with worry, Jane told the doctor how Keisha would sometimes cry in pain, would have such bad diarrhea that she was sometimes not making it to the bathroom in time, and had stopped growing. The doctor took one look at the clearly malnourished child and recognized why Lily would be so worried. The doctor carefully examined Keisha and then said to her mom, "Lily, your daughter has textbook findings of celiac disease. We should be able to quickly confirm this and get treatment under way." Sure enough, subsequent tests established that Keisha had classical celiac disease. Shortly after starting a gluten-free diet, Keisha quickly began to regain her health and once again became a vibrant and growing child.

When Symptoms Suggest Something Else: Looking at Non-Classical Celiac Disease

Non-classical celiac disease is the form of celiac disease characterized by the absence of (or minimal) small intestinal symptoms with the predominant complaints being related to some other organ. This is in distinct contrast to classical celiac disease wherein symptoms are primarily or, often exclusively, related to the small intestine and the associated malabsorption. Also, non-classical celiac disease is most commonly diagnosed in adults and relatively less often in children. However, even in children, the non-classical form is being seen more often, especially in older children.

Despite the lack of gastrointestinal (GI) symptoms, the small intestine *is* damaged if you have non-classical celiac disease.

Non-classical celiac disease is much more common in society than is classical celiac disease. (In fact, the non-classical form used to be called "atypical" celiac disease but was renamed because the *atypical* came to be a misnomer; it no longer made sense to call it "atypical" when it was the most typical form of celiac disease!)

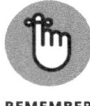

REMEMBER

Because non-classical celiac disease often centers on non-gastrointestinal symptoms, it's a diagnosis that may not be considered by doctors. For that reason, if you think you may have it (based on the features we discuss in the next section), feel free to mention the possible diagnosis to your physician. As always, we'll be happy to take the blame should your doctor — perish the thought! — take offense at your raising the issue.

Looking at GI symptoms of non-classical celiac disease

When present, GI symptoms may include mild indigestion, heartburn, abdominal cramps and bloating, diarrhea, and/or constipation. Because these GI symptoms are mild and so commonly seen in otherwise healthy individuals or people with any of a whole slew of different ailments, most physicians wouldn't — perfectly understandably by the way — readily consider celiac disease as the culprit. More likely, if you were having these GI symptoms, a doctor would entertain other diagnoses such as these:

>> **Irritable bowel syndrome:** A condition characterized by abdominal discomfort and altered bowel habits (frequently involving both constipation and diarrhea). (We discuss this condition in Chapter 12.)

>> **Gastro-esophageal reflux (GERD):** An ailment in which acid from the stomach goes back up into the esophagus. (We discuss this condition in Chapter 12.)

Examining non-GI symptoms of non-classical celiac disease

As we mentioned earlier in this section, non-classical celiac disease is characterized by a paucity or complete absence of gastrointestinal symptoms. Many different circumstances lead to the ultimate diagnosis of non-classical celiac disease. What they have in common is someone (be it a physician, a nurse, a dietitian, another healthcare provider or, importantly, a patient) thinking of the possibility.

Many different scenarios may lead — sometimes sooner, sometimes later — to a diagnosis of non-classical celiac disease, including when a person is discovered to have otherwise unexplained:

>> Anemia

>> Osteoporosis or low-impact fracture (we define these terms in the section "Osteoporosis") in adults; rickets in a child

>> Infertility

>> Erratic blood glucose levels in the setting of type 1 diabetes

>> Skin rash

>> Nerve damage

>> Bleeding

>> Calcium deficiency

>> Vitamin deficiency

>> Tooth (enamel) defects in a child

We discuss the first four of the listed items in detail in the following sections. We discuss the other listed items (and many of the other possible health issues that can lead to a diagnosis of non-classical celiac disease) in Chapters 7 and 8.

Anemia

The small intestine is damaged if you have non-classical celiac disease just as it is with the classical form. When the small intestine is damaged, it loses its ability to absorb into the body essential nutrients required to make red blood cells. The three most common types of anemia that are seen are those due to low levels of

>> Iron (anemia due to low iron is called *iron-deficiency anemia*)

>> Folic acid (or *folate*)

>> Vitamin B12

TIP

You can have a deficiency of iron, folic acid, or vitamin B12 without necessarily being anemic. In this case, it's only when these specific nutrients are measured on a blood test that the deficiency is identified.

Deficiency of iron, folic acid, or vitamin B12, regardless of whether it's associated with anemia, does not necessarily cause symptoms.

EXAMPLE

Vikas was a perfectly healthy 40-year-old man who, after seeing a notice in the local newspaper asking for blood donors, headed down to the local clinic. To his shock, as he went through the screening process done prior to giving a donation, he was told he would not be allowed to give blood because he was anemic. He had felt completely well. Following the clinic's advice, he went to see his family physician, who discovered that Vikas was low in iron. Tests to rule out bleeding were normal (low iron can be caused by blood loss), so further testing was undertaken and, lo and behold, it was determined that Vikas had low iron due to iron malabsorption due to celiac disease. He was treated with a gluten-free diet and, for a time, iron supplements, and his iron level gradually returned to normal. After his anemia had corrected, he returned to the blood donor clinic and was able to donate.

We discuss the subject of anemia and celiac disease in more detail in Chapter 7.

Osteoporosis

Osteoporosis is a condition where loss of bone strength and mass (amount) occurs. Having osteoporosis increases your risk of a fracture. As we discuss in Chapter 7, to have healthy bones, you must have not only sufficient amounts of calcium and vitamin D in your diet, but you must also have a healthy small intestine that can absorb these nutrients from the gut into your body. If you have celiac disease, you may not be able to properly absorb calcium and vitamin D, and as a result, you can develop osteoporosis.

Because osteoporosis causes — and this is a surprise to most people — no symptoms at all, it is typically undetected until it's is found either when a person is sent by their doctor for a routine osteoporosis screening (bone mineral density or BMD) test or when an individual sustains a low-impact fracture. In medical parlance, a *low-impact fracture* is defined as a fracture of a bone (excluding the small bones of the hands or feet) that occurs despite only minor trauma, such as a seemingly harmless fall.

When celiac disease is the cause of osteoporosis and fractures, this is the usual chain of events leading to the diagnosis of celiac disease:

1. An apparently healthy person has a seemingly harmless fall.
2. Despite the person having had only a minor fall, they sustain a low-impact bone fracture.
3. Surprised that such minor trauma has led to a fracture in a healthy person, a doctor questions whether the person has some underlying bone disorder, such as osteoporosis, that made that person susceptible to a fracture.
4. The doctor orders a BMD test to evaluate the patient's bones, and it comes back showing osteoporosis.
5. The physician questions why this healthy person would have osteoporosis and, aware that osteoporosis can be caused by malabsorption, orders tests looking for this condition.

6. Blood tests confirm evidence of malabsorption, and the doctor then runs further tests, including those for celiac disease, to determine why malabsorption is present. Lo and behold, celiac disease is found. (Sometimes, a doctor may order celiac blood tests during Step 5.)

As you might imagine, the poor person who, until the fracture, had thought themselves to be perfectly well is typically stunned to find out they have not just one, but *two* underlying conditions: osteoporosis *and* celiac disease. There is, however, one silver lining to this. Unlike other people with osteoporosis, a person in this situation has one additional, highly potent therapeutic weapon available to help rebuild bone strength; use of a gluten-free diet. The gluten-free diet heals the intestine, which will then allow for the resumption of normal absorption of calcium and vitamin D.

You may perhaps have noticed that in the preceding list we twice referred to a doctor questioning the unanticipated occurrence of a problem and then doing further tests that subsequently led to an unexpected discovery. Alas, not all physicians are so questioning. For this reason, many people with fractures don't have their osteoporosis discovered and, if the osteoporosis was due to celiac disease, don't have this discovered either.

TIP

You can be your best advocate, and you can help your doctor help you and others, in the following ways:

>> If you have celiac disease and you ever sustain a low-impact fracture, ask your doctor to test your bone density to determine if you have osteoporosis.

>> If you are not known to have celiac disease and you sustain a low-impact fracture, ask your doctor to test you for osteoporosis. If osteoporosis is found, ask your doctor to also test you for celiac disease.

>> Regardless of whether you have celiac disease, feel free to share with others the information discussed in this section. If you know someone who has had a fracture despite only minor trauma, mention to that person that you read how osteoporosis (and celiac disease) can cause this.

Infertility

Though not widely appreciated by the public, nor even by some doctors, there appears to be an association between infertility and celiac disease.

EXAMPLE

Talia was a 34-year-old woman who, despite years of trying to start a family, had been unable to conceive. She had had repeated meetings with her gynecologist and had been poked, prodded, and tested more than she could have dreamt possible, yet no cause for her infertility had been discovered. Her husband, too, had been tested, but nothing untoward showed up. Talia decided to do her own research online, and she discovered that there were cases where similarly infertile women had been found to have celiac disease and after being placed on a gluten-free diet, had successfully conceived. She approached her gynecologist with this information and was tested for celiac disease. Despite not having a single other symptom of the disease, her results came back positive. Talia met with a dietitian, began a gluten-free diet, and a few months later was back in the doctor's office. Before the doctor said a word, he knew that his patient was pregnant: Talia's ear-to-ear smile told the story. Indeed, the story continued as, over the next few years, Talia ended up having two further, successful pregnancies. She was so overwhelmed by both her joy and how she had discovered her own celiac disease that she ended up starting a local community celiac disease support group.

TIP

It pays to be your own advocate. If you have infertility and routine tests don't reveal a cause, ask your doctor to consider the diagnosis of celiac disease. It's possible that they had already considered and excluded it. Or it could be that because you hadn't had any of the symptoms of celiac disease that are most familiar to doctors (that is, gastrointestinal symptoms), the diagnosis of celiac disease hadn't been considered.

We further discuss the relationship of infertility and celiac disease in Chapter 14.

Erratic blood glucose control (in people with type 1 diabetes)

Type 1 diabetes is the form of diabetes that most commonly onsets in children or young adults and requires the immediate introduction of — and ongoing use of — insulin therapy. Controlling blood glucose levels in type 1 diabetes is a fine balance between many factors, including, most importantly, food intake, exercise, and the amount of insulin given. If these are out of sync, then blood glucose control can become erratic.

As we discuss in Chapter 8, because celiac disease causes malabsorption, it can lead to unstable blood glucose control in a person with type 1 diabetes. Fortunately, nowadays, diabetes specialists are usually familiar with this and routinely test for celiac disease in this situation. If celiac disease is discovered, following a gluten-free diet may result in improved blood glucose control. Because celiac disease presenting this way is unassociated with other symptoms of celiac disease, it's said to be the non-classical form of celiac disease that is present.

TIP

In the preceding paragraph we mentioned that diabetes specialists are *usually* familiar with the relationship between type 1 diabetes and celiac disease, which is to say that not all such specialists are especially aware of this connection. Also, not every person with type 1 diabetes is being followed by a diabetes specialist. For these reasons, if you have type 1 diabetes and your blood glucose control has become unexpectedly erratic, we recommend that you ask your healthcare provider if you've been tested for celiac disease. If you haven't been tested for celiac disease, and if no other apparent explanation exists for your problem, you should have this testing undertaken.

Hushed but Not Forgotten: Silent Celiac Disease

Silent celiac disease (also sometimes called *subclinical celiac disease*) has three key features. The affected person

>> Doesn't have symptoms (gastrointestinal or otherwise) of celiac disease and doesn't have other diseases or health problems that would provide clues they have celiac disease

>> Has typical blood test abnormalities of celiac disease (and, like the other forms of celiac disease, is associated with certain HLA genes, as we describe in Chapter 3)

>> Has small intestine biopsy findings of celiac disease

Uncovering silent celiac disease

As you may expect, because silent celiac disease is, by definition, not associated with symptoms, it's most likely to be discovered as an incidental and unexpected finding, such as when a person has a small intestine biopsy done during an endoscopy being performed for an entirely unrelated condition (such as having an ulcer) or is tested for possible celiac disease due to an associated condition or being a close relative of someone who is known to have celiac disease. (We discuss screening in detail in Chapter 6.)

Treating silent celiac disease: Should you or shouldn't you?

Arguments can be made both for and against treating silent celiac disease (with a gluten-free diet). In support of not treating it, one could point out the following things:

>> The person with silent celiac disease feels perfectly well; why, therefore, ask that person to initiate therapy for something that isn't bothering them? (That is, "if it ain't broke, why fix it?")

>> Following a gluten-free diet is not an easy thing to do; indeed, it's not only inconvenient, but it can also be frankly difficult. Why, therefore, recommend that a perfectly healthy person take on this burden?

>> Doctors don't have any long-term scientific data to show that treating silent celiac disease is of value in protecting and preserving health, so in the absence of this data, isn't it inappropriate to advocate treating it?

On the flip side of the argument, in support of treating silent celiac disease, one could point out that:

>> A person with silent celiac disease may feel completely well, but that isn't a reason not to treat them. Rather, this simply means that they were fortunate to be discovered before celiac disease had had time to make them sick. Treating them now will help keep them from later getting sick.

>> It's not rare that a person who had no awareness of having symptoms only recognizes with the benefit of hindsight, once they've been following a gluten-free diet for a time, that in fact *they had* been having symptoms. In other words, it was only after symptoms they'd had chronically (and therefore didn't even notice them anymore) went away that they realized they'd ever been there in the first place.

>> Following a gluten-free diet isn't easy, but getting sick and running into complications from untreated celiac disease is far worse.

We wish harder scientific evidence were available to tell us what advice we should give patients, but, well, it isn't. In the absence of this evidence, healthcare professionals — including us — need to rely on our best clinical judgment. We know how much damage can be done by celiac disease; indeed, we see it all the time. So even though we don't have foolproof evidence that patients with the silent form of celiac disease benefit from following a gluten-free diet, we prefer to err on the side of caution. For that reason, we advocate that if you have silent celiac disease, you follow a gluten-free diet. Most of our colleagues, by the way, offer similar advice to their patients.

Lurking in the Background: Potential Celiac Disease

Potential celiac disease has two key features. The affected person

>> Has typical blood test abnormalities of celiac disease (and, like the other forms of celiac disease, is associated with certain HLA genes as we describe in Chapter 3)

>> Does not have small intestine biopsy findings of celiac disease

The most important difference between silent celiac disease and potential celiac disease is that with the former, the small intestine biopsy is abnormal, and with the latter it is normal. Potential celiac disease is most likely to be discovered when someone has an blood test checked to evaluate symptoms and it's abnormal, or they participate in a celiac disease screening program and then go on to have a normal small intestine biopsy.

There is disagreement whether potential celiac disease is truly a form of celiac disease or rather an intermediate state. Celiac disease is, by definition, a condition in which the small intestine has certain characteristic abnormalities. Potential celiac disease, by definition, is characterized by a normal small intestine biopsy. For this reason, there is uncertainty about whether a person with potential celiac disease should be advised to start a gluten-free diet.

Deciding whether potential celiac disease should be treated

The arguments pro and con are much the same as we outline in the preceding section where we discuss silent celiac disease but with one major difference. If you have silent celiac disease, by definition, you have an *ab*normal small intestine biopsy. In other words, there is clear evidence that your celiac disease is causing damage to your body. If you have potential celiac disease, by definition, you have a *normal* small intestine biopsy and thus no evidence that celiac disease is damaging your body.

Because potential celiac disease is not associated with damage to the body — and because there is currently no proof that damage would develop in the future — justifying treatment for it is harder than justifying treatment for silent celiac disease (where, by definition, there is already evidence of damage). Nonetheless, some celiac disease experts believe potential celiac disease would eventually lead to damage and that it's better to treat it sooner than later. Other celiac disease experts believe that potential celiac disease may remain potential indefinitely; in fact, some people with potential celiac disease have a normalization of their antibody levels over time, even if they continue to eat gluten regularly. As such, these experts believe that placing someone on lifelong treatment (even one not involving medication) is inappropriate in the absence of hard scientific evidence that it's beneficial for this particular group of individuals.

An additional argument in favor of treating potential celiac disease is the possibility that the normal small intestine biopsies that were taken simply missed the abnormal intestine due to patchy disease or disease that could not be reached because it was further down the small intestine. In other words, the person labeled as having potential celiac disease actually has celiac disease. (Although we see the rationale for this argument, we believe that it's important to find damaged intestine — such as by using additional tests as we discuss in Chapter 3 — before labeling someone as having potential celiac disease.)

Our opinion, based on the current literature and our own experience, is that there is, at this point in time, insufficient justification to routinely treat people with potential celiac disease. We also feel, however, that it's imperative that a person diagnosed with potential celiac disease be monitored for the development of more overt disease (that is, one of the types discussed earlier in this chapter). The majority of our colleagues follow a similar approach. (We discuss monitoring of celiac disease in Chapter 13.)

2

Dealing with the Diagnosis of Celiac Disease

Chapter **5**

Celiac Disease and You

mazingly, 1 percent of people in the world have celiac disease. Unfortunately, many people living with celiac disease don't know they have it. They may not have obvious symptoms (we discuss symptoms of celiac disease in Chapter 2), or they may have symptoms for a long time and simply become accustomed to living with them. Or sometimes, a doctor hasn't thought of the diagnosis. The list of possibilities is far-reaching.

When celiac disease goes undetected and untreated, it can damage the body and even increase the risk of some cancers (see Chapter 9). We hope this book helps you recognize the signs and symptoms of celiac disease so that you will know when to speak to your healthcare provider about the possibility of celiac disease — even if it means bringing up the potential diagnosis with your doctor.

Being diagnosed with celiac disease is, in many ways, the start of a journey — with many twists and turns. In this chapter, we look at questions that typically come up after someone has been given the news. Questions like "What *is* celiac disease?" And "What causes it?" And "Why did I get it?" We also answer — with apologies to Tina Turner — "What's gluten got to do with it?" Last, we have a look at how your gut works normally and what happens when you have celiac disease.

Knowing What Causes Celiac Disease

In order for you to develop celiac disease, several factors must be present. (We illustrate these in Figure 5-1 and discuss them in detail in the sections that follow this one.) Some of these factors are inherited, and several play a role later in the process. Here are those key factors:

>> **Genes that put you at risk.** In order for you to develop celiac disease, you must have the genes that put you at risk of celiac disease. Without these "at-risk" genes, your risk of getting celiac disease is almost nonexistent.

>> **Ingestion of gluten.** Only the glutens found in some types of grains (including wheat, rye, and barley), when ingested, trigger the abnormal immune response present in celiac disease. If a person has never eaten gluten, they could never get celiac disease. This connection between gluten and celiac disease is why celiac disease is treated with a diet that does not contain gluten, the so-called *gluten-free diet*.

>> **Other environmental factors.** Something in the environment can trigger celiac disease, and researchers, not sure what it is (see "Environmental factors" later in this chapter). Some studies suggest that intestinal infections are a key environmental trigger, but it's unknown whether that's a cause in most people who develop celiac disease.

>> **A problem with your immune system.** To get celiac disease, a specific problem within the immune system has to develop in which, after you ingest certain types of grain proteins (*glutens*), your body's immune system behaves abnormally, including making antibodies against some of your own tissues. For this reason, celiac disease is classified as an *autoimmune* disease, meaning that the immune system attacks one's own body.

>> **A damaged small intestine.** This results from the abnormal immune response to gluten and is the characteristic underlying feature of celiac disease.

You can't change your genes, but you can change what you eat, and that is the basic tenet of treating celiac disease. By eliminating gluten from your diet, you interrupt the processes that we just listed so that the antibodies diminish, the inflammation gradually goes away, and your health is restored. We discuss the treatment of celiac disease in detail in Chapter 10.

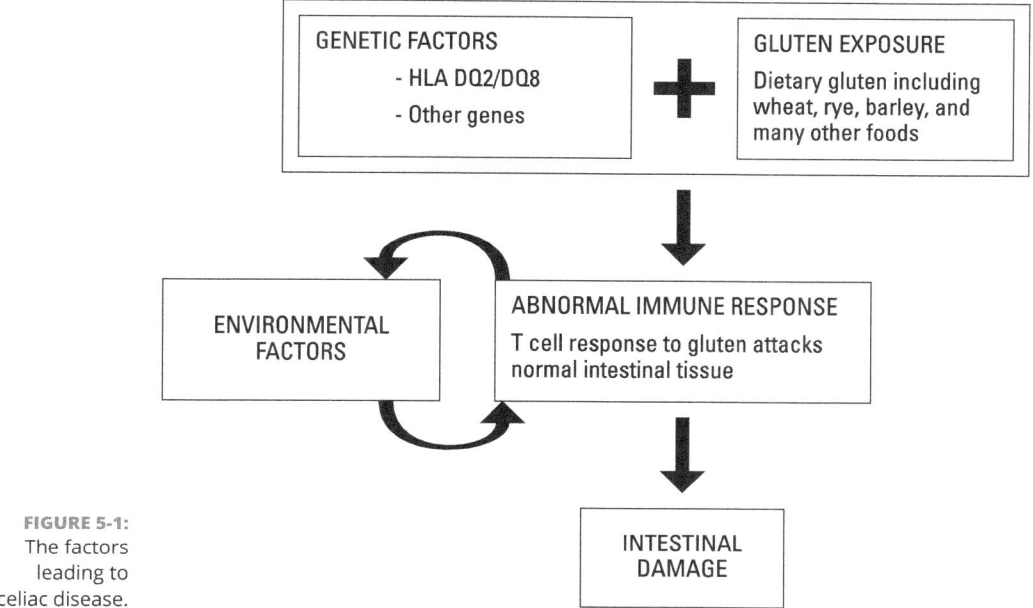

FIGURE 5-1:
The factors
leading to
celiac disease.

Genetic influences

Genes are those things found in cells' DNA that serve as a blueprint from which your body is built and develops. Your genes determine whether you're short or tall, blue-eyed or brown-eyed, and so on. Well before medical science knew about the specific genes that are associated with celiac disease, it was recognized that celiac disease runs in families. And even within families, there was additional evidence for a genetic influence because, doctors observed, both members within a set of identical twins (who, therefore, had the identical genes) were much more likely to have celiac disease than were members of a set of nonidentical twins (who share only half the same genes).

TECHNICAL
STUFF

Thanks to advances in medicine, a lot is now known about the genetics of celiac disease and, in particular, the important role of *human leukocyte associated* (HLA) genes. Depending on the type, there are many different types of HLA genes with widely varying roles in how the body functions (or malfunctions, as the case may be). The specific HLA genes involved with celiac disease are the DQ genes. (Despite their name, so far as we are aware, these genes don't make one long for soft ice cream; mind you, now that we think of it. . . .)

Virtually all people with celiac disease have either HLA DQ2 and/or DQ8 genes. Indeed, this association is so strong that if you have neither of these genes, you have almost no risk of ever developing celiac disease. Knowing this, doctors now use a test to detect HLA DQ2 and DQ8 genes to exclude the possibility of celiac disease in certain special situations. We discuss genetic testing further in Chapters 3 and 4.

The flip side, however, is not true: Because 40 percent of the North American population has these genes, yet only a very small percentage (2 or 3 percent) of this group develops celiac disease, other factors must be responsible for determining who gets celiac disease. We discuss this further in Chapter 15.

The immune system

The *immune system* is a complex set of cells and organs that protect the body from various types of illnesses. A major purpose of the immune system is to help fight off bacteria, viruses, parasites, and other infections. The immune system also helps get rid of dying cells and cancerous cells within our bodies. Every day, a slew of new research findings emerge about the incredibly important roles of the immune system in maintaining good health.

However wonderful the immune system is, sometimes, in fact, it does the wrong thing and turns against you by attacking your normal, healthy cells. Illnesses in which this behavior is a feature are called *autoimmune diseases*. Examples of autoimmune diseases are systemic lupus erythematosus (SLE), rheumatoid arthritis (RA), type 1 diabetes mellitus (all of which we discuss in Chapter 8), and, most important for this discussion, celiac disease.

Because celiac disease is an immune disease, we take a detailed look at the immune system in this section. Knowing the basics of how the immune system works helps you understand what happens when, as with celiac disease, it doesn't function properly. This information can be tough slogging, so we provide some handy dandy figures to help illustrate the key points we discuss.

The components of the immune system

The immune system consists of many types of cells and a number of different organs. It is made up of two branches:

TECHNICAL STUFF

>> **Systemic immune system:** Includes organs such as the thymus and the spleen; a variety of types of white blood cells that reside in the circulatory system of blood vessels; lymph glands (also known as lymph nodes); and lymph channels (that is, the pathways through which lymph fluid flows). This system is very important in protecting us against infections of the blood and also plays a role in autoimmune diseases.

>> **Mucosal immune system:** Consists of the immune cells present in the mucosal surfaces of the body. *Mucosal surfaces* are the linings of the respiratory tract, eyes, nose and sinuses, digestive tract, urinary tract, and the reproductive system. The mucosal immune system contains immune cells that are important in protecting us from infections of these parts of the body.

The immune system has a variety of different types of white blood cells, each with its own special function. Here we list some of these, and in the next section, we discuss what goes wrong when you have celiac disease:

>> **T cell lymphocytes (or just T cells for short):** Involved in recognizing and responding to sick cells, such as cells infected with a virus or cancerous cells.

>> **B cell lymphocytes:** Produce proteins called *antibodies.* Antibodies can attach to tiny molecules called *antigens*, which are present on the surface of germs and other substances, and allow the body to eliminate them.

>> **Neutrophils:** Help kill bacteria by releasing enzymes and toxins.

>> **Macrophages:** Eat (in a manner of speaking) other cells, including germs. They also act as a delivery service by taking certain proteins (antigens) that line the surface of various molecules and bringing them to T cells, where these lymphocytes can then act on them. (Sort of like an underworld boss's henchmen apprehending someone and bringing them to the boss to be worked over.) This is called *antigen presentation*.

>> **Eosinophils:** Involved in immune responses to parasites and are also important players in controlling the body's mechanisms associated with allergies.

>> **Basophils and mast cells:** Found either in the blood (basophils) or certain body organs, including the intestines (mast cells). Their main role is in generating an immune response to allergens and to certain parasites.

Now that you're armed with this information, we can show you what happens with your immune system if you have celiac disease.

The immune response

The *immune response* is the way in which the immune system reacts when exposed to tiny molecules called antigens. It is a wayward immune response to antigens that leads to diseases such as allergies and autoimmune diseases like celiac disease.

THE ROLE OF THE T CELL

In celiac disease, T cells play the greatest role in the abnormal immune response. In the case of celiac disease, gluten is the specific protein to which the immune system abnormally responds, and thus, it is gluten that triggers celiac disease. Gluten, which is present in certain foods, enters the mucosal lining of the small intestine, where macrophages then take it up. Through antigen presentation (see the preceding section, "The components of the immune system"), the macrophages "present" these foreign proteins to the T cells. The T cells generate an immune response to gluten that involves the production of inflammatory substances called *cytokines*, which damage the intestine.

THE ROLE OF TISSUE TRANSGLUTAMINASE (TTG)

With celiac disease, excess amounts of gluten enter the lining of the intestine. The gluten then encounters an enzyme called *tissue transglutaminase* (TTG) that has been released from intestinal cells that have already been damaged. When the gluten meets up with TTG, a very small piece of the gluten protein is broken off in a process known as *deamidation*. The deamidated gluten tenaciously attaches to and stimulates the T cells much more than regular gluten would. This is the last thing in the world you want to happen since it's the T cells that are already causing your gut to get damaged in the first place.

A vicious circle is now created (see Figure 5-2) in which gluten enters the lining of your intestine, T cells respond and release cytokines that cause damage; this damage leads to more gluten uptake, which in turn leads to deamidation that stimulates the T cells, which causes more cytokines to be released and causes more damage, and on and on. The net result is that the lining of your gut comes to resemble a war zone. At present, the only good way to bring the war to a halt is to remove gluten from the diet. We discuss the gluten-free diet in detail in Chapter 10.

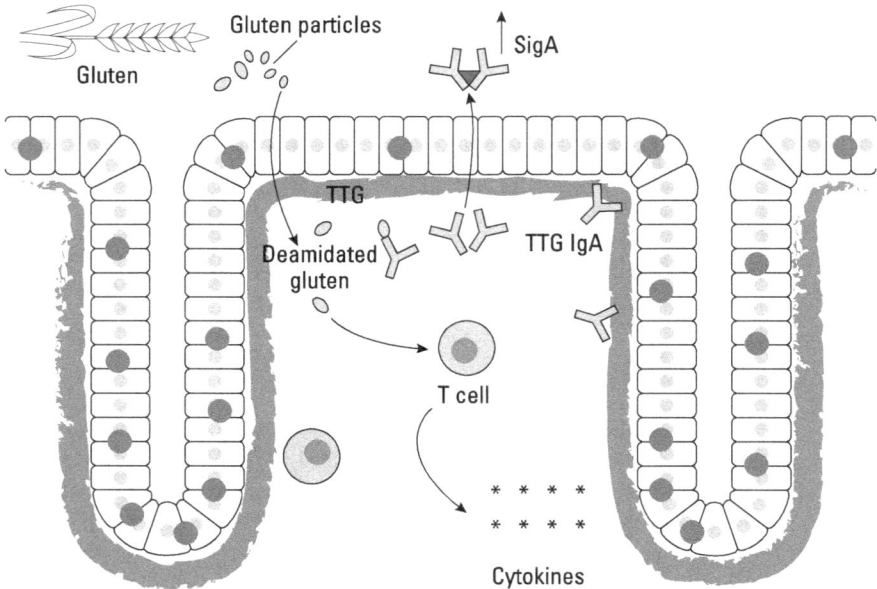

FIGURE 5-2:
The inflammatory changes in celiac disease.

Increased uptake of gluten by the small intestine

The *epithelial* cells that form the outermost layer of the small intestine are rather brilliant, at least when functioning normally. They know when to hold the line and when to allow things to get by. In terms of digestion, these cells keep germs and other foreigners out of the body while at the same time allowing absorption of nutrients into the body.

Many substances are not absorbed into the body through the cells per se, but rather, the minuscule spaces in between the cells. These spaces are known as *tight junctions* (see Figure 5-3). A variety of factors, including viral infections of the gut, anti-inflammatory medications, and intestinal diseases such as celiac disease, can cause these tight junctions to be, well, less tight, thereby allowing excess amounts and types of substances to gain entry into the body. This condition is referred to as *leakiness*. The increased leakiness (also known as increased *intestinal permeability*) seen with celiac disease is one way by which gluten may get a chance to start triggering the abnormal immune response that leads to the severe gut inflammation that we described in the preceding section.

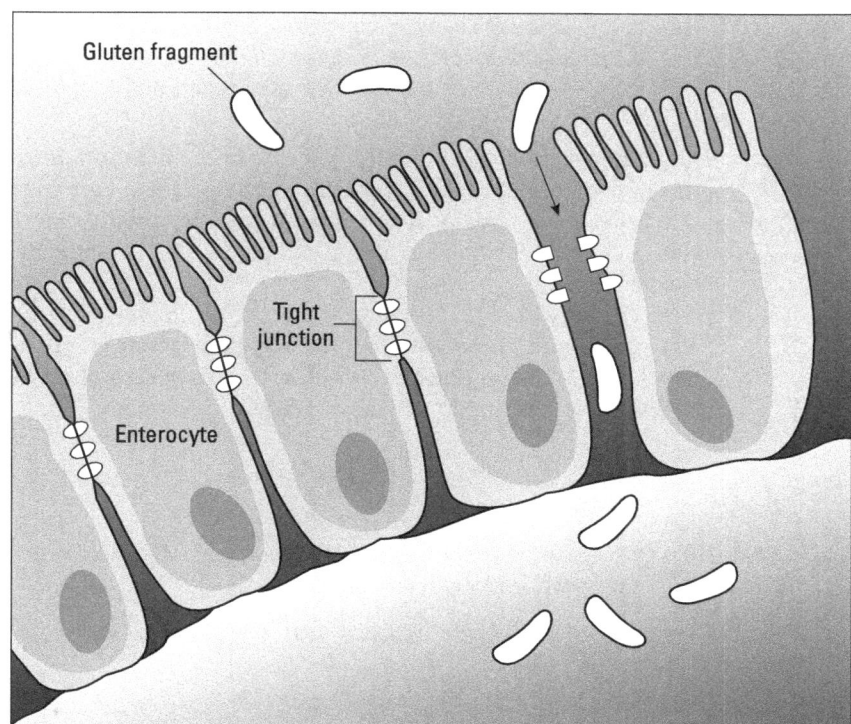

FIGURE 5-3:
Tight junctions.

Environmental factors

Anything apart from factors within your body that may cause illness is referred to as an *external* or *environmental factor*. As we mention earlier in this chapter, many people, although genetically at risk for getting celiac disease, never develop it, which tells doctors that other environmental factors must be responsible for celiac disease. Here are some additional clues that environmental factors are involved in celiac disease:

» **Geography:** Celiac disease is found in 1 percent of the population worldwide. Certain regions of the world have higher or lower prevalences, even while they have similar prevalences of the DQ2 and DQ8 genes. (Read more about the DQ genes in the "Genetic influences" section earlier in this chapter.)

» **Age:** Celiac disease is more common in young children today than it is in adults. Since celiac disease is considered a lifelong condition, there is likely something in the environment that is affecting children today that was not present among children generations ago.

» **An epidemic:** In the 1980s, there was a sudden increase in celiac disease among infants and young children in Sweden. This rise lasted for approximately ten years, and then, as quickly as it rose, cases dropped again. The causes of the epidemic are a matter of debate, though a main suspicion was the large amount of gluten in infant formula. (See the "Timing of gluten exposure in infancy" bullet later in this section, and Chapter 14.)

REMEMBER

Although consuming gluten leads to the inflammation found in the small intestine of people with celiac disease and results in the symptoms and other problems that are present, gluten in and of itself does *not* cause celiac disease. Gluten *triggers* or *causes flares* of celiac disease in people who are already predisposed to the condition.

So then, what is the environmental factor (or factors) that triggers celiac disease in genetically susceptible people? Alas, the answer is unknown. Also unknown are answers to other important questions, such as these:

» Why is celiac disease so much more prevalent now compared with 50 years ago?

» Whatever the factors responsible, why does celiac disease show up at different ages for different people?

» Why do these factors result in such varied ways in which celiac disease causes problems?

Although medical science doesn't have the answers to these questions, there's no shortage of theories. The following situations are potential factors that may play a role in why gluten triggers celiac disease:

» **Timing of gluten exposure in infancy:** It could be that the timing of when babies are first fed gluten-containing foods is an important environmental factor leading to celiac disease. We discuss this in detail in Chapter 14.

» **Excess hygiene:** The "hygiene hypothesis" proposes that the increasing number of people in industrialized societies with allergic and autoimmune diseases (such as celiac disease) is due in part to a relatively sterile environment (compared to other or previous societies). People in well-off societies have less exposure to germs and have fewer infections; the hygiene hypothesis suggests that this factor increases the chances of reacting to foods and other proteins in the environment and also to one's own antigens. This situation, in turn, can increase the chance of getting allergies, celiac disease, and other autoimmune diseases.

» **Infections:** It could be that during an episode of gastroenteritis (that is, an intestinal infection), the inflamed lining of the gut absorbs excess quantities of gluten, leading to an abnormal immune response which, in turn, causes celiac disease. (Although infections remain a possible factor in developing celiac disease, this does not seem to explain most cases.)

» **Stomach (gastric) surgery:** Sometimes, celiac disease shows up after patients have part of their stomach removed to treat an ulcer or to help severely overweight people lose weight ("bariatric surgery"). Why celiac disease shows up in these instances is unknown. Given the relative rarity of prior stomach surgery in people who are diagnosed with celiac disease, clearly this would be a factor in only a tiny proportion of cases.

» **Stress:** Various kinds of stress can influence many diseases, but typically by making a condition (such as high blood pressure) worse, rather than actually causing the condition to develop in the first place. Current medical research does not support previously held notions that stress is a cause of celiac disease; however, stress can make symptoms worse.

Understanding What Gluten Is

Almost everything humans eat is made from various types of proteins, carbohydrates, and fats. When considering celiac disease, the most important of these nutrients to know about is a protein called *gluten*. Gluten is a general name for the various *storage proteins* (also known as *prolamins*) found in grains. (Storage proteins are those proteins in grains available to provide nutrients for their future growth in the field.) Ingesting gluten triggers celiac disease and thus, gluten needs to be avoided if you have this condition.

As we discuss in Chapter 1, a Dutch physician observed that during World War II, when wheat was not available, previously ill children became healthier (and became ill again when wheat was reintroduced after the end of the war). This keen observation led to the eventual determination that celiac disease is triggered by exposure to gluten, which is a component of wheat and certain other grains.

TIP

Because the term *gluten* refers to a variety of different proteins, you may see it written in its plural form: *glutens.* However, most commonly it is used in the singular form.

Knowing where gluten is found

Gluten is present in many different types of foods and is also found in many commercial products (even some medicines!). Until not too long ago, it was very difficult to know if something did or did not contain gluten. Today, food and other product labels typically reveal this information. Food labels don't always indicate whether a food or product contains gluten, however. We discuss this and other gluten-free food and product issues in detail in Chapter 10. In this section, we list some commonly consumed foods and whether they contain gluten.

There are many naturally gluten-free foods, including dairy, seafood, meat, fruits, vegetables, and many grains. These naturally gluten-free foods can make up a delicious, healthy, and balanced diet. Table 5-1 will help you find your favorites.

Getting a handle on grains

Grains (cereals) are a major food staple in the human diet throughout the world. Not only are grains a key component of what people eat, but they have helped dictate how society has evolved. The ability to grow various foodstuffs — particularly grains — allowed and promoted the transition from hunter-gatherer societies to increasingly large and communal agricultural-based societies.

TABLE 5-1   General Foods to Include and Avoid on a Gluten-Free Diet

Type of Food	Foods to Include	Foods to Avoid

Grains and Grain-Based Products	Amaranth
	
	Arrowroot
	
	Buckwheat
	
	Cassava
	
	Corn
	
	Millet
	
	Oats (labeled GF)
	
	Potato (all varieties)
	
	Quinoa
	
	Rice (all varieties)
	
	Sorghum
	
	Tapioca
	
	Teff
	
	Pasta, breads, cereals, crackers, and cookies made from above grains
		Wheat: Kamut, semolina, spelt, triticale, farina, farro, emmer, einkorn, couscous
		
		Breads, cereals, pasta, cakes, cookies, and many snacks
		
		Barley
		
		  Flakes, flour, pearl
		
		  Malt: Flavoring, vinegar, extract, syrup
		
		  Beer, lager, ale
		
		Rye: Flour, bread, and flavoring
		
		Oats: Oats (not labeled GF)

Flours from Nontraditional Sources	Bean flour: Chickpea, lentil, soy Nut flour: Almond, chestnut, coconut Seed flour: Flaxseed	Wheat, rye, and barley-based flours
Dairy	Milk Cheese: Cottage, feta, blue cheese, cheddar, and so on Yogurt Kefir Ice cream Sour cream Whipped cream	Dairy with added cookie crumb or granola if not labeled GF

(continued)

TABLE 5-1 *(continued)*

Type of Food	Foods to Include	Foods to Avoid
Animal Protein	Meat	Imitation crab
	Eggs	Marinated, breaded, or coated proteins
	Fish/seafood	Be cautious with deli meats, sausages, salami, hot dogs, prepared meats
	Poultry	
Vegetable Protein	Beans/legumes	Seitan
	Hummus	Be cautious with tempeh and seasoned beans/nuts/seeds
	Tofu	Be cautious with protein powders
	Nuts/nut butters	
	Seeds/seed butters	
Fruits and Vegetables	All varieties	Be cautious with fruits and vegetables prepackaged in sauces
Fats and Oils	All varieties	Be cautious with baking spray
	Butter, margarine, oils	
Condiments, Sauces, Seasonings, Sweeteners, and Spices	Honey	Be cautious with
	Maple syrup	Cake icing
	Mayonnaise	Licorice
	Mustard (most are safe; read label)	Sprinkles
	Ketchup	Soy sauce
	Pasta sauce	Gravies, sauces, soups, and thickening agents
	Pickles, olives, relish	Spice blends, taco seasoning, marinades, pancake syrup
	Spices	
	Sugar	
	Sugar substitutes	
Alcohol	Alcohol	Beer, unless labeled gluten-free. (Note that "gluten-removed beer" is not gluten-free.)
	Distilled spirits	
	Hard cider	
	Wine	

Wheat, barley, and rye

Wheat is the major cereal grain consumed in many parts of the world, including North America, and, because wheat contains gluten, wheat is most responsible for triggering celiac disease in people living in these regions. Gluten found in wheat has two main components:

>> **Gliadins:** Responsible for dough's viscosity (thickness) and ability to be stretched. More important, in terms of celiac disease, it's the gliadins within gluten that are the specific trigger for celiac disease.

>> **Glutenins:** Responsible for dough's cohesiveness (tendency to stick together), strength, and elasticity.

The attributes of the gluten found in wheat (as we note in the preceding list) make wheat useful for making bread and also explain why making bread with gluten-free flours is difficult. We discuss tips for gluten-free baking in Chapter 10.

Barley contains a specific form of gluten known as *hordein*. Because barley contains gluten, it must be avoided by people with celiac disease.

Rye contains a specific form of gluten known as *secalin*. Because rye contains gluten, it, too, must be avoided by people with celiac disease.

Triticale is a blend of wheat and rye and is also to be avoided if you have celiac disease.

What about oats?

At one time, the consensus was that oats could trigger celiac disease, but a large number of studies in adults and children have now demonstrated that oats can, in fact, be safely consumed by people with celiac disease. There is, however, a *but*. Only oats labeled gluten-free are safe to eat if you have celiac disease. We include a list of brands of safe gluten-free oats in Appendix A.

WARNING

We do need to add one caveat to our "oats labeled gluten-free are okay to eat" comment. Some research suggests that a very small number of people with celiac disease do, in fact, react even to gluten-free oats.

Based on very good scientific studies as well as clinical experience showing oats to be well tolerated by both adults and children living with celiac disease, the current consensus among celiac disease experts is that if you have treated celiac disease and uneventfully eat gluten-free oat-containing foods, well, enjoy them. On the other hand, if you're having problems handling gluten-free oats, it may be best to discontinue consuming any and all oat products and consult your dietitian and physician for further advice.

Getting a grip on other grains

Most people are familiar with barley, rye, and wheat; however, there are a number of other, less well-known grains. Some of these contain gluten and therefore need to be avoided; others do not contain gluten and therefore can be safely consumed. Check Table 5-1 earlier in this chapter for grains to include and those to avoid.

Comparing Celiac Disease, Food Allergy, and Food Intolerance

To explain why they're on a special diet, many people with celiac disease understandably (and perfectly reasonably) try to make things easier for their friends, coworkers, and restaurant staff by just saying they are "allergic to wheat" rather than describing in detail what their condition is all about. Although saying you are allergic to wheat is perfectly fine and very useful when dining out or describing your dietary needs to other people, the statement is not perfectly accurate.

As we mention earlier in this chapter, celiac disease is an autoimmune disease, meaning that your immune system has turned against — and is attacking — your healthy tissues. Autoimmune diseases, including celiac disease, typically cause chronic problems, not sudden, life-threatening crises. Food allergies are caused by a different problem with the immune system and can lead to immediate, catastrophic situations. A food intolerance (such as lactose intolerance, which we discuss in detail in Chapter 11), on the other hand, is not related to the immune system and, although it leads at times to unpleasant symptoms, is not life-threatening in nature. We illustrate the key differences between these three conditions in Table 5-2.

TABLE 5-2   Comparing Celiac Disease, Food Allergy, and Food Intolerance

	Celiac Disease	Food Allergy (e.g., Peanut allergy)	Food Intolerance (e.g., Lactose intolerance)
Time to Onset after Consuming the Triggering Food	Days, months to years	Seconds to minutes	Minutes to hours
Common Symptoms	Variable, but often includes abdominal cramping, diarrhea	Shortness of breath, swelling of the lips and tongue, hives	Abdominal cramps, diarrhea
Immune Problem	T cell-mediated disease	Immediate hypersensitivity reaction	None

TECHNICAL STUFF

Technically speaking, a *food allergy* is a special type of immune reaction (called an *immediate hypersensitivity reaction*) that involves immune system cells called basophils and mast cells (these are special types of white blood cells involved with the body's allergic response and certain other conditions). An immediate hypersensitivity reaction results, upon exposure to a certain stimulus, in the immediate release into the bloodstream of a substance called *histamine,* which causes instantaneous — and sometimes life-threatening — symptoms such as shortness of breath, a swollen tongue, and a skin rash (hives). Perhaps you know people who are allergic to peanuts. They have this type of food allergy. People can also be allergic to wheat, which is different from celiac disease because the reactions to wheat are immediate and cause problems with breathing, hives, and swelling of the mouth and lips. Unlike in celiac disease, wheat does not cause intestinal damage in people with wheat allergy.

As you know from your own experiences living with celiac disease (or living with someone who has celiac disease), this is entirely different from what happens if a person with celiac disease consumes a gluten-containing food (such as wheat). Such instantaneous, life-threatening symptoms don't occur with celiac disease. As we discuss elsewhere in this chapter (see "Knowing How Things Work When You Have Celiac Disease"), the immune system plays a role in celiac disease, but it's of an entirely different nature.

The one exception to celiac disease and food intolerance being unrelated is if you have newly diagnosed and therefore untreated celiac disease, in which case, you may have temporary lactose intolerance. We discuss lactose intolerance in greater detail in Chapter 11.

Exploring Non-Celiac Gluten Sensitivity

Gluten sensitivity is not to be confused with the similar-sounding term, *gluten-sensitive enteropathy.* Gluten-sensitive enteropathy is simply a synonym for celiac disease. Gluten sensitivity, on the other hand, refers to the situation wherein a person who does *not* have celiac disease finds that ingesting gluten makes them feel unwell in one way or another.

Although much is yet to be learned about gluten sensitivity, two key points are well recognized:

>> Gluten sensitivity and celiac disease can cause *some* similar *gastrointestinal* symptoms such as nausea, abdominal discomfort or cramps, and diarrhea. Gluten sensitivity, however, does not cause the severe or specific problems

that can sometimes be seen with celiac disease, such as malabsorption and osteoporosis.

>> Whereas celiac disease causes demonstrable inflammation of the small intestine, gluten sensitivity does not damage the intestine or, for that matter, any other organs. In this sense, gluten sensitivity, even if it makes you feel unwell, does not carry the same potential dangers as celiac disease.

The cause of gluten sensitivity

Gluten sensitivity is neither a food allergy (like a peanut allergy) nor a T cell-mediated disease (like celiac disease). In fact, it is not necessarily gluten that is responsible for the symptoms of gluten-sensitivity in the first place.

If you are thought to have gluten sensitivity and have eliminated gluten from your diet and felt better thereafter, you may well be wondering how it could be that gluten wasn't actually responsible for your previous symptoms. (We'd sure wonder this if we were in this position.) Here's the explanation: Those who adopt a gluten-free diet can no longer eat a number of prepared foods (as these things contain gluten), and their diet starts to contain more *un*processed or natural foods. Going gluten-free gets rid of many additives, preservatives, fats, and other potentially unhealthy substances from the diet. Making this major improvement in your diet, it's no wonder that you would feel better! In other words, it's likely not the removal of gluten that made you feel better if you had gluten-sensitivity; it's eliminating all the other, unhealthy stuff that made the difference.

In some individuals with non-celiac gluten sensitivity, however, it may be gluten that is actually causing symptoms. Gluten can be hard to digest, and some medical studies have shown that diets high in gluten resulted in a larger output of stool compared to low-gluten diets. Perhaps this somehow results in the GI symptoms that are noted by people with gluten sensitivity. At present, this and other existing theories must be considered, well, just that: *theories*.

The potential hazards of treating presumed gluten sensitivity without first ruling out celiac disease

TIP

If, for any reason, you or a family member has symptoms that you believe are due to gluten, do *not* commit yourself or a family member to a long-term gluten-free diet without first seeing a physician to have an appropriate evaluation to determine whether celiac disease or some other potentially serious medical disorder is present.

Here are some of the many reasons why you or your family member should not follow a gluten–free diet without knowing what is being treated:

>> **A gluten-free diet may not be the correct treatment for the underlying medical problem.** A gluten-free diet, for instance, won't help inflammatory bowel disease (explained in Chapter 12).

>> **If you have been on a gluten-free diet for a number of months or more, it makes it more difficult to determine whether you have celiac disease (see Chapter 3).** Similarly, screening family members for celiac disease is more difficult if they are already on a gluten-free diet (see Chapter 6).

>> **A gluten-free diet is expensive, especially if the whole family eats gluten-free.** Why spend this extra money if you don't have to? Make sure at least someone in the family has a good reason to be eating gluten-free (be it celiac disease or gluten sensitivity) before committing to this expense.

>> **There is a risk of being less well nourished on a gluten-free diet.** Before you put yourself on a gluten-free diet, you should first meet with a registered dietitian to receive their expert advice. (See Chapter 11 for more on potential nutritional deficiencies due to celiac disease.)

>> **For medical insurance and tax reasons, it can be important to have a *proven* diagnosis of celiac disease.** Simply advising an insurer or tax department that you felt better not consuming gluten is unlikely to be sufficient to assist you with any insurance claims or applications for tax deductions. We discuss these issues in Chapter 13.

Understanding How the Normal Digestive Process Works

Digestion is the process of breaking down food and then absorbing its nutrients into your body. The digestive process involves a variety of organs (see Figure 5-4), each with special roles in helping transform the foods and liquids you consume into nutrients that are absorbed into the body and waste products that you excrete from your body. The organs involved with digestion are the

>> Gastrointestinal (GI) tract

>> Liver

>> Pancreas

This section covers how each of these organs assists with digestion.

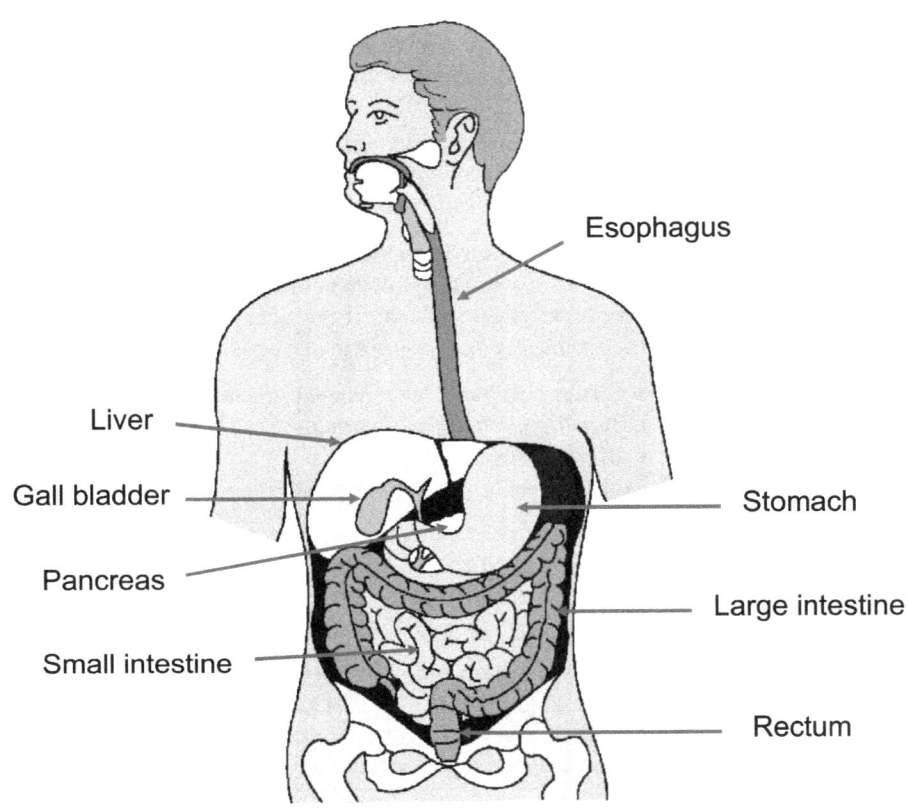

Esophagus

Liver

Gall bladder

Pancreas

Small intestine

Stomach

Large intestine

Rectum

FIGURE 5-4:
The digestive
system.

WHAT A PIECE OF WORK IS THE HUMAN BODY

Like many people, we marvel at the incredibly complex functioning of the most sophisticated computer in existence, the human brain. And, like many others, we also marvel at how, over a lifetime, the human heart will pump 3 billion times, and a person's kidneys will filter 1 million gallons of blood. Mind-boggling numbers indeed. But, equally incredible, although not getting nearly so much glory, is the work that the digestive system does as, over a lifetime, it looks after more than 100 tons (200,000 pounds; about 91,000 kilograms) of food and liquid you've swallowed! (In case you're wondering — and we suspect you aren't — that's equivalent to eating 20 elephants or, less tasty we presume, 10 city buses, not, ahem, including passengers.)

Getting down the gastrointestinal tract

Since digestion starts — and finishes — in the gastrointestinal tract (the "gut"), let's begin our journey here.

Normal anatomy of the gastrointestinal tract

The GI tract starts with the mouth, where food and liquids enter the body, and ends at the anus, where the wastes of what you eat — along with other things like dead bacteria and cells that line the gut — exit as stool. (*Stool* is the medical term for a bowel movement. Last time we checked — clearly we had too much time on our hands — there were well over 50 nonmedical synonyms for stool, many of which you may have some familiarity with, but of course we wouldn't know.)

For the purposes of discussion, the GI tract can be divided into three sections:

>> Mouth

>> Esophagus and stomach

>> Small intestine and large intestine (including the rectum)

In the following sections, we look — figuratively speaking — into each of these parts of your anatomy.

Looking at what the mouth, esophagus, and stomach do

The main job of the mouth is to chew food so you can swallow it. The mouth accomplishes this feat by using the teeth, tongue, and saliva (produced by the salivary glands):

>> **Teeth:** Help you chew food down into small pieces that are more easily swallowed.

>> **Tongue:** Allows you to taste the food you eat; if something tastes good, you are, of course, more likely to ingest it (and thus, derive nourishment from it).

>> **Saliva:** Aids in the digestive process, both by moistening food (which makes it easier to swallow) and by initiating breakdown of food through the action of saliva's digestive enzymes. We further discuss the role of digestive enzymes in the section, "Understanding what the pancreas and liver do."

When you swallow, food moves from your mouth into your esophagus. The esophagus is a flexible, muscular tube through which the food passes as it travels from your mouth into your stomach.

The stomach is a workhorse. This muscular organ helps digest food in two ways:

>> **Churning food:** Repeated, forceful contractions, which turn food into smaller pieces.

>> **Producing acid:** Helps break down proteins and other food components.

It takes up to several hours for the contents of the stomach to empty into the small intestine after a regular meal.

Recognizing the importance of the small intestine

Since celiac disease causes most of its havoc by damaging the small intestine, we look at this organ in detail. In this section, we discuss the features of a healthy small intestine, and later in this chapter (see "Knowing How Things Work When You Have Celiac Disease"), we look at abnormalities that can develop.

The small intestine (also known as the small bowel) is a long, coiled tube that, if stretched end to end, would measure over 20 feet. (Please don't try this at home!) The small intestine is the most vital part of the digestive process because this is where virtually all nutrients are extracted from food. The small intestine also helps regulate the body's fluid balance because it's responsible for absorbing most of the fluids you drink, along with those produced by the digestive tract, totaling about 6 to 8 liters a day. You cannot survive without your small intestine, and if this part of the digestive tract is damaged or partially removed, then you're at risk of malnutrition and dehydration, depending on how much small intestine function you are missing.

The small intestine consists of three sections (see Figure 5-5):

>> **Duodenum:** This first part of the small intestine measures just less than 1 foot in length (the jejunum and ileum are each considerably longer). The very first part of the duodenum is called the duodenal bulb. The stomach empties its contents into the duodenum. Digestive enzymes are made in the pancreas, and bile is made in the liver and empties through a duct into the duodenum. Iron and calcium are some of the few nutrients that are absorbed into the body from this part of the small intestine.

>> **Jejunum:** This second part absorbs the major food components, including proteins (in the form of small molecules like peptides and amino acids), carbohydrates (as small sugars such as glucose), fats (as triglycerides), and a variety of vitamins and minerals.

>> **Ileum:** The third part of the small intestine plays a role in absorbing vitamin B12 and bile salts, which are important in fat absorption.

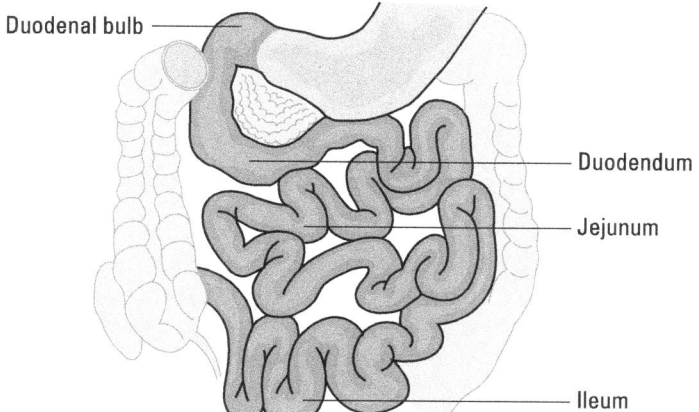

FIGURE 5-5:
The parts of the
small intestine.

The small intestine has millions of small, finger-like projections called *villi* that extend inward from the lining of the small intestine and greatly increase the amount of surface area available to interact with food and extract nutrients (see Figure 5-6). Villi increase the surface area of the small intestine in much the same way that the many branches on a tree increase the amount of a tree's surface area compared to having one long trunk.

The villi, in turn, are lined by even smaller projections called *microvilli* (also shown in Figure 5-6). Microvilli help with digestion because they further increase the surface area in the small intestine; also, they contain many digestive enzymes. Because microvilli are numerous and are packed closely together like a hairbrush with many densely packed bristles, the microvilli form what is called a brush-border.

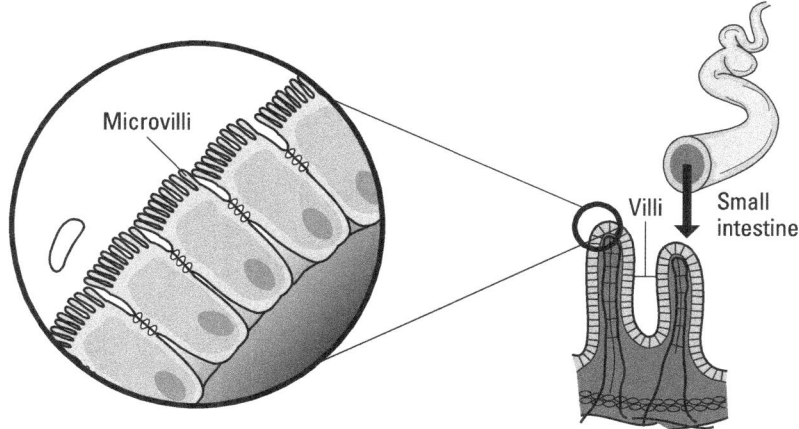

FIGURE 5-6:
The villi and
microvilli of the
small intestine.

The villi and microvilli increase the absorptive surface of the small intestine to about 350 square feet, the equivalent size of a small studio apartment in New York City!

Knowing what the large intestine and rectum do

The large intestine (also known as the colon) is the wide, 5-foot-long part of the gastrointestinal tract that connects the small intestine to the anus. The colon turns about 1 to 2 quarts of very liquid bowel contents it receives from the ileum into about one-third of a quart of solid stool each day. Prior to having a bowel movement, stool is stored toward the end of the large intestine, an area called the *sigmoid colon*. (Sigmoid means "S-shaped.") Just prior to defecating, stool passes from the sigmoid colon into the very last part of the large intestine: the rectum. It's the presence of stool in the rectum that gives you the urge to go to the bathroom. The very last part of the process is the subsequent passage of stool from the rectum through the anus into the toilet.

TIP

Although lots of people think the only normal pattern is passing a stool once a day, the normal range is actually anywhere from two or three a day down to three times a week.

Understanding what the pancreas and liver do

The pancreas is a 10-inch-long organ located in the upper part of the abdomen and behind the stomach. The pancreas produces digestive enzymes that travel down a duct from the pancreas and empty into the duodenum. These enzymes break down foods into microscopic sizes, which then allows them to be absorbed into the body across the lining of the small intestine (primarily the jejunum). The other essential function of the pancreas is to produce hormones, such as insulin, that help to control metabolism. These hormones are released from the pancreas directly into the blood. (For example, insulin helps regulate blood glucose; having insufficient insulin causes diabetes.)

The liver produces bile, which is transported through the bile ducts into the small intestine, where it helps digest fats. Bile can be stored in the gallbladder, which acts as a reservoir of bile between meals.

Knowing How Things Work When You Have Celiac Disease

In the previous sections, we look in detail at the normal anatomy and functioning of the digestive system. In the following sections, we look at the small intestinal abnormalities that are present in celiac disease. (The remainder of the digestive system is typically unaffected.) We can group these into two categories: abnormalities of structure and abnormalities of function.

Changes to the structure of the small intestine

The beautifully intricate and amazing structure of the small intestine is the very first thing to be injured if you have celiac disease. With celiac disease, the duodenum and jejunum are damaged; the ileum, however, is not usually affected. These are the stages in which damage to the small intestine happens after gluten exposure:

1. White blood cells, called *lymphocytes* (these are part of the immune system), accumulate in abnormal numbers in the tips of the small intestine's villi. Because of their location in the surface layer (*epithelial layer*) of the small intestine, these lymphocytes are called *intra-epithelial lymphocytes* or *IELs*.

2. The spaces (*crypts*) below the villi become proportionately longer (something called *crypt hyperplasia*).

3. The villi become shorter, or blunted, which is known as *partial villous atrophy*. (*Partial* because the blunting is not complete. *Atrophy* means "wasting away" or shrinking.)

4. The villi become so severely damaged that they are completely flattened; this condition is called *total villous atrophy*.

Figure 5-7 illustrates the various stages of intestinal damage in celiac disease.

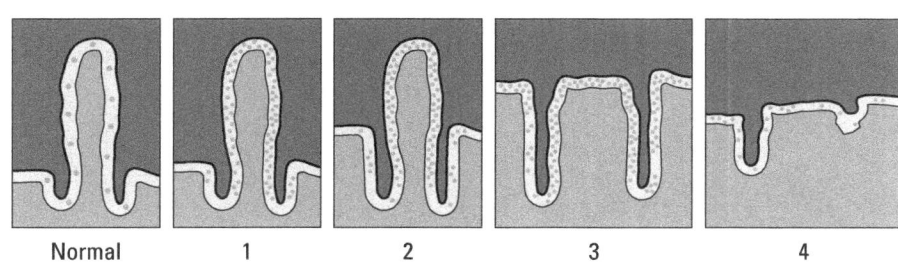

FIGURE 5-7:
The stages of intestinal damage in celiac disease.

Normal   1   2   3   4

Changes to the function of the small intestine

In the section, "Recognizing the importance of the small intestine," we discuss the importance to digestion of the huge surface area provided to the small intestine by the millions of villi (and microvilli). As you might expect, because celiac disease causes these villi to shrink — sometimes to the point of not even being identifiable — and because significant inflammation is now present in the small intestine, this organ's ability to function is severely compromised. Problems with small intestine function may include

- » Reduced ability to absorb fluids (and increased fluid production by the small intestine), which, if sufficiently severe, results in diarrhea.

- » Malabsorption of important minerals (such as iron and calcium) and vitamins (such as vitamin D and folic acid). Malabsorption can lead to anemia, osteoporosis, and other ailments.

- » Malabsorption of nutrients such as protein, which, in turn, may lead to progressive weight loss.

We discuss these and other potential complications from celiac disease in Chapters 7, 8, and 9. Now, lest you feel overwhelmed and discouraged by the problems we've pointed out in this chapter, be sure to read Part 3 of this book because that's where you'll find out what you need to know to correct these problems or avoid them in the first place.

Chapter **6**

Screening for Celiac Disease

f celiac disease caused every person with the condition to develop a shiny green foot, figuring out who does and who does not have the condition would be a piece of cake and as simple as having you take off your shoe. No diagnostic uncertainty. No tests necessary. But things are seldom that simple. As we discuss in Chapter 2, there is no symptom (or group of symptoms) that is unique to celiac disease. For that reason, when someone has suspicious symptoms — such as unexplained diarrhea, fatigue, or weight loss — further investigations, such as those described in Chapter 3, are required.

But what if you have no symptoms at all? Should you still be tested to see whether you have celiac disease? The quick answer is "it depends." The longer answer is, well, the entirety of this chapter. So read on . . .

Knowing When to Screen Someone for Celiac Disease

Screening for a disease is the term used when a doctor tests someone who doesn't have evidence of a disease to see if, nonetheless, they do in fact have it. In other words, screening is looking for a condition before it turns into a problem.

You may be surprised to learn that throughout your life, you've been screened for various diseases. Screening begins at birth when all infants are tested for hearing loss. As the years roll by, doctors perform other screening tests, including, depending on a person's age and gender, those for diabetes, high cholesterol, high blood pressure, breast cancer, colon cancer, and cervical cancer, to name but a few.

Two main criteria must be met in order to justify screening someone for celiac disease:

>> **A reasonable probability exists that testing will show you do indeed have celiac disease.** If the odds of your having celiac disease are close to zero, performing testing for this disease is, as you may expect, rarely going to be helpful.

>> **Determining that you have celiac disease is meaningful.** In other words, justification to test you for celiac disease only exists if, upon finding out you do indeed have the condition, you begin following a gluten-free diet. Also, the diet would need to be of health benefit to you.

We discuss controversies surrounding celiac disease screening in the sidebar, "To screen or not to screen, that is the question."

Determining Who Should Be Screened for Celiac Disease

A number of factors put you at increased risk of having celiac disease and, there-fore, may make screening you for celiac disease more appropriate.

These factors are the most important *general* situations that may make screening you for celiac disease appropriate (we discuss specific situations in a moment):

>> **If you have a close relative with celiac disease.** A close relative is consid-ered a *first-degree relative*, that is, a parent, sibling, or child with celiac disease.

>> **If you have a disease that often occurs together with celiac disease.** An example of such a so-called *associated disorder* is having another autoimmune disease, such as type 1 diabetes. We discuss this and other associated conditions in Chapter 8.

>> **If you have a disease that can be caused by celiac disease, such as osteoporosis or iron deficiency.** We discuss these conditions further in Chapter 7.

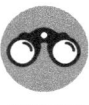

EXAMPLE

Jacob, a 25-year-old man, had been having problems with abdominal cramping and heartburn. Tests were run and a diagnosis of celiac disease was made. His perfectly healthy sister, Tara, having heard about her brother's diagnosis, saw her own physician, who tested her for celiac disease by sending her for appropriate investigations. As it turned out, she also had celiac disease. Both Jacob and Tara had celiac disease, but it was Tara who, being free of symptoms or other evidence of celiac disease, had been *screened* for the condition.

TO SCREEN OR NOT TO SCREEN, THAT IS THE QUESTION

In North America, people are screened for celiac disease only if it is thought they are at significant risk of having the condition. Several reasons exist for doing this *selective screening* rather than screening everybody (so-called *universal screening*), including

- The costs of the screening tests.

- Concerns about diagnosing a condition that may never cause clinical problems. (In other words, "if it ain't broke, don't fix it.")

- Identifying a problem for which the affected person is, perhaps, not interested in being treated.

Screening for diseases is important when the disease is contagious or if having the condition diagnosed and treated helps prevent deterioration in one's health, reduced quality of life, premature death, or any combination of the preceding. Because celiac disease is not contagious, it does not usually shorten lifespan significantly, and people with celiac disease who are symptom-free and only diagnosed by screening might never get sick from it. Screening everyone for the condition is not recommended in most countries. However, this remains a controversial area among experts in the field of celiac disease and, understandably, is also sometimes a point of contention among many individuals and their family members who have suffered from a delayed diagnosis of celiac disease.

The debate continues as to whether screening for celiac disease is justified on a widespread basis in the general population. Conversely, determining whether screening an individual on a case-by-case basis is a different matter because, for a specific individual, a doctor can generally estimate whether there is a sufficient probability of celiac disease that testing the person for it is appropriate.

Screening and genetic ancestry

Because of their genetic ancestry, some people (such as those from East Asia) are at lower risk of having celiac disease. Nonetheless, because North America has a long history of immigration from all corners of the world, determining which Americans are genetically at risk is not easy. For this reason, people who, based purely on their ancestry, might be considered to be at low risk for celiac disease are sometimes screened for this condition anyhow.

Screening and symptoms

TIP

We recommend you discuss with your doctor whether you should be screened for celiac disease if you have any of the following (all of which we discuss in Chapters 7 and 8), *particularly when other known causes of these conditions or symptoms cannot be identified*:

» Alopecia (loss of hair)

» Dry eyes and mouth

» Aphthous ulcers ("chancre sores") of the mouth

» Erosions of dental enamel

» Thyroid disorders

» Indigestion or heartburn

» Type 1 diabetes mellitus

» Liver and biliary tract problems (such as abnormal liver enzyme tests or autoimmune liver disease)

» Anemia

» Irritable bowel syndrome symptoms (bloating, cramps, altered bowel habits)

» Gynecological problems, such as not having begun having periods despite reaching an appropriate age, having periods stop before reaching menopausal age, or early menopause

>> Obstetrical problems, such as the inability to get pregnant, frequent miscarriages, and delivering premature babies

>> Osteoporosis, unexpected broken bones

>> Neurological problems, such as neuropathies, difficulties with balance, and migraine headaches

>> Behavioral disorders, including hyperactivity, difficulty concentrating

>> Mood and thinking problems such as depression, irritability, or forgetfulness

>> Growth and development problems in infants and young children, including lack of growth, insufficient growth, and unexplained weight loss

>> Fatigue, if chronic

>> Down syndrome or Turner syndrome

TECHNICAL
STUFF

One could consider looking for celiac disease in such instances as case finding rather than screening, since many, if not most, of the disorders listed above can be associated with celiac disease and since, by definition, screening is typically considered to be testing for a condition in the absence of any evidence that it is present. But hey, we don't want to get overly nitpicky here.

The preceding list is long and admittedly somewhat intimidating: What person, after all, hasn't had at least some of the features that we noted? Indeed, the number of situations in which celiac disease could be considered is rather mind-boggling. Turning things on their ear, one could reasonably ask, "Who should *not* be tested for celiac disease?" The truth of the matter is that the answers to the questions of who to screen and who not to screen simply aren't known. We think a reasonable compromise is for you to be tested if you have features in the preceding list *and* they are persisting or unexplained by other, more obvious causes.

Screening, personal choices, and one's stage in life

That the person being screened should want to be screened goes without saying. Undergoing screening tests may not be a huge ordeal, but some people would rather not undergo these tests, thank you very much. Also, some people don't want to be treated for the condition being searched for, in which case there's no point searching for the condition in the first place. Some benefit must be derived from finding out that you have celiac disease, and some value must be obtained by being treated with a gluten-free diet.

Understanding How Screening for Celiac Disease Works

Screening for celiac disease is performed in two ways:

>> **Genetic testing** is performed on either a blood sample or on cells obtained from the inside of the cheek (obtained by a painless "scraping" of the inside of the cheek). If the test is positive, further investigations are then undertaken. We discuss this further in the section "Genetic testing."

>> **Antibody testing** is performed on a blood sample obtained from the person being screened. If the test is negative (that is, the antibody is not present), the test is repeated every few years. Lifelong rescreening applies primarily to first degree relatives of celiac disease patients, although if celiac disease has not developed by later in life, a case could be made that enough is enough and screening may then be discontinued. (Having said that, because celiac disease can present in every decade of life, experts don't really know when screening should stop in someone who has the HLA DQ2 and/or DQ8 genes that make them at risk of developing celiac disease.)

Genetic testing

Your genes lay out your body's blueprint. Your genes determine whether you have dark hair or blond hair, are short or tall, and so forth. As we discuss in Chapter 2, the genes most associated with celiac disease are called HLA DQ2 and DQ8.

If you have the HLA DQ2 and/or DQ8 genes, this does *not* mean that you are certain (or even likely) to have celiac disease, but it does mean that you are at increased risk. Therefore, if you have these genes, additional tests (including antibody testing and, if positive, endoscopy with small intestine biopsy) are needed to determine whether celiac disease is present. The main benefit of having genetic screening is that if you don't have the HLA DQ2 or DQ8 genes, you are almost without risk of ever getting celiac disease, and so further screening is not necessary.

Antibody testing

As we discuss in Chapter 3, several blood tests are available that check whether you have antibodies to various proteins that are associated with celiac disease. Of these, the most accurate one to help diagnose (or, if absent, exclude) celiac disease is the IgA antibody to tissue transglutaminase (TTG IgA).

REMEMBER

The TTG antibody is not a perfect test and can be falsely elevated; for example, it can be positive even in people without celiac disease. Therefore, if your TTG Ab result is positive, this result does not automatically mean you have celiac disease, and you may still need a biopsy of your small intestine performed. (See Chapter 3.)

Asymptomatic Celiac Disease Detected by Screening

When an asymptomatic individual (that is, someone who has no symptoms) undergoes screening and is found to have celiac disease, they have either the silent or potential forms of celiac disease. We discuss these and the other types of celiac disease in Chapter 4.

The long-term outlook for people diagnosed with silent or potential celiac disease is unknown, and some controversy exists as to whether such individuals should be treated with a gluten-free diet. On the one hand, after starting the gluten-free diet, some people discover they indeed had symptoms (fatigue, constipation, bloating); they had considered the way they felt as "normal." Some studies demonstrate an improved quality of life after asymptomatic celiac disease is detected by screening and treated by a gluten-free diet. However, some people report increased burden of the diet and disease.

Given this conflicting information, doctors are often understandably hesitant to screen everyone at risk of celiac disease, seeing as the discovery of these asymptomatic forms of celiac disease doesn't always clarify what should be done, if anything.

Chapter **7**

Conditions Caused by Celiac Disease

As we explain in Chapter 5, celiac disease damages the small intestine and, as a result, decreases the absorption of nutrients into the body. This is called *malabsorption*. If you have malabsorption, the nutrients from the food you eat are not fully absorbed and are lost from your body with your stool. The extent of the damage to the intestine will affect how much and which specific nutrients are lost. As your intestines heal, your absorption of nutrients will increase. This chapter looks at this subject in detail. It also examines several other conditions that are related to celiac disease but where the connection to malabsorption is less clearly established.

As you read through this chapter, keep in mind that each person is unique and the various conditions may not affect everyone. Also, keep in mind that these conditions are treatable. And speaking of treatment, in Chapter 13, we look at how often you should have laboratory tests done to monitor your body's levels of many of the things we discuss here.

Vanishing Vitamins

For the most part, the vitamins that people require for good health are readily available and consumed as part of a healthy diet. However, if you have celiac disease, you may have some degree of malabsorption leading to potentially insufficient levels of these vitamins in your body. As a result, your health can suffer. In this section, we look at the various vitamin deficiencies that can be seen with celiac disease and foods rich in the vitamins to add to your gluten-free diet.

Considerations about taking vitamin supplements

Regardless of whether you have celiac disease, if you are currently taking, or are considering taking, vitamin supplements, just like taking a prescription or over-the-counter medicine, taking vitamin supplements should be done with proper caution. Consider the following things:

>> You should have blood work done to see if you actually need any vitamin supplements.

>> If you are deficient, you only need to take the specific vitamin you need.

>> Remember, even vitamins at high doses or when you don't need them can become toxic.

TIP

When it comes to all things nutrition, we encourage you to speak to your dietitian about your vitamin requirements and how best you can ensure you meet these through your healthy, gluten-free eating and, if necessary, by taking supplements.

REMEMBER

In this section, when we discuss the various vitamins, we encourage you to think about including the foods rich in these vitamins in your routine gluten-free diet. As these vitamins can come from the diet, routine use of vitamin supplements is not necessary for most people.

Vitamin A

Vitamin A is found in

>> Liver, beef, chicken

>> Eggs, cheese, milk, butter, margarine

>> Carrots, sweet potatoes, spinach, and other green vegetables

>> Mangoes, oranges

Deficiency of vitamin A can lead to

>> The inability to properly see in dim light (night blindness). If not treated, with time, this can progress to complete blindness.

>> Poor bone development and impaired growth in children.

>> Reduced functioning of the immune system, thus increasing one's susceptibility to infections.

>> Dry hair, dry and itchy skin, fragile and easily broken fingernails.

>> Miscarriages and reduced ability to breastfeed.

Most people, even those with celiac disease, living in developed societies like North America, rarely develop vitamin A deficiency. However, if your eyesight in low-light conditions is not what it should be, let your doctor know. They can send you for a blood test to measure your vitamin A level.

Vitamin B9 (folate or folic acid)

Vitamin B9, more commonly known as *folate* or *folic acid*, is found in

>> Green, leafy vegetables (such as spinach, swiss chard, cabbage, kale, cauliflower, broccoli, and Brussels sprouts)

>> Citrus fruits

>> Beans

>> Animal products

A deficiency of vitamin B9 can lead to

>> Anemia (see "Low Blood: Anemia" later in this chapter for more information).

>> Premature atherosclerosis ("hardening of the arteries"), which, in turn, increases the risk of heart attack and stroke. (This is not yet fully proven.)

>> Pregnancy complications, including damage to the fetus's developing spinal cord.

>> Soreness and inflammation of the tongue.

TIP

Contrary to what many people think, vitamin B9 deficiency does *not* cause nerve damage.

Folic acid deficiency is often found in people with celiac disease, since gluten-free breads and pastas are often not fortified with folic acid like wheat-based products are. If you're deficient in folic acid, in addition to following a gluten-free diet, you should ensure that your diet is rich in foods containing this vitamin. Most people with low folate acid levels have no symptoms, but this should be treated so as to prevent the potential consequences of long-term deficiency. If necessary, your healthcare provider will recommend a folic acid supplement and monitor your bloodwork.

Vitamin B12

Vitamin B12 is found in

» Animal products

» Dairy products

Because vitamin B12 is found only in animal products, deficiencies can be found in people who follow a vegan diet (a diet that eliminates all animal products).

Deficiency of vitamin B12 can lead to

» Anemia (see "Low Blood: Anemia" later in this chapter)

» Nerve damage leading to an unsteady gait

» Impaired thinking, memory, and change to one's personality

» Soreness and inflammation of the tongue

Vitamin B12 is absorbed into the body from the end part of the small intestine (the terminal ileum; see Chapter 5 for an in-depth discussion of the small intestine). Because this area of the bowel is seldom damaged by celiac disease, vitamin B12 deficiency is uncommon. If you do have a vitamin B12 deficiency, then the treatment would include adding foods that are rich in this vitamin or taking an oral vitamin B12 supplement. In some cases, vitamin B12 needs to be given by periodic injection.

Vitamin D

Vitamin D is found in

>> Fatty fish

>> Eggs

>> Vitamin D–fortified dairy products

Sunlight is the primary source of Vitamin D for most people. Sun exposure allows a person's skin to naturally make its own vitamin D (though we don't recommend spending lots of time in the sun, given the risk of burns in the short term and skin cancer in the long term). Because so few foods naturally contain vitamin D, it is added to many food products (such as milk).

A vitamin D deficiency can lead to

>> Osteoporosis in adults, rickets in children, and bone pain. (We discuss osteoporosis and rickets later in this chapter.)

>> Calcium deficiency.

>> Decreased immune function.

Many other ailments, including some types of cancer, heart disease, diabetes, and multiple sclerosis, also seem to occur more often in people with vitamin D deficiency, although supplementation is not thought to prevent these conditions.

Although vitamin D deficiency occurs commonly in the general population, it is more common in people with celiac disease. In addition to following a gluten-free diet, treatment consists of taking vitamin D supplements and, when necessary, calcium. The dose of vitamin D that you require needs to be individualized, but usual doses, depending on your dietary intake, range from 400 to 1,000 units per day.

TIP

As they get older, many people, with or without celiac disease, do not have sufficient intake of vitamin D in their diets or sufficient sun exposure to make enough vitamin D. Also, the skin's ability to make vitamin D deteriorates as one ages. For this reason, routine use of vitamin D supplements is sometimes advised by healthcare providers for their patients in this situation. Be sure to ask your healthcare provider whether you should routinely take vitamin D (and calcium).

Vitamin E

Vitamin E is found in

>> Green, leafy vegetables (such as spinach, swiss chard, cabbage, kale, cauliflower, broccoli, Brussels sprouts)

>> Asparagus, avocado

>> Oils (vegetable, soybean, canola, corn, cottonseed)

>> Nuts and seeds

>> Milk, eggs

A vitamin E deficiency can lead to

>> Anemia

>> Nerve damage

>> Muscle injury

Most people are unlikely to ever develop vitamin E deficiency, and routine testing of this vitamin is not part of standard blood work.

Vitamin K

Vitamin K is found in

>> Green, leafy vegetables (such as spinach, swiss chard, cabbage, kale, cauliflower, broccoli, Brussels sprouts)

>> Avocado

>> Kiwifruit

The human gut, through the action of the bacteria that normally reside in the small intestine (part of the *microbiome*, the name for the collective group of microbes that live within our gut), also manufacturers some vitamin K from other nutrients that are eaten.

Deficiency of vitamin K can lead to

>> Impaired ability of the blood to clot (coagulate); this can result in easy bruising and bleeding from the gums, bladder, gut, and other organs.

>> Impaired bone growth and strength. (Why vitamin K deficiency leads to bone problems is not fully sorted out.)

It's highly unlikely you will be deficient in vitamin K, and neither routinely testing for this nor the use of vitamin K supplements is necessary. Having said that, if ever you notice unexpected or undue bleeding, it is imperative that you — or *anyone* for that matter — seek urgent medical attention.

Missing Minerals

Like vitamins and other nutrients, minerals are also absorbed into your body in the small intestine. Again, as your intestine heals, your absorption of nutri-ents improves.

REMEMBER

In this section, when we discuss the treatment of mineral deficiencies, our recommendations should always be considered as *supplementary* to a balanced and varied gluten-free diet.

Calcium deficiency

Calcium is found in

>> Milk products including milk, yogurt, ice cream, and certain cheeses

>> Tofu

>> Canned salmon or sardines containing bones

>> Dark green vegetables, dried beans

Calcium is also often added to foods such as some brands of orange juice, as well as almond, rice, and soy beverages.

A calcium deficiency can lead to

>> Osteoporosis and, in children, rickets. (We discuss these conditions later in this chapter.)

>> Muscle spasms.

>> Seizures (also known as convulsions or epilepsy).

>> Fatigue, irritability, anxiety, and depression.

Calcium deficiency due to celiac disease is most often manifests as interfering with normal bone growth and strength.

Measuring calcium is complicated because the circulating level of calcium in the blood only tells part of the story; most calcium is stored in the bones. In fact, high levels of calcium circulating in the blood is sometimes a sign that bone calcium stores are being depleted. Still, healthcare providers routinely monitor blood calcium (and vitamin D) levels in people with celiac disease. If you are deficient in calcium, treatment consists of taking calcium supplements, usually in a dose ranging from one to several grams per day, depending on your bone density, blood test results, and your dietary intake. Also, to maintain good bone health, many women — regardless of whether they have celiac disease — are recommended to take calcium supplements, particularly if their dietary intake is inadequate. Speak to your dietitian to find out your particular requirements.

TIP

Low calcium due to celiac disease rarely occurs in isolation; more commonly, it occurs in the context of low levels of vitamin D. Therefore, supplements of both calcium and vitamin D are typically required in this situation.

WARNING

If you're taking a calcium supplement, it's important to take it without food, and especially not with calcium-rich foods or an iron supplement. Only a small percentage of calcium is absorbed at one time, so separating it from calcium-rich foods maximizes the amount of calcium you get from both the foods and the supplement. Also, calcium and iron are absorbed in the same area of the small intestine and therefore compete for absorption, so it's best to keep them in separate doses.

Iron deficiency

Iron is found in

>> Red meat

>> Tuna, salmon

>> Chicken and other poultry

>> Clams, oysters, mussels

>> Lentils, beans, chickpeas

While wheat-based products are required to be supplemented with iron (so-called "iron-fortified" foods) to make up for the iron lost during processing, gluten-free products are not required to be supplemented.

TIP

Iron found in red meat, fish, poultry, and seafood is more readily absorbed into the body (more *bioavailable*) than iron found in vegetables, fortified foods, or in oral iron supplements.

An iron deficiency can lead to

>> Anemia (discussed in detail in the later section "Low Blood: Anemia").

>> Fatigue. Iron deficiency can cause fatigue even if anemia is not present.

>> Tongue pain, dry mouth, and hair loss. These occur infrequently.

Iron deficiency occurs commonly in people with celiac disease. In fact, the detection of anemia (due to iron deficiency) is often the first clue that a person has celiac disease.

Successfully treating iron deficiency

The mainstays of treating iron deficiency due to celiac disease are to follow a gluten-free diet, to ensure one's diet contains sufficient iron, and, for most people, to take an iron supplement. We list iron-rich foods earlier in this section; for a full discussion of a gluten-free diet, go to Chapter 10. Here are key points regarding oral iron supplements:

>> **Three types of oral iron supplements are available:** *ferrous fumarate, ferrous gluconate,* **and** *ferrous sulfate.* Although a virtually infinite number of oral iron preparations are sold on the market, they all contain just one of these three types of iron).

>> **Each of the available iron supplements contains different amounts of iron.** When reading the labels on iron supplements, be sure to differentiate the total iron content of a pill from the *elemental iron content*. It's only the elemental iron content that's meaningful.

>> **Coated or sustained-release iron supplements are less effective than regular iron supplements.** Iron is absorbed best from the duodenum and the first part of the jejunum (refer to Chapter 5 for a discussion of these parts of the small intestine), but coated and sustained-release iron formulations are absorbed further down the gut. This mismatch means that these iron preparations are less well absorbed into the body.

>> **They work less well when taken at the same time as food.** Certain constituents of food (such as phosphates) attach to the orally taken iron and interfere with its absorption into the body. This is particularly true of milk, eggs, coffee, tea, fiber, and cereals. In general, it is best to take oral iron supplements on an empty stomach (see later in this list).

>> **They shouldn't be taken at the same time as antacids.** Antacids interfere with the absorption of oral iron supplements; therefore, take your iron at least two hours before, or at least four hours after, taking an antacid.

>> **Taking vitamin C (ascorbic acid) or drinking a glass of citrus juice (like orange juice) at the same time as your iron pill will help the iron get absorbed into your body.** If you're taking vitamin C, a dose of 250 mg is recommended.

>> **Iron supplements can cause gastrointestinal side effects.** GI side-effects due to oral iron therapy are quite commonly seen. Symptoms include nausea, abdominal discomfort, constipation, and, sometimes, diarrhea. If you are having GI side effects from your oral iron pills, speak to your doctor or dietitian, who may recommend the following:

- *Reducing your dose and then gradually building the dose back up.* Using a low dose and then gradually increasing the dose may be better tolerated by the gut.

- *Taking your iron with food rather than on an empty stomach.* Oral iron taken with food causes fewer GI side effects than when it is taken on an empty stomach. On the other hand, when taken with food, the iron is less well absorbed. One way around this is to take a higher dose of the iron with food.

- *Changing to a different iron preparation.* Ferrous gluconate *may* cause fewer GI side effects than the other types of oral iron. This, however, is arguable since the amount of elemental, as opposed to *total,* iron in ferrous gluconate pills is considerably less than is found in ferrous fumarate or ferrous sulfate. In other words, it may be the amount of iron, not the type of iron, that is responsible for the side effects.

- *Taking liquid iron supplements if you are unable to tolerate any of the available iron pills.* Liquid iron is called *ferrous sulfate elixir.*

What about iron given by injection?

Because iron taken by mouth is often not well-tolerated, the question comes up whether iron can be given by injection instead. Indeed, there are iron preparations, expressly designed for this purpose. Such injections are sometimes used to treat iron deficiency in special situations and can prove invaluable for those specific scenarios.

Other mineral deficiencies

In addition to the minerals discussed previously, small amounts of copper, magnesium, selenium, and zinc are also required for good health. It is rare for people to be deficient in these elements; therefore, routine testing or supplementing for these is uncommon unless a person has severe diarrhea or evidence of marked malnutrition.

Low Blood: Anemia

Anemia is defined as an insufficient number of red blood cells. To make red blood cells, the bone marrow requires iron, folic acid, and vitamin B12. If you are deficient in these nutrients, anemia may result. Since the main job of red blood cells is to carry oxygen to the body's various organs, if you're anemic, your heart, muscles, and other organs are deprived of this vital substance. As a result, you may experience symptoms such as fatigue, shortness of breath, and reduced stamina when exercising.

TIP

If you experience the symptoms we just mentioned, be sure to ask your doctor whether they have recently checked your blood hemoglobin level and, if not, ask for the test.

Anemia due to low iron ("iron deficiency anemia")

As we discuss earlier in this chapter, iron deficiency occurs commonly in celiac disease. When iron deficiency leads to anemia, the condition is called *iron deficiency anemia*. Because iron deficiency anemia is common in celiac disease, we look at it in detail in this section.

How is iron deficiency anemia diagnosed?

Iron deficiency anemia is diagnosed when blood tests show that a person has both anemia and low iron.

TECHNICAL STUFF

Several different types of blood tests are used to determine whether someone is iron-deficient. Each of these tests has its pros and cons. The most accurate test to determine if you lack sufficient iron is the *ferritin*. Having a low ferritin indicates you are deficient in iron. Nonetheless, a normal ferritin doesn't guarantee that you are *not* iron-deficient, so other tests or a combination of tests are sometimes used.

Ensuring your celiac disease isn't overlooked if you have iron deficiency anemia

If your celiac disease has not yet been diagnosed, and your doctor determines that you have iron deficiency anemia, celiac disease will likely not be high on the radar, and you'll be at risk of having the real cause of your anemia (that is, your celiac disease) overlooked. Why? Because your iron deficiency anemia may be thought to be due to one of the more common causes, such as menstrual blood loss in a woman or colon cancer in an older person of either gender, rather than caused by undiagnosed celiac disease.

Following are a few scenarios where iron deficiency anemia is commonly misattributed. If ever you — or a loved one — are in this situation, you can raise the possibility of celiac disease.

THE WOMAN WHO HAS PERIODS

Many, many women who have periods have iron deficiency anemia because of the iron lost with their periods (blood is rich in iron). Because this occurs so often, most doctors who discover one of their female patients who menstruates has iron deficiency anemia will, perfectly appropriately, simply prescribe iron therapy.

The key to avoiding having the diagnosis of celiac disease overlooked is this: If your iron deficiency anemia is being treated with iron supplements — and assuming you've been taking them as prescribed — yet you continue to be iron deficient, ask your doctor about the possibility that the real problem is malabsorption of iron due to celiac disease.

THE OLDER PERSON

Iron deficiency anemia in the elderly is often due to bleeding from the intestine, invariably in such tiny quantities that it's not visible. This is called *occult GI blood loss*. (Occult as in *hidden*.)

Because occult GI blood loss is often due to serious diseases, a thorough search for the cause must be undertaken. This search typically involves having a colonoscopy (where the doctor performing the test will look for a variety of abnormalities, the most important of which is colon cancer). If the colonoscopy is normal, the next step is typically to have an upper endoscopy (that is, a scope of your esophagus, stomach, and duodenum; we discuss this procedure in Chapter 3), where the doctor will look for problems such as cancer, ulcers, and abnormal blood vessels.

Save yourself an extra endoscopy! If, as part of investigations to determine if you're having occult GI bleeding, you're scheduled for an endoscopy, in advance of having the procedure done, ask the doctor doing the test to do a small intestine biopsy while they're at it. Otherwise, the endoscopy may end up needing to be repeated later on if, once GI bleeding has been excluded, the diagnosis of celiac disease is only then being entertained.

How is iron deficiency anemia treated?

The treatment of iron deficiency due to celiac disease is to follow a gluten-free diet, to ensure your diet includes sufficient dietary iron and, if necessary, take oral iron supplements. We discuss this topic in detail in the earlier section "Iron deficiency."

Hassan, a 35-year-old plumber, was seeing his family physician for a regular checkup. He had routine blood tests performed and, to the doctor's and Hassan's surprise, these revealed that Hassan had anemia. Further blood tests revealed that the cause of the anemia was low iron. The doctor sent Hassan for a colonoscopy to make sure he wasn't losing blood from the large intestine. The test was normal. Similarly, an endoscopy found Hassan's stomach and small intestine to look normal. The doctor performing the endoscopy thought to perform small intestine biopsies, and these came back showing typical features of celiac disease. As a result, the doctor then checked a tissue transglutaminase IgA, and it was elevated. The diagnosis of celiac disease was then confirmed, and Hassan was sent to a dietitian, placed on a gluten-free diet and iron supplements, and in a few months, his iron level and hemoglobin were both back to normal. At no time had Hassan experienced symptoms.

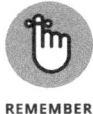

As Hassan from the preceding anecdote discovered, you can have celiac disease even if you feel completely well, and iron deficiency anemia may be the first clue to the diagnosis of celiac disease.

If you have an iron deficiency due to celiac disease and you are then treated with a gluten-free diet, once your iron levels are back to normal, ongoing iron supplements are typically no longer required. There are, however, two main exceptions to this: if you're a vegetarian, especially a vegan (as we discuss in Chapter 11, such individuals can have difficulty consuming sufficient quantities of dietary iron), or a woman who experiences heavy periods. For these people, ongoing use of oral iron supplements may be necessary.

Anemia due to low levels of folic acid

Like iron deficiency, folic acid (folate) deficiency is also common in people with celiac disease. Anemia from folic acid deficiency, however, occurs far less often than anemia due to iron deficiency.

TECHNICAL
STUFF

In your Internet travels, you may come across the term *megaloblastic anemia.* This refers to anemia due to either folic acid or vitamin B12 deficiency.

Malabsorption from celiac disease can lead to folic acid deficiency and, hence, anemia because of insufficient absorption of this nutrient into the body, which in turn occurs because of inflammation in the small intestine. If you have celiac disease, your doctor will likely be routinely monitoring your hemoglobin and folic acid levels. (We discuss ongoing monitoring of celiac disease in Chapter 13.)

Anemia due to low levels of vitamin B12

Anemia due to low levels of vitamin B12 occurs *un*commonly in celiac disease. Unlike iron and folic acid, vitamin B12 is absorbed into the body from the end part of the small intestine (the terminal ileum), an area of the bowel seldom damaged by celiac disease.

We discuss the symptoms of — and the treatment of — vitamin B12 deficiency earlier in this chapter; see "Vitamin B12."

TECHNICAL
STUFF

In your investigations, you may come across the term *pernicious anemia.* Like celiac disease, pernicious anemia is also an autoimmune disease; however, the mechanism by which it leads to vitamin B12 deficiency is very different. Still, some people with celiac disease also have pernicious anemia; people with one autoimmune condition are more likely to have another.

Skeleton Isn't Just an Olympic Sport: Celiac Disease and Your Bones

Although people often tend to think of their bones as being inanimate, in fact, bones are incredibly dynamic, with new bone constantly being formed and old bone constantly being removed. During childhood, the amount of new bone being formed is much greater than the amount being removed, and, as people age (particularly as we reach our later years), the converse is true.

Since, as we discuss earlier in this chapter, celiac disease may cause malabsorption of calcium and vitamin D (both of which are essential for healthy bone development and maintenance), this condition puts you at risk of bone problems. We discuss these bone abnormalities in this section.

Osteoporosis

Osteoporosis is a condition in which you lose bone mass (quantity) and strength. If you have osteoporosis, you are at increased risk of having a hip fracture or a fracture of a bone (vertebrae) in your back. Though osteoporosis is very common even in otherwise healthy people, having celiac disease increases your risk further.

Testing you for osteoporosis

The standard test to detect osteoporosis is a form of X-ray called a *bone mineral density* (BMD) test. This is commonly referred to as a *DEXA scan*, which is an acronym for *dual energy X-ray absorptiometry,* a fancy medical term describing an X-ray of the bones to measure their thickness. During this fast and painless procedure, measurements of bone density are made in both the back (the lumbar spine) and the hip (the femur; that is, the thigh bone).

Most people in North America are sent by their primary care provider for routine DEXA testing once they reach the age of 65 (for women) or 70 (for men); however, if you have celiac disease, you're at risk of developing osteoporosis at a considerably younger age. For this reason, if you have celiac disease, discuss with your doctor whether you should have your DEXA test performed earlier. Many celiac specialists recommend getting a bone density test done after an individual is diagnosed with celiac disease. There is some uncertainty on whether it should be done at diagnosis or after a year on the gluten-free diet to allow the bone density to improve before first measuring it.

Treating your osteoporosis

Treatment for osteoporosis due to celiac disease includes the following:

>> **Following a gluten-free diet.** Like other complications related to celiac disease, the first step in successfully treating your osteoporosis is following a gluten-free diet. Doing so helps ensure you properly absorb the calcium and vitamin D you ingest.

We strongly advise that *everyone* with celiac disease see a registered dietitian to receive expert guidance regarding a gluten-free diet; seeing a dietitian becomes even more important if you have osteoporosis. If you have celiac disease, your dietitian is the best person to help you determine how to get the right amount of calcium, magnesium, and vitamin D in your diet and how much, if any, supplements you should take.

>> **Consuming sufficient amounts of calcium.** You should ingest 1.5 grams of calcium per day if you have osteoporosis. Most people don't get this amount from their diet, so calcium supplements are typically necessary to make up the shortfall.

>> **Consuming sufficient quantities of magnesium.** Magnesium is involved in regulating how calcium is absorbed into the body. Therefore, it's important to consume sufficient quantities of magnesium.

>> **Consuming sufficient quantities of vitamin D.** You should ingest approximately 1,000 units of vitamin D per day. As with calcium, most people require vitamin D supplements to reach this amount.

>> **Prescription medication.** Depending on the severity of your osteoporosis, you may benefit from taking prescription drugs such as *bisphosphonates*. Your family doctor is typically the first person you should speak to regarding whether you should take prescription drugs for your osteoporosis.

TIP

The preceding recommendations regarding diet, calcium, and vitamin D intake are also the most effective strategies to prevent osteoporosis from developing in the first place. As we discuss in Chapter 11, the quantity of vitamin D and calcium you need to ingest to help prevent osteoporosis depends on your age and other factors. We recommend you speak to your dietitian and physician to find out the best amounts for your specific situation.

TIP

If you have osteoporosis, your doctor should periodically send you for follow-up DEXA testing to ensure you are responding sufficiently well to the therapies we just discussed.

Rickets

Whereas osteoporosis (see the preceding section) is a condition wherein adults lose bone they've previously acquired, *rickets* is a disease of childhood in which bone is not properly or sufficiently made in the first place.

Just like you need sufficient amounts of raw materials (brick, mortar, and so on) to make a brick house, so too do children need the right amounts of calcium and vitamin D to create a healthy skeleton. If a child has undiagnosed or untreated celiac disease, they may not be able to properly absorb these nutrients into the body and consequently may develop rickets.

The skeletal abnormality most likely to develop depends on the age of the affected child; toddlers, for example, may develop outward bowing of the legs (unimaginatively — but aptly — referred to as *bow legs*), and older children may develop inward bending of the legs (*knock knees*).

Impaired bone development isn't the only feature of rickets. Other findings include

>> Bone pain.

>> Muscle weakness.

>> Dental problems (such as poor enamel).

>> Seizures. These are most likely to occur in infants with rickets and are related to low calcium levels.

If a child has rickets, it's usually detected when either a parent notices the child is not developing normally and therefore brings the youngster to the doctor (who confirms the observation) or when a physician examines a child brought in for a routine checkup.

TIP

If your child has celiac disease, the doctor will know that celiac disease can cause rickets and will monitor your child for this. A child with celiac disease who carefully follows a gluten-free diet and ingests the right amounts of the right nutrients (which your dietitian can teach you all about) as part of a healthy diet can expect to develop perfectly healthy bones.

The treatment of rickets due to celiac disease consists of a gluten-free diet and sufficient ingestion of calcium and vitamin D. The required amounts of calcium and vitamin D depend on the age of the child and the severity of the problem. As always, it's essential that you and your child meet with a dietitian to receive expert advice tailored to your specific situation. Fortunately, if rickets is detected and treated sufficiently early (especially if the child's bones are still developing), an excellent response to therapy is typically seen and, ultimately, the child's bones can return to normal.

Osteomalacia

Osteomalacia, like osteoporosis, is a condition in which the bones are "weak" and prone to fracturing. Also, both conditions have reduced bone density. The main difference between the two conditions is that in osteoporosis, the internal architecture of the bones is preserved, whereas in osteomalacia, the bone is soft due to low bone mineralization. By way of analogy, imagine a thick wall built of reinforced concrete. If this wall had osteoporosis, the concrete would be too thin but otherwise preserved. If this wall had osteomalacia, the main problem would be that the internal reinforcing rods were soft and pliable at the time the wall was first constructed.

Osteoporosis and osteomalacia share much in common, such as vitamin D malabsorption being an important cause, and treatment including taking supplemental vitamin D and calcium. One significant difference between the two conditions is that although osteoporosis does not cause symptoms (unless it causes a fracture), osteomalacia can be associated with bone pains and tenderness, and muscle weakness. Also, osteomalacia often requires treatment with higher doses of vitamin D than does osteoporosis.

Oral Health

Celiac disease can affect various parts of the mouth, including the teeth, tongue, and gums.

Dental health

Enamel is the hard, white outer coating of the teeth. People with celiac disease may develop dental problems as a result of defects in the enamel.

EXAMPLE

When Miriam noticed her five-year-old son, Leo, had yellowed teeth, she became concerned and took him to the dentist. The dentist asked her if she had taken tetracycline during her pregnancy (a known cause of this), but she hadn't. Had he been receiving excess fluoride (another known cause)? Nope. The dentist referred Leo to a pediatric gastroenterologist, and, several investigations later, the diagnosis of celiac disease was confirmed. Leo had not had even a single other symptom.

When celiac disease causes damage to the enamel, the affected teeth are typically located symmetrically within the mouth (that is, the same teeth on both sides of the mouth are affected). Also, the teeth most likely to be injured are the incisors. (The incisors are the pointed teeth toward the front of the mouth.) The enamel can be injured in several different ways, including discoloration (with the teeth turning cream-, yellow-, or brown-colored) or development of white spots.

The exact cause of the damage to the enamel is unknown, but it is likely not simply a problem with insufficient absorption of nutrients — such as calcium — from the gut. Treatment with a gluten-free diet helps prevent further dental problems, but, unfortunately, the established enamel defects do not resolve.

The rest of the mouth

These are other things that can go wrong in the mouth if you have celiac disease:

>> Your tongue can become sore or have a burning feeling. (Similar symptoms can also be seen if you have low levels of iron, folic acid, or vitamin B12.)

>> Canker sores (*aphthous ulcers*) can develop.

>> You may develop sore, cracking of the skin at the corners of the mouth (a condition called *angular stomatitis* or *angular cheilitis*).

>> Your mouth may feel dry. This may be due to decreased saliva production; however, in some people, this symptom is present despite normal amounts of saliva.

Fortunately, all these problems usually improve soon after you start a gluten-free diet.

Infertility and Complications of Pregnancy

Having celiac disease may make it more difficult for a couple to conceive; that is, celiac disease may increase the risk of infertility. Also, once pregnant, a woman with celiac disease may be at increased risk of having a miscarriage. These risks are most likely to apply to people with *untreated* celiac disease.

Although the explanation(s) for the increased risk of infertility and miscarriages are not fully sorted out, factors may include reduced levels of important nutrients and abnormal hormone levels. In active celiac disease, there may be less frequent ovulation. Additionally, both men and women with celiac disease are at increased risk of other hormonal disorders — such as thyroid disease — that can impact normal reproductive function.

We discuss these topics in detail in Chapter 14.

Hyposplenism and Increased Risk of Infection

Until not too long ago, the spleen was thought to be an unimportant organ. In fact, it is now known that the spleen has a number of important functions in maintaining good health, one of which is to help protect against serious infections from a bacterium called *pneumococcus*.

There is some (limited) evidence that if a person has active celiac disease, their spleen may not function normally (a condition called *hyposplenism*) and as a result that person would be at increased risk of infections from the aforementioned pneumococcus germ. For this reason, some experts recommend that people with celiac disease be given a pneumococcal vaccination to lower the risk of getting this infection.

Chapter **8**

Conditions Associated with Celiac Disease

Having celiac disease doesn't make you an unhealthy person. Indeed, once you found out you had celiac disease, you may have become more knowledgeable about your health and more aware of good nutrition than most people around you. You likely also discovered that you can eat a wide variety of naturally gluten-free foods, exercise regularly, and, basically, do anything you want to do.

Having celiac disease may increase your risk of having certain other types of health conditions. Some of these are directly related to celiac disease, and others are simply associated with celiac disease. In Chapter 7, we look at those conditions that are directly related (such as active celiac disease causing malabsorption of iron, which in turn leads to anemia). In this chapter, we look at those conditions, such as type 1 diabetes, that are associated with celiac disease.

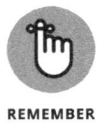

REMEMBER

We discuss a number of different health conditions in this chapter. Although disparate in many ways, they do have one important thing in common: No definitive proof exists that following a gluten-free diet will improve any of these conditions except dermatitis herpetiformis; instead, you need to rely on other, effective therapies to improve these conditions.

Understanding What "Associated" Means

You may be at increased risk compared to someone without celiac disease of developing certain health problems associated with celiac disease. But importantly, the odds remain high that you will never get any of these conditions.

Distinguishing between those things in life that are directly related and those that are simply associated can be a challenge. Here are examples to help clarify the distinction. If you use a hammer and you hit your thumb, the action and outcome are directly related. The hammer directly caused your thumb injury. In contrast, if you have red hair and skin freckles, your red hair did not cause you to have skin freckles; the two traits are simply associated.

REMEMBER

There is a lot of uncertainty about why certain conditions are associated with celiac disease. In this chapter, we explore some theories. It's important to keep in mind that just a condition being associated with celiac disease does not necessarily mean that it's due to celiac disease or related to the gluten-free diet. Some of these associated conditions are very common in the general population, and it may be a coincidence that someone has celiac disease and these other conditions. Researchers are exploring the reasons why these conditions are more common in people with celiac disease than chance would dictate.

Skin Deep: Dermatological Conditions

There are several skin conditions that are associated with celiac disease. We explore these conditions in this section.

TIP

If you have not been diagnosed with celiac disease and you have a skin rash that you think may indicate you have celiac disease, we recommend that before you start yourself on a gluten-free diet in the hope this will help your skin condition, you first speak to your doctor. As we discuss in Chapter 3, if you are on a gluten-free diet, figuring out whether you do or don't have celiac disease is more difficult.

Dermatitis herpetiformis

TECHNICAL STUFF

Dermatitis herpetiformis (DH), literally translated, means "skin inflammation resembling herpes." Despite the name, DH is not caused by the herpes virus and, apart from some similarities in the way the rash looks, has no other relationship to herpes.

Decades ago, it was thought that up to 15 percent of people with celiac disease either have or at some point develop DH. But in recent years, for unknown reasons, this skin condition has become much less common; we estimate that fewer than 5 percent of people with celiac disease develop this condition. Conversely, virtually everyone with DH has, if looked for sufficiently thoroughly, some evidence of celiac disease. As you may expect, therefore, those people who are genetically at risk of celiac disease are the same people at risk of DH. (We look at the genetics of celiac disease in Chapter 5.) Although DH can be found at any age, you are most likely to first develop it if you are between the ages of 15 and 40.

Celiac disease and DH share so much in common that DH is sometimes referred to as "celiac disease of the skin." Nonetheless, even if a person has both conditions, the severity of the two conditions is not necessarily similar. You can have severe GI symptoms from celiac disease but only mild skin problems from DH, or you can have very mild (or even nonexistent) GI symptoms from celiac disease and have severe skin issues from DH.

TIP

Today, every doctor has at least some familiarity with celiac disease, but many physicians are not familiar with DH. For this reason, if you have celiac disease and you also have a skin rash — especially if it has gone undiagnosed or persists despite treatment — there's no harm in asking your doctor (even your dermatologist) whether you might have DH.

Knowing the features of DH

DH is a form of skin rash. Although there can be many exceptions, DH generally has the following features:

>> The areas most likely to be affected are the elbows, knees, and buttocks (less often, the shoulders, scalp, face, and back). The oral or genital areas are only occasionally involved. DH doesn't affect the palms or soles.

>> It consists of groupings of small, flesh colored-to-pink, blister-like sores that are raised above the surface of the skin.

>> The rash is intensely itchy. Intense as in "I'm scratching so hard I'm worried I'm going to peel my skin right down to the bone." Before the itching develops, the small blisters or bumps may have a burning feeling.

Because the itch is so intense, and because the affected person understandably tends to scratch so vigorously, the typical appearance of DH can become obscured by the effects of the scratching itself. This is one of the reasons that doctors — even dermatologists — may (mis)diagnose the rash as being something else altogether, like eczema, mosquito bites, allergies, or even psoriasis.

Diagnosing DH

As with most other diseases, the first step in diagnosing DH is having a doctor who considers the possibility. In determining whether you have DH, your doctor will do these key things:

>> **Talk to you.** The doctor needs to determine when your rash started, what it feels like, whether it's getting better or worse, and so on. Also, if DH is suspected, your doctor will want to know whether you have celiac disease or symptoms suggesting that you might (see Chapter 2).

>> **Examine you.** Your doctor will need to carefully inspect your skin, looking particularly for what the skin rash looks like and where on your body the rash is located.

>> **Send you for blood tests.** As with celiac disease, the most important of these tests looks for the presence of tissue transglutaminase antibody (see Chapter 3). This antibody is present in the majority of people with DH. Because a skin biopsy, as we mention in the next bullet, is the only definitive way to diagnose DH, a dermatologist may elect to forego this or other blood tests in lieu of proceeding directly with a biopsy.

>> **Have a skin biopsy performed.** The *only* way that DH can be definitively diagnosed is with a skin biopsy. Everything else we mention in the preceding bullets is complementary to this. These are the most important features of having a skin biopsy:

  ● A skin biopsy is a fast and safe outpatient procedure.

  ● To get a high-quality specimen, the biopsy needs to be done by a doctor who is skilled at performing the procedure.

  ● The biopsy should, ideally, be taken from normal-appearing skin adjacent to a newly developed blister.

  ● The dermatologist sends the biopsy specimen to the laboratory, where it's analyzed by a pathologist. The pathologist looks at the pattern of cells in the biopsy sample and also looks specifically for a substance unique to DH called *granular IgA antibodies*, which, if present, clinch the diagnosis.

TIP

No test is perfect. Therefore, if you have other features of DH, yet your skin biopsy does not confirm this, you should either have the biopsy repeated or, alternatively, your doctor should have the specimen reviewed by another pathologist.

Understanding why celiac disease is associated with DH

At first look, it may seem peculiar that a condition — celiac disease — that affects the intestine is associated with a condition — DH — that affects the skin. The quick and dirty explanation is that the same antibodies cause both conditions in response to the same trigger (gluten). The more difficult part here is to figure out why these antibodies target such different parts of the body. Most likely, this is because both the skin and the bowel contain certain proteins (called *antigens*) that are similar enough that the antibodies can't tell them apart and target them regardless of their location. However, only a fairly small percentage of people with celiac disease get DH.

How DH is treated

Although much is unknown about DH, what is, however, abundantly clear is how to make it better. Don't consume gluten. Period. That much is simple. What is far less simple is trying to predict how long it will take from the time that you eliminate gluten until your skin rash goes away. Here are a couple of general expectations:

>> Most people notice some initial improvement within a few weeks of adopting a gluten-free diet and have almost complete resolution of their DH within a few months.

>> The longer and more severe the DH, the longer it takes to start to improve and, ultimately, resolve. In the most severe cases, it can take well over a year before things are entirely back to normal.

If your symptoms are bothersome enough, while you await the benefits of your gluten-free diet to take hold, there are medications you can take to make you feel better, faster. We look at these next.

REMEMBER

Although medications are helpful in the treatment of DH, they do not treat the underlying immune problem that causes this disease. The only therapy that targets the underlying problem is the gluten-free diet. When you use these medicines, you must continue to follow your gluten-free diet.

DAPSONE

Dapsone is an oral medication. It reduces the inflammation present in the skin sores and, as a result, helps improve the rash and ease the itch of DH.

Although generally well-tolerated, dapsone can have serious side effects, such as anemia, decreased white blood cell production (which increases the risk of infection), kidney damage, and nerve damage. For these reasons, your doctor needs to use the lowest effective dose of dapsone for the shortest possible period. Nonetheless, some people — particularly those with severe DH — can take a very long time to sufficiently respond to a gluten-free diet and therefore may need to take the medicine for as long as 6 to 12 months before the dose can be reduced. Occasionally, a person simply has such refractory DH that they need to stay on dapsone indefinitely (though, again, this should be in the lowest possible dose).

TOPICAL MEDICATIONS

Two types of topical medication can be tried to treat DH, but they're not routinely used:

>> **Corticosteroid-containing creams** work by reducing the amount of inflammation in the affected skin. (Corticosteroids are potent anti-inflammatory medications.)

>> **Immune-modulating creams** (such as drugs called tacrolimus and pimecrolimus) modulate (hence the name for this drug class) part of the immune system and, by doing so, help to suppress the immune reaction in the affected skin. As a result, inflammation is reduced.

Vitiligo

Vitiligo is a chronic condition in which a person loses pigment from various areas of the skin; as a result, the affected areas turn white. The hands, abdomen, chest, and sometimes face can be involved. In extreme cases, virtually the entire body can turn white. Although vitiligo is not a threat to one's physical health, the cosmetic appearance, depending on the extent of one's natural skin color, may be significant.

Vitiligo is an autoimmune disease — that is, a condition in which the immune system targets its own tissues. Sometimes multiple autoimmune diseases tend to occur in the same person; this likely explains why people with celiac disease (which is also an autoimmune condition) are more prone to vitiligo.

There's no cure for vitiligo, and it seldom requires treatment beyond sunscreens, makeup, or skin stains; however, ultraviolet light or prescription drug therapy (such as with corticosteroids) is sometimes used.

Psoriasis

Psoriasis is a chronic skin condition in which areas of the body (most commonly the scalp, elbows, knees, and back, though other areas can also be affected) become red and scaly. These sores are called *plaques*.

Psoriasis, like celiac disease, is an autoimmune condition, and people with celiac disease have higher rates of psoriasis compared to the general population.

If your psoriasis is mild, the only treatment typically required is a topical therapy such as vitamin D or corticosteroids. There are a great many different types of topical corticosteroid medication; your family physician or dermatologist will recommend the one they feel will work best for you. For people with more extensive psoriasis, physicians prescribe *biologics,* drugs that are engineered to target one or more components of the immune system.

Eczema

Eczema, also known as *atopic dermatitis*, is a chronic skin condition, often onsetting in childhood, characterized by itchy, thickened skin most commonly affecting creased areas of the body, such as the neck, the front of the elbows, and the backs of the knees. Affected somewhat less often are the face, wrists, and forearms. Other areas of the body can also be involved.

Eczema is a very common condition in the general population and, like the other skin conditions we've described, it's more common in people with celiac disease.

In terms of celiac disease, the most important thing to know about eczema is that dermatitis herpetiformis (see "Knowing the features of dermatitis herpetiformis") can be misdiagnosed as eczema.

TIP

If you have celiac disease and you're diagnosed with eczema, the odds are good that you have this condition. Nonetheless, there is no harm in mentioning to your doctor that you have celiac disease and asking if the possibility exists that your skin rash actually represents dermatitis herpetiformis.

Depression and Anxiety

Feeling sad is a normal part of life. Sadness is a temporary feeling typically related to an identifiable and specific cause, be it something as relatively minor as arguing with a friend or as devastating as the loss of a loved one. *Depression*, on the other hand, is an overwhelming and persisting feeling of despair often not clearly related to a triggering event. Depressed people often sleep poorly, feel tired, have a decreased appetite and weight loss, and, in some cases, may be suicidal.

Although the exact reasons that people with celiac disease are at increased risk of depression are not known, several factors may account for at least part of the explanation:

>> Prior to being diagnosed with celiac disease, you may have felt unwell for a long time. Indeed, you may have suffered for years from indigestion, abdominal cramps, diarrhea, fatigue, and other symptoms before their cause was discovered. Feeling chronically ill can understandably take a heavy emotional toll.

>> Before your celiac disease was diagnosed, you may have attributed — or your family, friends, or doctor may have attributed — your gastrointestinal or other symptoms to emotional causes such as stress. Perhaps you came to "beat yourself up" over having symptoms that were inaccurately thought to be due to emotional "weakness."

>> After being diagnosed with celiac disease and starting on a gluten-free diet, you may have concluded this treatment was overly restrictive and interfered unduly with your ability to share in the pleasures of family celebrations, parties, and other events where food is often front and center.

>> Celiac disease may cause decreased absorption of certain nutrients. One theory holds that this may lead to decreased levels of the brain's chemical messengers (neurotransmitters) and that this chemical imbalance is a factor in causing depression.

>> The inflammation in the body that results from celiac disease may, in itself, affect mood and thinking.

Anxiety is even more common than depression. Again, some anxiety can be a normal response to stressful circumstances, but when it becomes debilitating and interferes with the ability to carry out day-to-day activities, professional guidance is required. Treatment can include various kinds of therapy, medications, or a combination.

Like depression, anxiety is more common in people with celiac disease as compared to the general population. In some people, anxiety is closely related to the day-to-day realities of living with celiac disease. For example, some may worry about getting sick from an accidental gluten exposure or about being stuck at a social function without safe food options. Some people may develop anxiety reading about the various ways that celiac disease can affect the body; we hope that this book (which lists all of these conditions) provides a measured discussion and reassurance and doesn't exacerbate anxiety!

REMEMBER

If you're suffering from depression or anxiety, it's essential that you seek help. Although your family and friends may offer invaluable support, you should let your doctor know how you're feeling so that they can provide you with — or arrange for — the medical care you require.

WHAT CAUSES CELIAC DISEASE NEUROLOGICAL PROBLEMS?

In some circumstances, the connection between neurological problems and celiac disease is direct. For example, in rare, severe cases of malabsorption, a person with untreated celiac disease can develop a very low calcium level (*hypocalcemia*) and, as a result, have a seizure.

In other cases, the link is less clear but can be inferred. For example, some infants with untreated celiac disease, although having normal routine blood tests, are slow to develop mentally (something called *developmental delay*) but improve nicely once they're treated with a gluten-free diet. This outcome suggests they were suffering from a deficiency of nutrients, but of such a small (though significant) magnitude that blood tests were unable to detect it.

Another mechanism has also been described. It could be that neurological problems in some people with celiac disease develop not from malabsorption but from a defect in the immune system itself. Celiac disease is an autoimmune disorder (see Chapter 5) leading to inflammation in the lining of the intestine (and, in the case of dermatitis herpetiformis, in the skin). Cases have been described where people with celiac disease and brain malfunction had evidence of autoimmune damage in the brain. Whether this was the cause of their neurological problems or was coincidental is unknown.

Getting a Head Start: Neurological Manifestations

As with other ailments we discuss in this chapter, the link between celiac disease and certain neurological disorders is unclear and may simply reflect the coincidental occurrence of relatively common disorders. Having said that, some neurological conditions possibly do occur more commonly if you have celiac disease. We discuss these in this section.

Migraine headache

Migraine headaches are typically felt as throbbing, intense headaches that occur on one side of the head and can range in severity from mild to disabling. The headache is often accompanied by nausea and vomiting. Migraine headaches are often foreshadowed by a warning (*aura*) symptom (or symptoms) such as seeing flashing lights or geometric patterns. Some people experience the aura without the headache.

If your migraines are infrequent, the usual treatment strategy is to take a non-steroidal anti-inflammatory drug (such as ibuprofen) or a *triptan* (a class of drugs used specifically for migraines) when an episode is coming on. If your migraines are more frequent, taking a preventative medicine (such as a drug like propranolol from the beta-blocker family) is often advised.

Peripheral neuropathy

TECHNICAL STUFF

The peripheral nervous system is that collection of nerves that carries messages between the central nervous system (the brain and spinal cord) and your organs, such as the muscles and skin. So, for example, if you move your fingers to turn this page, it's your peripheral nervous system that's receiving the instructions from your central nervous system and "telling" the muscles in your hand and fingers what to do. Conversely, if you turn this page and get a paper cut, it's your peripheral nervous system that carries the pain message from your finger to your central nervous system.

Peripheral neuropathy is a condition wherein nerves within the peripheral nervous system are damaged. Depending on which part of the peripheral nervous system is damaged, symptoms can vary from numbness, burning, or other types of pain in the fingers or toes to weak muscles.

An association exists between celiac disease and peripheral neuropathy. Though the reason is unknown, this may be due to chronic inflammation or deficiencies in certain vitamins such as B12. As we discuss in Chapter 7, vitamin B12 is an important nutrient to keep nerves healthy. If, as occasionally happens, celiac disease damages the end part of the small intestine (the terminal ileum) — where vitamin B12 is absorbed into the body — you will be at risk of vitamin B12 deficiency and, as a result, peripheral neuropathy.

TIP

If you have symptoms like those we have just described, ask your doctor to check your vitamin B12 level. This is done on a blood sample.

Ataxia

TECHNICAL
STUFF

Ataxia is the medical term for imbalance and incoordination. It occurs when there is damage to the parts of the nervous system that control balance, position, and movement.

An (extreme) example of ataxia is the difficulty moving both feet. More commonly, people may have more subtle degrees of ataxia. It can be due to vitamin B12 deficiency, but can also exist even in the absence of any identified vitamin deficiencies.

TIP

If you have ataxia, ask your doctor to check the vitamin B12 level in your blood.

Epilepsy (seizures)

Epilepsy is a condition in which episodes of abnormal electrical discharge occur in the brain. Depending on the area involved, these electrical discharges can lead to abnormal movements or behaviors. There are a variety of types of epilepsy. The one most familiar to people is grand mal seizures, in which an affected individual suddenly and with little or no warning loses consciousness, has thrashing movements of their arms and legs, incontinence, and then a period of confusion lasting up to a few hours before returning to normal.

Evidence exists that epilepsy is slightly more common in people with celiac disease. This is an area where continued research will help clarify the association. At this point, the reasons for this association are thought to be related to the immune system and triggered by gluten, somehow affecting the brain in a way that makes it more prone to seizures.

There is one rare but well-understood way that celiac disease can be associated with epilepsy: Celiac disease can cause malabsorption of calcium and magnesium, leading to deficiency of these minerals; if sufficiently severe, you can have a seizure. Fortunately, this degree of calcium and magnesium deficiency seldom happens. Doctors routinely check calcium and magnesium levels (on a blood test) in people with unexplained seizures.

Attention-Deficit/Hyperactivity Disorder

Attention-Deficit/Hyperactivity Disorder (ADHD) is a condition in which the affected person has difficulty paying attention, tends to be overly active, and often acts impulsively. ADHD is typically diagnosed in childhood; however, increasing numbers of adults are also being diagnosed. The cause (or causes) of ADHD remains an area of intense study. There's a potential link to celiac disease, but it's still not well established.

For people with both celiac disease and a prior diagnosis of ADHD, some report that treating celiac disease with the gluten-free diet seems to positively affect ADHD symptoms. This has led people without celiac disease to try the same thing, but there is no convincing evidence that the use of a gluten-free diet is helpful for the treatment of ADHD in people without a diagnosis of celiac disease.

Autism spectrum disorder

Autism spectrum disorder is a condition in which the affected person has difficulties communicating and interacting socially.

There is limited research on the potential link between celiac disease and autism. Thus far, research has indicated no benefit of the gluten-free diet. Some earlier scientific studies had suggested that children with autism were more likely to have celiac disease, but more recent evidence does not support there being this association. Currently, it's not recommended that children with autism be routinely screened for celiac disease, nor is it advised that children with autism be placed on a gluten-free diet on speculation that it will be of benefit. Of course, if someone with autism is experiencing symptoms suggestive of celiac disease, testing is warranted, and it's particularly important to do this testing before starting a gluten-free diet (see Chapter 3).

Hormonal Health: Endocrine Disorders and Celiac Disease

The *endocrine system* refers to the body's complex network of glands that produce ("secrete") hormones. Hormones control an array of bodily functions, including growth, metabolism, and sexual and reproductive function, to name but a few.

As you discover in Chapter 5, celiac disease is an autoimmune disease. So, too, are a variety of endocrine disorders. If you have one autoimmune disease, you may be at increased risk of having others, including some types of endocrine diseases. We look at these types in this section.

Type 1 diabetes

Diabetes mellitus (virtually always abbreviated simply as "diabetes") is a disease in which one has elevated blood glucose (blood sugar) levels due to insufficient insulin or ineffective insulin or both. There are two main types of diabetes mellitus:

>> **Type 1 diabetes** is an autoimmune disorder that typically first occurs in children, teens, or young adults, and always requires insulin therapy.

>> **Type 2 diabetes** is not autoimmune, typically develops in middle-aged or older individuals, and can often be managed by diet and exercise — without insulin.

If you have type 1 diabetes, you have about a 5 percent to 10 percent lifetime risk of being found to also have celiac disease (compared to the general population risk of about 1 percent).

Exploring how celiac disease affects diabetes

People with type 1 diabetes need to administer insulin either through an injection or an insulin pump before they eat. The dose of insulin is proportionate to the amount of carbohydrate in the meal or snack. (Carbohydrates make blood glucose go up; insulin helps bring it down or helps prevent the blood glucose from going up in the first place.) This treatment strategy (called *carbohydrate counting* or *carb counting* for short) generally works very well but is dependent on the ingested carbohydrates being predictably absorbed into the body. Undiagnosed or insufficiently treated celiac disease (with its attendant effect on carbohydrate — and other nutrient — absorption into the body) — may confound this predictability and lead to erratic blood glucose levels. Some patients with type 1 diabetes have found that once their celiac disease has been diagnosed and controlled, blood glucose control also improves.

Divina was a 22-year-old patient with type 1 diabetes. Her blood glucose control had been typically excellent over the years, but for the past six months, her control had become increasingly erratic to the point that Divina felt she was on a perpetual roller coaster. She felt otherwise completely well; her diet hadn't changed, her exercise pattern had remained consistent, and her insulin therapy hadn't altered. Further investigations were undertaken, including blood tests and a small intestinal biopsy (see Chapter 3). The results came back showing that Divina had celiac disease. When Divina started a gluten-free diet, her blood glucose returned to being in good control.

TIP

If you have type 1 diabetes and your blood glucose control is erratic for no clear reason, discuss with your diabetes specialist whether you should be tested for celiac disease.

Screening for celiac disease if you have type 1 diabetes

As we discuss in Chapter 6, screening for a disease means testing for it in the absence of any evidence that it's present. A common example of screening is having your blood pressure checked even when no suspicion exists that it's high; doctors do this as part of a routine checkup.

Because your risk of having celiac disease is much greater if you have type 1 diabetes, some experts advocate that all people (especially children) with type 1 diabetes be tested for celiac disease. Other experts advise that, because it isn't proven that treating entirely asymptomatic people with celiac disease improves their long-term health, such testing should only be done on people — including those with type 1 diabetes — who are having symptoms or other evidence (such as erratic blood glucose levels) that they may have celiac disease.

The American Diabetes Association (ADA) has published recommendations regarding screening for celiac disease in children and adolescents with type 1 diabetes. The ADA recommends that they be screened for celiac disease soon after the diagnosis of type 1 diabetes has been made and, if celiac disease isn't found, that screening be redone two and five years later, even if the person is asymptomatic (that is, not having any symptoms to suggest they have celiac disease).

Thyroid disease

The *thyroid gland* is a small organ located low down in the neck in front of and beside the windpipe (the *trachea*). The thyroid makes thyroid hormone, which is involved with controlling and regulating many different processes within the body. Indeed, if a body part moves (think bowels), squeezes (heart), bleeds (uterus), pulls (muscles), grows (nails), or pretty much performs any other bodily function, then the thyroid typically plays at least some role.

WHY BLOOD GLUCOSE CONTROL IS ERRATIC IF YOU HAVE DIABETES AND UNTREATED CELIAC DISEASE

When a person with no health problems ingests carbohydrates (some examples being bread, potatoes, grains, cereals, rice, and some dairy products like milk and yogurt), the carbohydrates are quickly absorbed into the body and converted to a sugar molecule called glucose. The pancreas recognizes that additional glucose has entered the bloodstream and instantly releases precise quantities of insulin, which allows the glucose to move, in just the right amounts, from the blood into the body's cells.

A person with diabetes who's being treated with a quick-acting form of insulin taken with meals does so in a dose designed to match the expected amount of carbohydrate about to be absorbed into the body. If you have undiagnosed celiac disease, however, malabsorption may cause only a portion of the ingested carbohydrate to be absorbed. As a result, a mismatch occurs, with too much insulin having been given for the amount of glucose present in the blood. As a result, low blood glucose (*hypoglycemia*) occurs. Fortunately, once your celiac disease is discovered and treated, your bowel will heal, and the carbohydrates you ingest will once again be consistently and predictably absorbed, with, in most cases, an attendant return of more predictable insulin requirements.

The thyroid gland is commonly affected by autoimmune disease and, as multiple autoimmune diseases may to occur in the same individual, if you have celiac disease (which is an autoimmune condition) you are at increased risk of having one of these conditions. Autoimmune thyroid disease is the most common autoimmune disease, and more than 10 percent of people with celiac disease have one of the two thyroid conditions we discuss in this section.

Graves' disease

Graves' disease — so called because it was first described by Dr. Robert Graves, not because it is a grave disease — is an autoimmune condition (called *hyperthyroidism*) in which antibodies attack the thyroid and cause it to overfunction and produce too much thyroxine hormone, which speeds up the body's metabolism.

These are some common symptoms of hyperthyroidism:

» Excess sweating

» Fatigue

>> Feeling overly hot

>> Frequent bowel movements (sometimes to the point of having diarrhea)

>> Palpitations

>> Thyroid swelling (goiter)

>> Tremor

>> Weight loss

From the preceding list, you can see that some of the symptoms of hyperthyroidism are also symptoms of celiac disease. Specifically, both conditions can cause frequent stools, weight loss, and fatigue. For this reason, if you have celiac disease and you develop these symptoms, you may understandably be inclined to attribute them to your bowel disease and question whether you've inadvertently been ingesting gluten. This makes perfect sense, but if the real problem is that you've developed hyperthyroidism, this will be overlooked. Therefore, if you develop these symptoms, mention them to your physician so that you can be assessed and, if indicated, tested for hyperthyroidism.

The diagnosis of hyperthyroidism is usually easily confirmed by measuring your thyroid hormone levels on a blood test and by performing a nuclear medicine test called a *thyroid scan*. Treatment options include the use of medications to reduce the production of thyroxine hormone, a dose of radioactive iodine which destroys some of the thyroid gland, or surgery.

Hashimoto's thyroiditis

Hashimoto's thyroiditis is an autoimmune condition in which antibodies attack the thyroid and, often, cause it to underfunction; a condition called *hypothyroidism*.

These are some common symptoms of hypothyroidism:

>> Brittle hair

>> Constipation

>> Dry skin

>> Fatigue

>> Thyroid swelling (*goiter*)

>> Weight gain

TIP

If you develop these symptoms, be sure to see your doctor so that they can check to see whether you may have hypothyroidism.

The diagnosis of hypothyroidism is easily made by measuring your thyroid hormone levels on a blood test. Hashimoto's thyroiditis is similarly easily diagnosed by finding certain thyroid antibodies on a blood test.

Hypothyroidism is treated with oral thyroid hormone supplements. If you're on the right dose of thyroid hormone (this is readily determined by measuring your thyroid hormone levels on a blood test), your symptoms of hypothyroidism will all gradually resolve. If, however, they persist despite normal thyroid hormone levels, then your doctor will need to look for a non-thyroid cause.

Adrenal insufficiency (Addison's disease)

Adrenal insufficiency (typically referred to as Addison's disease, though technically Addison's disease is but one form of adrenal insufficiency) is a condition in which the adrenal glands (small, paired organs that are located just above the kidneys) become damaged. This typically happens as part of an autoimmune process and results in the adrenal glands' being unable to make sufficient quantities of certain types of hormones, called *corticosteroids*.

Two types of corticosteroids are available, and, depending on which type is lacking, different symptoms result:

» *Glucocorticoid* deficiency leads to

- Weight loss

- Fatigue

- Nausea

- Abdominal pain

- Malaise (meaning you feel generally poorly)

» *Mineralocorticoid* deficiency leads to

- Increased thirst

- Craving for salty foods

- Dehydration

- Low blood pressure

  Low blood pressure has a range of severity. If it's mild, it may only cause lightheadedness or faintness, especially when you first stand up. Severe low blood pressure, however, can be life-threatening.

WARNING

Because both celiac disease and adrenal insufficiency are autoimmune diseases, and because having one such condition increases the risk of having another, if you have celiac disease, you may be at increased — though still small — risk of developing Addison's disease.

If you think of the symptoms you had prior to your celiac disease having been discovered and treated, you may recall having had some of the same symptoms — such as weight loss, fatigue, nausea, abdominal pain, and malaise. That doesn't mean you have Addison's disease; indeed, if your symptoms went away once you got going on your gluten-free diet and you've been fine since, it is highly unlikely you have Addison's disease. Nonetheless, you are at increased risk of developing Addison's disease, so it's important that you seek medical attention to have the cause determined if you develop the symptoms we mention in the preceding list — especially if they are severe or persisting.

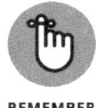

REMEMBER

The symptoms of Addison's disease can be quite nonspecific. For this reason, doctors typically look for more common causes to explain them. This may lead to a delay in the diagnosis, with the correct cause not being determined for some time.

The diagnosis of Addison's disease is confirmed by blood tests showing decreased glucocorticoid levels (specifically, cortisol), and, sometimes, an imbalance of sodium and potassium levels. Treatment consists of taking (oral) supplements of the missing hormones.

Disjointed: Rheumatologic Disorders

Rheumatologic disorders are those ailments affecting the musculoskeletal system (the muscles, joints, cartilage, and other parts of our anatomy responsible for motion). Because immune problems cause many rheumatologic diseases, and because the immune system is directly involved in how the entire body functions, many rheumatologic diseases also affect the internal organs.

Connective tissue disorders

Connective tissue disorders comprise a wide range of diseases in which connective tissues (such as tendons, ligaments, and cartilage) become inflamed and damaged. Connective tissue diseases are typically considered under the umbrella of "arthritis" ailments; however, joint pains, per se, are not necessarily prominent. Because connective tissue diseases are typically due to an autoimmune process and because autoimmune conditions tend to occur in groups, if you have celiac disease (which is an autoimmune disease), you may be at increased risk of also having certain types of connective tissue disease. We discuss these conditions in the following sections.

Sjogren's syndrome

Sjogren's syndrome is an autoimmune condition in which there is a reduced ability to produce certain bodily fluids, especially saliva and tears. We first look at the various ways in which Sjogren's syndrome can affect someone and, following that, we look at helpful ways to reduce symptoms.

TIP

Like many other conditions we discuss in this chapter, if you have celiac disease, you may be at increased risk of Sjogren's syndrome, but your overall risk of acquiring this is still low.

INSUFFICIENT ABILITY TO MAKE SALIVA

Like many things in life, the ability to make saliva is one of those things people don't think about much, if at all, until it's gone. And when it's gone, it can cause big problems, including

>> **Difficulty chewing food:** Imagine chewing a cracker with no saliva in your mouth.

>> **Difficulty swallowing:** Imagine now swallowing that same cracker without any moisture in your mouth.

 If chewing and swallowing are sufficiently severe, you may find eating so onerous that you actually start to eat less and, as a result, lose weight.

>> **Increased risk of oral diseases, such as the following:**

- *Dental cavities (caries):* This point is a surprise to most people. As it turns out, saliva is an essential element in protecting your teeth from damage.

- *Gum disease:* Inflammation and infection can occur, leading to loss of teeth.

- *Yeast infections within the mouth (candidiasis):* With this problem, you may find your mouth feels uncomfortable, burns, or even feels painful. If you look in the mirror and stick out your tongue, it can look redder than normal or, conversely, can have white patches.

Other oral problems include difficulty speaking for long periods of time and altered food taste.

INSUFFICIENT ABILITY TO MAKE TEARS

Many people think of tears as being primarily related to shows of emotion, but tears are also a key element of the eyes' defense shield, protecting these vital structures from being damaged. If you don't make sufficient tears, you are prone to

>> **Eye irritation:** Eyes have a constant sensation of grittiness, as if some sand got in your eye and, try as you might, you can't get rid of it. This symptom is usually worse as the day progresses. Eye irritation due to Sjogren's syndrome comes on gradually over years.

>> **Ulceration of the cornea:** The cornea is the clear outermost part of the eye through which light first passes as it first enters your eye. If your cornea becomes ulcerated, it can lead to sight-threatening complications.

Surprisingly, even people with profoundly dry eyes typically retain the ability to cry.

INSUFFICIENT ABILITY TO MAKE VAGINAL SECRETIONS

As the glands responsible for providing moisture to the vagina are frequently involved, women with Sjogren's syndrome are prone to vaginal dryness. Vaginal dryness is a common cause of painful sexual intercourse (*dyspareunia*).

INSUFFICIENT ABILITY TO MAKE UPPER AIRWAYS SECRETIONS

The upper airways are those parts of the respiratory system well above the lungs, such as the nose and sinuses. When Sjogren's syndrome affects these parts of one's anatomy, a dry cough can develop.

TREATING SJOGREN'S SYNDROME

A mainstay of treating Sjogren's syndrome is to maintain moisture in the various parts of the body that have become dry. Good oral hygiene is also imperative. There are many therapies available to treat Sjogren's syndrome, including the use of medications. We recommend you speak to your healthcare provider about these. (Typically, this condition is looked after by a *rheumatologist*, an arthritis specialist.) Here, we list a few basic elements of treating this condition:

>> Avoid drugs (such as decongestants) that can exacerbate oral dryness.

>> Avoid unduly lowering the humidity in your house. Use a humidifier if your house is overly dry.

>> Use artificial tears.

>> Sip water regularly, use artificial saliva preparations, and suck on sugar-free lozenges. (Sugar-free so as not to promote dental cavities.)

>> Maintain excellent oral hygiene. Brush and floss after every meal. See your dentist regularly. Ask your dentist about dental fluoride treatment.

>> Use a vaginal lubricant during intercourse.

Lupus (systemic lupus erythematosus or SLE)

Lupus, *or SLE*, is an autoimmune connective tissue disease in which there is inflammation of the joints and, potentially, many internal organs, including the lungs, heart, and kidneys. Having celiac disease may increase your risk of also having lupus; importantly, however, your overall risk of acquiring this condition remains low.

Because lupus is often characterized by nonspecific symptoms, a number of which are common to celiac disease, there is a real possibility that you may pass off symptoms you are experiencing as being due to your celiac disease when, in fact, they are due to lupus.

Lupus can cause many, many, different symptoms — far more than we can cover here. These are, however, some of the most common symptoms for you to be aware of:

>> **Fatigue:** This is the most common symptom of all and can be severe.

>> **Joint pains:** This most commonly affects the joints in the fingers, wrists, ankles, and the balls of the feet.

>> **Skin rash:** The most common type of rash affects the nose and cheeks and is in the shape of a butterfly; this type of rash is unsurprisingly referred to as a *butterfly rash*. Another common type of rash is one that develops in sun-exposed areas upon, well, exposure to the sun.

TIP

If, despite carefully following your gluten-free diet, you have symptoms such as those we just described, be sure to see your physician to have the cause — be it lupus or something else altogether — sorted out. Don't assume that just because you have celiac disease that it may be the cause of any symptoms.

There is no cure for lupus. The treatment focuses on managing the symptoms, reducing inflammation, and using medication to control the immune system. Lifestyle measures include using sun protection, routine activity, rest, stress management, and a balanced, healthy diet.

Fibromyalgia

Fibromyalgia (also known as *fibromyalgia syndrome* or *FMS*) is a very common condition that causes various musculoskeletal aches and pains, yet is unassociated with evidence of inflammation or other form of injury to muscles, joints, or other organs. Indeed, fibromyalgia is as remarkable for what it is (a constellation of aches and pains) as for what it isn't (inflammation or apparent damage to the body).

The relationship between celiac disease and fibromyalgia is far from clear and could just be a chance association, but there does appear to be a slight increased likelihood of having FMS if you have celiac disease. (If a person with FMS has intestinal troubles, it's much more likely that these intestinal symptoms are due to irritable bowel syndrome than celiac disease. We discuss this further in Chapter 12.)

These are some of the most common features of fibromyalgia:

>> Three times more common in women than men.

>> Diffuse, unremitting, waxing, and waning pain, most commonly in the neck, back, chest, arms, and legs.

>> Fatigue and/or lack of feeling refreshed after sleeping.

>> Mood problems (such as depression or anxiety), cognitive issues (such as poor short-term memory), or headaches.

>> Tender points

   Despite having what can be very bothersome — even disabling — symptoms, the affected person typically looks well and, when examined by a doctor, the only significant finding is that of discomfort when the doctor presses on certain muscles and tendons, collectively referred to as *tender points*.

>> Normal laboratory tests and X-rays.

Although fibromyalgia has no cure, a variety of therapies are available to help ease fibromyalgia symptoms, including

>> Patient education (our all-time favorite treatment for so many different ailments) — which in and of itself is associated with lessening of symptoms.

>> Antidepressant medication.

>> Analgesics (that is, painkillers).

>> Anticonvulsant medication (that is, anti-epilepsy drugs). Despite the name, these types of medicines are often used, with varying success, to treat a wide variety of ailments, including FMS, where pain is a feature.

Raynaud's phenomenon

Raynaud's phenomenon is a condition in which the fingertips or toes temporarily turn white upon exposure to cold (such as taking something out of the freezer). The cold exposure causes small arteries in the digits to go into spasm, which blocks the flow of blood (causing the white appearance).

Raynaud's is often present in people with connective tissue diseases (see the earlier section "Connective tissue disorders") and also occurs in people who use vibrating machinery such as jackhammers. Some evidence exists that people with celiac disease are more prone to Raynaud's phenomenon.

The mainstay of treatment is to avoid cold exposure by, for example, making sure to dress warmly, wearing gloves in cold weather or when taking items out of the fridge or freezer, and so on. There are also medications available to help prevent attacks; the most commonly used ones belong to a class of drugs called *calcium channel blockers*.

Liver and Bile Duct Conditions

Having celiac disease may increase your risk of developing certain disorders of the liver and the bile ducts. We discuss these disorders in this section.

TECHNICAL
STUFF

The liver performs a number of essential functions, including (but not limited to) assisting with digestion (by making bile acids that help to digest fat), making clotting factors to prevent bleeding, and storing and manufacturing glucose. Suffice to say that a healthy liver is integral to good health and just as much a vital organ as the heart. The *bile ducts* are those tubes that take bile acids from the liver and deliver them to the small intestine.

Abnormal liver enzyme levels

If you have newly diagnosed celiac disease, there's a decent likelihood that your liver enzyme levels (specifically the transaminase levels) will be mildly elevated on a blood test. Elevated liver enzyme levels do not necessarily mean that you have significant liver disease. Indeed, these enzyme levels typically return to normal within months of starting a gluten-free diet.

TIP

If you are newly diagnosed with celiac disease and your doctor advises you that your liver tests are mildly abnormal and recommends further investigations be undertaken, there's no harm in asking whether it would be safe to simply wait to recheck the tests a few months after you've gotten on track with your diet. Depending on the state of your health, the degree of abnormality of your liver tests, and so on, it may or may not be appropriate to adopt this "wait and see" approach.

If you and your doctor elect to wait and retest later, and your liver tests do not improve despite your following a gluten-free diet, you then need to be checked for liver disease. One of the most common causes of elevated liver enzymes, and unrelated to celiac disease, is so-called "fatty liver" (which goes by a variety of other, more formal medical terms, including *metabolic dysfunction-associated steatohepatitis (MASH)*. In the next few sections, we look at liver diseases that are related to celiac disease.

Common to all these liver conditions is the need for blood tests as well as imaging studies, such as an abdominal ultrasound to look at the structure of the liver and bile duct system. (To see an illustration of the digestive system, see Chapter 5.)

Primary biliary cholangitis

Primary biliary cholangitis (PBC) is an autoimmune disease that leads to permanent scarring of the liver. It derives its name from *primary* (meaning of unknown cause), *biliary* (pertaining, in this case, to the damage to the bile ducts within the liver that occurs with this disease), and *cholangitis* (meaning inflammation of the bile ducts). PBC is the most common of the serious liver diseases found in people with celiac disease.

Some of the more common symptoms of PBC are

>> Fatigue

>> Itchy skin (*pruritus*)

>> Jaundice (yellowing of the skin and eyes)

Treatment is geared toward controlling symptoms, treating complications as they arise, and using medicines to stop worsening liver injury from occurring. This last strategy is often successful, but not always. Should liver scarring (*cirrhosis*) develop, the remaining therapeutic option is to have a liver transplant, which is not only life-enhancing, but also life-saving.

Autoimmune hepatitis

Autoimmune hepatitis is a chronic autoimmune disease characterized by liver inflammation. It goes by many aliases, including *active chronic hepatitis* and *autoimmune chronic active hepatitis*.

Like primary biliary cholangitis (see the immediately preceding section, "Primary biliary cholangitis"), autoimmune hepatitis does not always lead to progressively worsening liver damage. Indeed, many affected individuals remain free of symptoms for many years. Some people, however, have severe autoimmune hepatitis with rapid deterioration in their condition.

If you have autoimmune hepatitis, you are at a small increased risk of having celiac disease. The converse, however, is not true; that is, the vast majority of people with celiac disease never develop autoimmune hepatitis.

Not everyone with autoimmune hepatitis requires treatment. For instance, if the condition is very mild, some patients do not require therapy. For more active cases, potent medicines are used to suppress the inflammation present in the liver.

Primary sclerosing cholangitis

Primary sclerosing cholangitis (PSC) is a disease of unknown cause that leads to progressively worsening narrowing and, ultimately, destruction of the bile ducts. (Bile ducts carry bile from the liver to the small intestine.) This, in turn, leads to severe liver damage.

Most patients with PSC initially have no symptoms. As the condition worsens, symptoms then develop — the first ones typically being fatigue and skin itching (pruritus). Fevers and night sweats are also common early symptoms.

As is true of PBC (covered in the previous section, "Primary biliary cholangitis"), treatment of PSC is geared toward controlling symptoms, treating complications as they arise, and using medicines to try to stop worsening liver injury from occurring. Unfortunately, despite therapy, the disease tends to progress, leading to severe liver damage requiring liver transplantation.

Chromosomal Disorders

DNA is the substance in the body's cells that provides the genetic blueprint that is directly responsible for some traits (such as hair and eye color) and also plays a role in establishing the risk for certain diseases, such as heart disease, high blood pressure, diabetes, celiac disease, and many other conditions. DNA is contained in a person's 23 pairs of chromosomes. Chromosomes, in turn, are made up of many small regions called genes. Certain chromosomal (meaning, related to the chromosomes) and genetic (related to the genes) disorders are associated with celiac disease. We discuss these disorders in the following sections.

Down syndrome

Down syndrome is a condition in which a person has an extra chromosome number 21. Normally, people have 23 pairs of chromosomes (numbered 1 through 23). A person with Down syndrome, however, has three chromosome 21 instead of the normal two. Although the way in which Down syndrome affects people varies, some of the more common features include distinct facial characteristics and intellectual disability. People with Down syndrome have a higher risk of celiac disease — it is found in about 5 percent to 10 percent of people with Down syndrome.

Making a diagnosis of celiac disease in a person with Down syndrome can be challenging because the affected person may not necessarily be able to readily describe their symptoms. For this reason, if you have a loved one with Down syndrome who develops persisting or worsening symptoms of celiac disease, such as weight loss, abdominal pain, or diarrhea, we recommend that you let the doctor know and ask that celiac disease be considered as a possible cause.

Williams syndrome

Williams syndrome is a genetic condition caused by the deletion of part of chromosome number 7. Characteristics of Williams syndrome include distinct facial features, heart and blood vessel abnormalities, and intellectual disability (though relatively strong musical skills). Celiac disease is present in approximately 10 percent of people with Williams syndrome, and detecting symptoms can sometimes be challenging due to limited communication, similar to those with Down syndrome.

Turner syndrome

Turner syndrome is a genetic condition in which a female is missing all (or part of) one of her two X chromosomes. A person with Turner syndrome is likely to be short and have other distinct physical traits. She is also at increased risk of having celiac disease. About 10 percent of people with Turner syndrome also have celiac disease. Because of this increased risk, if you have Turner syndrome and you develop symptoms suggestive of celiac disease (see Chapter 2), be sure to notify your physician.

IgA Deficiency

IgA (short for *Immunoglobulin A*) is a group of antibodies that help fight infection. Some people are genetically deficient in IgA. The great majority of these people never have any ill effect from it, but a small percent do have an increased number of respiratory and digestive tract infections.

As we discuss in Chapter 3, people with celiac disease face a double-edged sword: Not only are they at increased risk of IgA deficiency, but having this deficiency further complicates matters because it makes it harder to diagnose celiac disease. (The best blood test — the IgA tissue transglutaminase antibody — to assist with diagnosing celiac disease is unhelpful in the setting of IgA deficiency, so other diagnostic measures, such as the IgG tissue transglutaminase antibody or the IgG deamidated gliadin antibody, need to be performed instead.)

Chapter **9**

Celiac Disease and Cancer

H aving celiac disease may increase your risk of developing certain types of cancer. Being aware of this risk allows you to follow precautions to reduce your risk of developing cancers related to celiac disease and also to monitor yourself for clues that cancer may have developed. In this chapter, we look in detail at these issues.

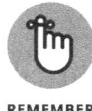

REMEMBER

As you read this chapter, there are two very important things to remember:

» **Having an *increased* risk is not the same as having a *high* risk.** The vast majority of people with celiac disease never develop any of the cancers we discuss in this section.

» **There is evidence that the risk of developing the cancers we discuss is reduced if you have celiac disease by following a gluten-free diet.** Indeed, within a few years of being on this diet, your risk will decrease and may return to that of someone who has never had celiac disease.

One rather unexpected and pleasantly surprising finding about celiac disease and cancer deserves special mention here. Some studies suggest that celiac disease actually *reduces* the risk of a few malignancies, including breast cancer and, possibly, lung cancer. One reason for the lower risk of lung cancer may lie in the observation that people with celiac disease are less likely to smoke. That's certainly a welcome finding! Clearly, there is a lot yet to learn about the relationship between celiac disease and cancer.

Assessing How Great the Increased Risk Is

Your risk of developing any type of cancer as a direct result of your celiac disease is very small. In this section, we explore the topic of cancer risk.

TECHNICAL STUFF

When doctors talk of a person being at increased risk of having a particular disease, they are actually referring to two different types of risk: *relative risk* and *absolute risk*.

The differences between these are important (much undo fear is created because of the overly loose use of the term "risk"), as we describe here:

>> **Relative risk:** *Relative risk* is the risk, or likelihood, of one thing happening compared to the risk of something else happening. For example, the relative risk of a person with celiac disease developing a type of cancer called non-Hodgkin lymphoma (which we discuss later in this chapter) compared with the risk of this same cancer developing in someone who does not have celiac disease is about two- or threefold. In other words, the fact that you have celiac disease means you have approximately two to three times greater likelihood of developing this type of cancer compared to the population at large.

>> **Absolute risk:** *Absolute risk* is the risk of something happening without comparing it to another risk. If we again look at the risk of developing the non-Hodgkin lymphoma cancer mentioned earlier, if you have celiac disease, your absolute risk of developing this cancer is somewhere between *2 and 3 percent* over the course of your lifetime, which is a low risk.

Looking at both relative and absolute risk at the same time, for non-Hodgkin lymphoma, if you have celiac disease, your relative risk of developing this cancer goes up by about two or three times, which means that your absolute risk goes from less than one in a hundred to one in forty. Clearly, despite the higher risk, the odds are high that you're not going to develop this cancer. Basically, if something happens rarely — like this type of cancer — even if the risk goes up, it's still unlikely to happen.

TECHNICAL STUFF

Of course, even though you are at low risk, this is clearly not the same as being at no risk, and cancer due to celiac disease does happen. In the remainder of this chapter, we look in detail at the key information you should know about the various celiac disease–related cancers, starting with those factors that influence your risk of developing cancer.

Putting cancer risk in perspective

Looking at all people with celiac disease and all types of cancers, studies have found a consistent signal of an increased relative risk, but this translates into a small absolute risk. One nationwide study done in Sweden followed all people with celiac disease in that country for more than a decade, and cancer developed in about 8 percent of people with celiac disease, as compared to about 7 percent of people of similar ages without celiac disease. This means a few things:

>> If you imagine 125 people with celiac disease and 125 people without celiac disease, there would be just one extra case of cancer in the group with celiac disease.

>> The great majority of people with celiac disease followed for more than a decade did not develop cancer.

>> Even among those with celiac disease who developed cancer, most were not due to celiac disease affecting their cancer risk.

Possible reasons for an increased risk of cancer

Despite the fact that the risk is small, it exists, and some studies have found that this risk is higher in people with poorly controlled celiac disease or longstanding untreated celiac disease. Why does celiac disease increase the risk of some cancers? The quick answer is that medical science simply doesn't know. Having said that, there is no shortage of theories, such as these:

>> The chronic overstimulation of the immune system caused by celiac disease may promote the development of cancer cells and/or interfere with the immune system's normal ability to destroy cancer cells or potentially cancerous cells.

>> Celiac disease causes malabsorption of important substances, possibly including cancer-fighting nutrients and vitamins. As a result, you have fewer of these substances to help protect you from cancer.

>> Celiac disease may make the intestine more susceptible to absorbing into the body potentially carcinogenic/toxic substances present in the foods you eat.

>> The inflammation in the body caused by celiac disease may, in itself, be toxic on some tissues and cause them to become cancerous.

Looking at the Types of Cancer Where There Is Increased Risk

There are several types of cancer for which people with celiac disease may be at increased risk. Here we list them, and in the following sections, we look at the more common types in detail:

>> **Enteropathy-associated T cell lymphoma (EATCL)** is a rare form of cancer affecting the small intestine. It's the cancer most closely linked to celiac disease.

>> **Certain other types of lymphomas** can occur, including other T cell as well as B cell lymphomas (we discuss T and B lymphocytes that give rise to these cancers in Chapter 5).

>> **Small intestine adenocarcinoma** is a rare cancer of the small intestine.

In your research online, you may come across discussions about a variety of other cancers that are said to occur more commonly if you have celiac disease. The reason why different sources say different things lies in the fact that scientific studies can vary considerably in the way they are performed and the groups of people they evaluate; as a result, different studies often arrive at different conclusions.

Enteropathy-associated T cell lymphoma

Of the various cancers associated with celiac disease, enteropathy-associated T cell lymphoma is the cancer that is most closely linked. Nonetheless, regardless of whether you have celiac disease, it occurs only rarely (that is, your absolute risk for this cancer remains tiny, less than one in a thousand). Because this is the type of cancer most closely linked to celiac disease, we look at it in detail in this section.

TECHNICAL STUFF

There are two different abbreviations for this one condition:

>> **EATCL** for enteropathy-associated T cell lymphoma. This abbreviation is the one most often used, and it's the one we use in this book.

>> **EATL** for enteropathy-associated T cell lymphoma.

Enteropathy-associated T cell lymphoma derives its name from *entero* (meaning intestinal), *pathy* (short for pathology or abnormality) *associated* (having to do with), *T cell* (T cells are the specific type of white blood cells [*lymphocytes*] that are involved), *lymphoma* (meaning a cancer that begins in cells of the immune system). You can readily see why it's called EATCL instead!

TIP

You may also come across the term *non-Hodgkin lymphoma*. Non-Hodgkin lymphoma (abbreviated NHL) is the name for a group of different types of lymphomas that share certain features in common. EATCL is a member of this group.

TECHNICAL
STUFF

Like virtually every other cell type in the body, cells in the immune system can become cancerous (and, as mentioned, these types of cancers are called lymphomas). EATCL is a type of lymphoma that starts in the intra-epithelial lymphocytes (IELs), which are located in the lining of the small intestine. A hallmark of celiac disease (and present in virtually all cases) is an increased number of these cells. In those rare cases where these cells become cancerous, it is thought to be a result of their being excessively stimulated by the overly active immune system in the small intestine that occurs if celiac disease is insufficiently treated.

Symptoms of EATCL

These are the most common symptoms of EATCL:

>> Abdominal pain (typically felt as a dull ache or fullness)

>> Diarrhea

>> Fever

>> Loss of appetite (anorexia)

>> Malaise (that is, feeling generally unwell)

>> Weight loss

At one time or another, you (and everyone else) have likely experienced most, or even all, of the symptoms in the preceding list. Most likely, they quickly passed on their own. With EATCL, however, the symptoms don't pass. Day after day after day, you continue to feel unwell, your weight may progressively fall, fevers may persist, and so forth. If ever you are in this situation, you should contact your doctor to be checked out. It may turn out to be nothing; however, it could also be that something is seriously wrong, be it EATCL or some other, significant ailment. EATCL can also lead to perforation (a hole or tear) in the wall of the intestine. If this happens, you can experience sudden, severe abdominal pain that requires immediate medical attention.

Other features of EATCL that a doctor looks for when they suspect you have this condition are

>> An enlarged liver.

>> A mass (that is, a growth) in your abdomen.

>> Swollen lymph glands. Although EATCL begins in the lymph cells in the small intestine, it often spreads to lymph glands elsewhere in the body, including those that a doctor can feel in locations such as the groin.

Tests to investigate suspected EATCL

If your doctor suspects you have EATCL, you will be sent for a number of different tests, both to establish the diagnosis and, if present, to determine its extent. Tests may include the following:

>> **An ear, nose, and throat examination** to look for swollen lymph glands in these areas of your body.

>> **A CT ("CAT") scan of your chest.** A CT scan is a type of X-ray and is done, in this context, to look for evidence of lymph gland cancer within your chest.

>> **A CT scan of your abdomen** to look for this cancer within your abdomen. This test sometimes includes having you swallow barium (a chalky liquid) before the CT scan is performed. The barium shows up white on the X-ray and allows fine details of your small intestine's appearance to be better visualized. This combined barium/CT scan procedure is called *CT enterography*.

>> **A PET scan** to look for this cancer throughout your body. This test is a type of CT scan that detects *metabolism*, the way your cells process nutrients. Lymphoma cells exhibit increased metabolism, so a PET scan is a way to visualize lymphoma.

>> **Capsule endoscopy** to look for cancerous growths within your gastrointestinal tract. (See Chapter 3 for more on capsule endoscopy.)

>> **Endoscopic procedures** to directly visualize the area where a tumor is suspected. (For more on endoscopic procedures, see Chapter 3.)

>> **A biopsy** of the suspected cancerous tissue.

Like virtually any other cancer, a diagnosis of EATCL should only be made if a tissue sample (biopsy) of the suspected cancer has been obtained and, when analyzed by the pathologist, is found to show certain specific features of this disease. In some cases, a biopsy sample of suspected EATCL can be obtained by performing an endoscopy; in other cases, abdominal surgery may be required.

Treatment of EATCL

EATCL is treated with surgery and chemotherapy (that is, drugs) to try to shrink the cancerous tissue. Unfortunately, this treatment often has limited effectiveness, and the prognosis is poor.

Other lymphomas

Of the various cancers associated with celiac disease, EATCL (see the preceding section) has the strongest association with celiac disease. However, other types of non-Hodgkin lymphomas are somewhat more likely to occur in celiac disease. These include other non-intestinal T cell lymphomas as well as B cell lymphomas, including diffuse large B cell lymphoma.

These lymphomas can be associated with swollen lymph glands. Symptoms such as fever, drenching sweats, and weight loss may also develop. The mainstay of therapy is chemotherapy. Radiation therapy is also often used. If a large tumor mass is present, this may require surgery to remove it.

Small intestine adenocarcinoma

Small intestine adenocarcinoma is a form of cancer of the *epithelial cells* that make up the top layer of cells lining the small intestine. This cancer is uncommon in the general population. Having celiac disease seems to increase the risk of this cancer. This increased risk may be related to the known cancer risk associated with chronic inflammation in the body (as is seen if celiac disease is untreated or insufficiently treated).

The most common symptoms of small intestine adenocarcinoma are abdominal pain and weight loss. Sometimes, the tumor can lead to bleeding, in which case you would start to pass blood with your stools. Everyone gets abdominal pain of one type or another from time to time; however, if you get abdominal pain that is particularly bad or that persists (especially if you are also losing weight), see your doctor.

Small intestine adenocarcinoma can often be treated by surgically removing the diseased part of the intestine.

Other cancers and celiac disease

In addition to the cancers we've already discussed, various medical studies suggest there may be a small increase in some other types of cancers if you have celiac disease.

Cancer of the oral cavity, esophagus, pancreas, liver, and bile ducts

The risk of cancer of the oral cavity, esophagus, pancreas, liver, and bile ducts may be increased, though the certainty of this link varies based on the cancer type. Cancer of the pancreas typically causes rapid and profound weight loss, as well as upper abdominal and back pain. Liver cancer and bile duct cancer are commonly discovered after someone becomes jaundiced (presence of a yellow tinge of the skin and the whites of the eyes).

Cancer of the colon (large intestine)

There is conflicting information regarding the risk of colon cancer if you have celiac disease. Some medical studies suggest your risk goes up if you have celiac disease, and some studies suggest your risk goes down. The fact that such opposite research results have been found suggests that, if an increased risk of this cancer does exist, it must be very small. (If the risk of a disease is dramatically increased, typically different studies carried out in different populations should consistently show at least some degree of increased risk.)

TIP

Colon cancer is quite a common cancer in the general population. We recommend that *everyone* age 45 and older — whether they have celiac disease or not — get checked out for colon cancer. If you are at increased risk of colon cancer because colon cancer developed in a first-degree family member (your parents or siblings) at a relatively young age (under age 60), then you should start having your checkups earlier than 45 years of age.

Breast cancer

Several studies suggest that the risk of a woman developing breast cancer is decreased if you have celiac disease. Of course, this is not a reason to ignore your breast health. Your primary healthcare provider or gynecologist can tell you the best screening schedule for you to follow.

Screening for Cancer

Screening for a disease is searching for a condition in the absence of evidence, such as symptoms, to suggest its presence. Examples of screening for cancer in the general population are performing a preventive colonoscopy or (in women) a mammogram.

Knowing that certain cancers occur with increased frequency in people with celiac disease, the question arises whether these cancers should be routinely screened for in this population. To justify screening for a celiac disease–related cancer, the probability of having the cancer would have to be sufficient to justify the time, labor, costs, hassles, discomfort, and, importantly, the risks of the screening tests themselves. These risks include those inherent to any procedure (for example, radiation risk of a CT scan) but also the consequences of false positive results, which can lead to further invasive procedures as well as a lot of anxiety prior to learning that it was all a "false alarm."

At present, routine screening for celiac disease–related cancers is not thought to be justified. Screening is, however, warranted for certain individuals, such as those with refractory celiac disease (see Chapter 12), where the risk of cancer becomes sufficiently high as to make screening appropriate. Screening procedures would include a doctor interviewing you to review how you're feeling and then examining your abdomen and checking for swollen lymph glands. A capsule endoscopy, an ultrasound of the abdomen, and other tests may also be done.

Preventing Cancer

As we mention at the outset of this chapter, there is scientific evidence that people with celiac disease can reduce the likelihood of developing some celiac disease–associated cancer by following a gluten-free diet, and that doing so reduces the risk to the same level as someone without celiac disease within a few years.

The most likely reason why following a gluten-free diet provides this protection (in people with celiac disease) lies in the now well-established link between chronic inflammation in the body and cancer. Active celiac disease is, by definition, a condition in which there is inflammation. Following a gluten-free diet eliminates this inflammation and, hence, reduces your cancer risk.

REMEMBER

For most individuals with celiac disease, the likelihood of getting cancer is only slightly increased (compared to someone without celiac disease); therefore, special screening and prevention strategies are seldom necessary. If you have celiac disease, the best possible thing for you to do to protect yourself from cancer is to follow the same healthy-living strategies as the general population.

Here are some ways to protect yourself from getting gastrointestinal cancer (and many other health problems while you're at it):

>> Avoid tobacco products of any kind.

>> Drink alcohol in moderation.

>> Get regular physical exercise.

>> Maintain a healthy weight (Chapter 11 has pointers).

>> Eat a balanced, varied diet that is not too high in fat, red meat, and processed foods and that contains fiber, fruits, and vegetables.

3

Treating Celiac Disease

IN THIS PART . . .

Dive into the basics of the gluten-free diet.

Explore other nutritional considerations.

Follow up after the diagnosis.

IN THIS CHAPTER

» **Examining the what, where, how, and why of a gluten-free diet**

» **Knowing how to shop gluten-free**

» **Mastering the art of cooking gluten-free**

» **Discovering how to eat out gluten-free**

» **Identifying hidden sources of gluten**

Chapter **10**

Treating Celiac Disease with a Gluten-Free Diet

The key to successfully treating your celiac disease is changing your diet. Because consuming gluten is what triggers celiac disease in predisposed individuals, the treatment relies on *eliminating* — not just reducing — gluten from your diet.

A diet in which gluten is eliminated is unimaginatively, but fittingly, called a *gluten-free diet.* (Oh, wouldn't it be a joy if doctors could always be so plain-spoken!) The silver lining of having celiac disease is that the treatment is simply to follow a gluten-free diet — that's it. No medications necessary — just delicious gluten-free food. The power to manage your celiac disease is all yours.

Following a gluten-free diet can be challenging because so many of the foods people routinely eat contain gluten; also, it's not always readily apparent whether a food contains gluten in the first place.

In this chapter, we look at the ins and outs of following a gluten-free diet, how to find gluten-free foods when you're doing your grocery shopping, and how to take those purchases and turn them into tasty and healthy gluten-free meals. We also look at hidden sources of gluten, for which you'll need to be on the lookout to avoid inadvertently consuming gluten.

Going Gluten-Free

So you've just been to your doctor and been told you have celiac disease and need to go on a gluten-free diet. As you left the office, you may well have asked yourself, "What *is* a "gluten-free diet?" and "What am I supposed to do?" You may have felt confused, frustrated, and anxious all at once. Unfortunately, some busy doctors sometimes don't say much more than tell their newly diagnosed patients to look up this diet on the Internet. Looking up medical information on the Internet can be confusing for patients and their families because there is so much information available, and it often offers very contrasting — or even contradictory — advice. As we tell all our patients with celiac disease (and many other diseases, too), and as we discuss in Chapter 1, the Internet is a wonderful resource but is also a sometimes dangerous place from which to glean medical information (which is, by the way, a major reason we wrote this book).

Knowing what "gluten-free" means

As we discuss in Chapter 2, glutens are proteins found in grains such as wheat, rye (in which gluten is in the form of a protein called *secalin*), and barley (in which gluten is in the form of a protein called *hordein*). Other names for wheat include bulgur, couscous, durum, einkorn, emmer, farina, farro, kamut, semolina, spelt (dinkel), and triticale. In North America and most of the Western world, the major source of gluten is wheat because this is the most commonly eaten cereal grain.

The key to staying healthy with celiac disease is following a gluten-free diet. This means avoiding any and all gluten.

REMEMBER

Gluten can be found in many different types of packaged and processed foods. Therefore, to succeed with your gluten-free diet, you need to carefully check the labels of any food products you buy or cook with to ensure they don't contain gluten. This is the single biggest challenge in living gluten-free.

In the United States, labeling for the eight main food allergens — milk, eggs, peanuts, tree nuts (almonds, Brazil nuts, cashews, hazelnuts [filberts], macadamia nuts, pecans, pine nuts [pignolias], pistachio nuts, and walnuts), fish, shellfish, soy, and wheat — began in 2006. Labeling for gluten-free was finalized in August 2014, assuring that manufacturers must comply with the FDA guidelines for the voluntary "Gluten-Free" label.

We wholeheartedly support this important labeling when a product contains these substances. Most people consider it a mixed blessing, however, when a manufacturer indicates not that *the product* contains one of these food ingredients, but that it was produced *in a facility* that processes these food ingredients.

On the one hand, it makes sense to exercise this extra caution, for example, if there's a chance that consuming a food item (which may be contaminated with an allergen) could cause a serious or even fatal reaction. On the other hand, it means this same warning is present when there is only the most remote likelihood of causing any sort of problem at all. By way of example, imagine purchasing a salsa containing tomatoes, onions, peppers, cilantro, garlic, lemon juice, vinegar, salt, and spices. As expected, and as appropriate, neither wheat nor gluten is listed. Indeed, gluten was assuredly not present. However, printed below this list of ingredients was the statement "Made on shared equipment with wheat, milk, eggs, peanuts, tree nuts, soy, fish, and shellfish." In other words, this product, which clearly didn't contain gluten, was now flagged (likely for legal reasons alone) as potentially containing wheat. What are you to do in this situation?

TIP

When you encounter this predicament, we suggest using common sense when deciding whether to purchase such an item. Contamination by gluten is highly unlikely to occur if a product is *naturally* gluten-free. In contrast, if you're considering whether to purchase a *baked good* (which, therefore, is at higher risk of contamination with gluten) made without gluten but in a facility that produces foods containing gluten, then we suggest taking a pass on the item.

DEFINING A GLUTEN-FREE DIET, ACCORDING TO INTERNATIONAL STANDARDS

Different countries have different standards as to what constitutes a gluten-free diet. In July 2008, an international codex standard was implemented to define gluten-free as containing not more than 20 milligrams of gluten per kilogram of food or less than 20 parts per million (ppm). The international codex standard also defines "reduced gluten" foods as containing between 20 and 100 ppm of gluten.! In the United States, products labeled "gluten-free" must comply with the standard of less than 20 ppm.

Knowing whether you need to eliminate other things besides gluten

Wheat and other grains contain many different proteins. Of these, glutens are the ones responsible for the problems seen with celiac disease. The other proteins found in these foodstuffs seldom cause health problems, regardless of whether you have celiac disease.

Just because you have celiac disease does *not* mean that you are also prone to having food allergies. Indeed, very few individuals have both celiac disease *and* a true food allergy. Similarly, if you have celiac disease, you are *not* at an increased risk of other food intolerances (with the exception of lactose intolerance — see Chapter 11 — which can be present in some patients who have yet to begin their gluten-free diet). Therefore, the only restriction for most individuals with celiac disease is to avoid gluten.

TIP

Life with celiac disease is complicated enough; don't make things more difficult on yourself by looking for things other than gluten to eliminate from your diet.

Many people with untreated celiac disease observe what they interpret to be intolerance or sensitivity to many different types of foods, but once they eliminate gluten from their diet, these other problems melt away. In other words, it had been gluten *alone* to which they had truly been intolerant, as it may be difficult to identify which food was the trigger.

If you have celiac disease and have successfully removed all gluten from your diet, yet you continue to have gastrointestinal (GI) symptoms (such as abdominal cramps and diarrhea), speak to your doctor about whether you may also have some other GI disorder, such as irritable bowel syndrome or functional dyspepsia.

To find out more about the differences between food allergies, food sensitivities, and gluten's effect if you have celiac disease, have a look at Chapter 5.

Examining the reasons for a gluten-free diet

As we discuss in Chapter 2, gluten is the driving force in the immune response that leads to intestinal damage in celiac disease. Without gluten in the diet, even someone with the genetic predisposition to celiac disease would never develop the condition.

Once gluten is no longer present in the diet, the immune reaction it triggered quickly starts to settle, and the intestine starts to heal. However, if you then consume even a small amount of gluten, you reactivate the immune system problem that led to your original intestinal damage; in other words, you'll immediately start to undo the healing process. The response is dose-dependent, so more gluten or more frequent gluten causes more damage. Moral of the story: Avoid eating gluten-containing foods and avoid cross-contact with crumbs.

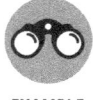

EXAMPLE

Richard was a 49-year-old man who was referred to a gastroenterologist for ongoing management of his celiac disease. At the time of their first meeting, Richard told the doctor that he was following a gluten-free diet and that he felt perfectly well. When the doctor examined him, they didn't find anything amiss. Nonetheless, subsequent blood tests came back abnormal, revealing both a positive tissue transglutaminase antibody (see Chapter 3) and iron deficiency anemia (Chapter 7) — findings that were in keeping with an active immune response from celiac disease. An endoscopy and small intestine biopsy confirmed the previous test results. When the doctor's results were shared with Richard, he sheepishly reported that he "loved pasta" and just "couldn't stay away from it." The doctor explained the hazards of ongoing consumption of gluten (as is found in pasta) and had Richard meet with an expert dietitian who reinforced this message. Regrettably, Richard ignored the advice, and it was only when he then became ill with worsening anemia, shortness of breath, and fatigue that he finally took things to heart, eliminated gluten from his diet (including changing to gluten-free pasta), and gradually improved. Richard's parting words from their most recent visit: "I guess I'm lucky that I eventually smartened up. It could've been a lot worse. Heck, I could have gotten osteoporosis or," he hesitated, "even cancer."

Understanding the downsides of a gluten-free diet

Following a gluten-free diet is not an easy task. However, an expert dietitian can help make the transition to a gluten-free diet easier. Figuring out which foods are gluten-free and which are not is a big task for most people with newly diagnosed celiac disease and can be downright overwhelming at times. And because the person with celiac disease isn't necessarily the one who buys the family's groceries or does the family's cooking, these challenges fall on other shoulders, too.

Living gluten-free requires knowledge, motivation, and perseverance. Here are some of the hurdles you will confront:

>> **Preparing gluten-free meals:** Gluten-free food preparation involves some trial and error and can be disappointing at times.

>> **Eating out of the home:** Whether you eat at the homes of friends and relatives, school and work events, or parties, while traveling, or in any of

the vast number of other situations in which you find yourself eating away from home, you can find yourself exposed to gluten even when you don't intend to.

» **Social pressures:** It isn't always easy to contend with friends or relatives who say "Oh, just a bit won't hurt you" or, in the case of a child with celiac disease, the situation where other children make fun of them for not eating birthday cake at a friend's party (instead, having brought their own gluten-free treat).

» **Being tempted to revert back to gluten-containing foods:** As Richard discovered in an anecdote earlier in this chapter, it can be darn hard to say goodbye to your favorite foods.

Most people with celiac disease complain about missing a few key foods, such as bread, pizza, and pasta, when they start a gluten-free diet. In spite of the many recent advances in the types and quality of gluten-free food availability, the truth of the matter remains that gluten-free products are often simply not as tasty as their gluten-containing counterparts. Adding insult to injury, gluten-free products such as cookies, breads, cakes, and other baked goods are generally more expensive than their gluten-containing equivalents. Indeed, a study conducted by the Celiac Disease Center at Columbia University in New York reported that gluten-free versions of products like bread, pizza, and crackers are nearly three times as expensive as regular products. In fact, several studies from around the world have reported limited availability of gluten-free products and costs as much as two to four times higher than gluten-containing foods.

Now, lest we leave this section on a dour note, we must add this: Despite all the hurdles we've just listed, the vast majority of patients with celiac disease and their families adjust very well to a gluten-free diet. Indeed, as the family watches a previously ill loved one with recently diagnosed celiac disease recover good health, following a gluten-free diet becomes, if not necessarily a pleasure, at least a true labor of love.

Getting help

Learning the ins and outs of a gluten-free diet takes time and, most importantly, a reliable source of information. It is, therefore, essential that you meet with an experienced and knowledgeable registered dietitian (nutritionist) to receive expert guidance. Most physicians have neither the time nor the necessary knowledge to provide this counseling. A dietitian can help you find gluten-free substitutes for your favorite foods and has the training to make sure your new diet is healthy, tasty, and gluten-free.

SAVING ON YOUR TAXES IF YOU'RE LIVING GLUTEN-FREE

Having celiac disease can be considered for a tax deduction in Canada and the United States. The eligibility requirements and the amount you can deduct vary depending on the jurisdiction in which you live, but in this sidebar, we look at some general policies that are typically in place.

To qualify for a tax benefit, you need a letter or a completed form from a physician certifying your diagnosis of celiac disease. This typically requires that you've had a small intestine biopsy that showed changes of celiac disease.

Eligibility for a possible tax benefit typically applies only to the individuals in the household who have celiac disease, not to other members of the family.

Your annual income, deductions, plus other medical expenses are factors that determine whether keeping track of the cost of being gluten-free and submitting this information is worth doing. In the United States, if your total medical expenses for the tax year exceed 7.5 percent of your adjusted gross income, you can write off certain expenses associated with celiac disease. You can find more information about deducting the costs of food as they apply in the United States at www.irs.gov/pub/irs-pdf/p502.pdf.

Here are some expenses that qualify as additional costs of living gluten-free:

- Differences in the costs of buying gluten-free foods compared to their gluten-containing equivalents. You will need proof of the costs of comparable products that are not gluten-free.

- Extra automobile mileage to obtain gluten-free foods. Keep a log of miles incurred for such outings.

- Shipping charges for mail orders for purchasing gluten-free ingredients, foods, cookbooks, and so on. Itemize these and make a note of what the comparable costs would have been had you instead bought similar, but gluten-containing items. The tax department may want this information.

- Special items that are not used except in gluten-free cooking, such as xanthan gum.

Be sure to always save any and all receipts for these purchases. The tax department requires these to support your medical expense claims.

An important takeaway is that if you have a lot of annual medical expenses, keeping track of the costs of gluten-free items and the associated costs is probably worthwhile; otherwise, it may not be worth all the extra time and effort.

Not all dietitians know as much about celiac disease as would be ideal. Therefore, instead of finding a dietitian online, we recommend that you ask your celiac disease specialist or family physician for a referral. Additionally, many of the celiac support groups have lists of celiac specialist dietitians.

If you have private health insurance, check with your insurer to see whether your policy covers the costs of dietary counseling. In Canada, there is typically no charge for obtaining nutrition counseling as long as it's provided in a hospital-based clinic.

Shopping Successfully for Gluten-Free Foods

The first rule of thumb in going gluten-free is giving up foods that come in cans, boxes, jars, and other packages. Eating naturally gluten-free foods such as fruits, vegetables, legumes, nuts, meat, poultry, fish, seafood, dairy products, and certain grains such as rice, quinoa, and certified oats will ensure you are not inadvertently consuming gluten. These basic items should become the staple foods of your diet. (Because processed foods are typically not as healthy as non-processed foods, avoiding these is a good idea not only for those with celiac disease but for everyone.)

If you're going to shop successfully for gluten-free foods, you need to know which foods contain gluten and which do not. As we discuss in Chapter 2, rice, corn, certified oats, soy, millet, teff, sorghum, buckwheat (kasha), quinoa, and amaranth do not contain gluten. These grains are available as flours or can be used to make flours that are helpful when baking gluten-free goods. Other items that can be milled into flour and are gluten-free include the following:

>> Chickpeas (garbanzos)

>> Job's Tears (Hato Mugi, Juno's Tears, River Grain)

>> Lentils

>> Peas

>> Ragi

>> Tapioca

>> Wild rice

Corn flours such as masa and hominy are also gluten-free.

When you do have to purchase foods that come in cans, jars, packets, and boxes, learning how to read the list of ingredients on the food label is crucial to determining whether the product contains gluten.

As we mention earlier in this chapter in the section "Knowing what 'gluten-free' means," similar to the situation with peanuts and other foods to which one may be allergic, manufacturers who cannot guarantee that an item is entirely gluten-free must indicate this on the food label using phrases such as "Made on shared equipment used for wheat" or "Facility processes wheat." That's good. What's bad is that foods that are intrinsically gluten-free must, nonetheless, have a food label that implies the manufacturer cannot guarantee the absence of gluten if even the remotest chance exists that during their processing they may have become contaminated by some other gluten-containing product. This is designed to ensure safety, but we think there is, at times, excess caution (perhaps for legal reasons) and that all this sometimes does is make it harder to shop. Indeed, many theoretical situations of gluten contamination during the manufacturing process in reality are highly unlikely to lead to a significant level of gluten in the food product.

Here is a list of certain common, gluten-containing ingredients found in prepared foods. *Avoid* foods with these ingredients:

>> **Barley malt, malt extract, malt syrup, and malt vinegar:** These malt-based products all contain gluten (in the form of hordein) as they are derived from barley.

>> **Soy sauce manufactured from wheat:** Soy sauce made from *non-gluten-containing food sources* is, however, permitted. More and more gluten-free labeled soy sauce brands are available; however, you will still come across soy sauce labels that don't indicate whether the product contains gluten. In this case, you can contact the manufacturer of the particular brand to find out.

>> **Modified food starch if it's derived from wheat:** Modified food starch made from corn, rice, potato, or tapioca is safe to consume. If the label simply says "starch" (rather than "modified food starch"), then that food starch is cornstarch and is allowed. Other sources of starches must be identified in North America.

>> **Brewer's yeast:** Brewer's yeast is not gluten-free. Baker's yeast and yeast extract are gluten-free and are permitted.

One item that generates some controversy as to whether it's gluten-free is certified gluten-free wheat starch. This is used in European gluten-free products and is considered gluten-free, but there are concerns about whether all traces of wheat protein are removed during the processing. There are several gluten-free flour blends available now that have certified wheat starch in them. Many patients report that they make the best challah and other breads. We encourage you to talk with your gastroenterologist and dietitian before using them.

Cooking Gluten-Free Food

Cooking gluten-free may feel challenging at first, but once you're familiar with the new ingredients and products, it's easy and delicious. Indeed, millions of families successfully do this every day. Here are key elements and some tips to help you succeed with gluten-free cooking:

» The following foods are naturally gluten-free and thus serve as an excellent foundation from which to make a meal: all meat, poultry, fish, seafood, eggs, vegetables, potatoes, and rice.

» Avoid flour as a thickener. Instead, substitute a gluten-free item such as cornstarch, tapioca starch, or, when the dish calls for it, cream or butter. Although you may be tempted to use a can of mushroom soup as a thickener, avoid doing so unless the manufacturer specifically states on the food label that the soup is not thickened with flour; if the soup contains flour, as it typically does, then it contains gluten.

» Substitute gluten-free pasta in classical family favorites such as macaroni and cheese or lasagna.

» Leave out the croutons in salads and instead use nuts, sunflower seeds, or gluten-free croutons to add crunchy and tasty items.

» If a dish calls for breadcrumbs, substitute with gluten-free crackers or gluten-free bread crumbs, gluten-free panko, or even gluten-free corn-flake crumbs.

» A nut-butter-sugar crust for a cheesecake base is a very tasty substitute for a graham cracker crust.

REMEMBER

Using naturally gluten-free ingredients is the best way to create tasty, nutritious, and healthy meals.

TIP

MEAL PREPARATION TIPS

Whether you have celiac disease yourself or someone in the family does, here are some tips and tricks to make meal preparation a bit easier:

- The center of the meal can be a naturally gluten-free food, such as beans, chicken, or beef, served with fresh salad or other vegetables. You can add rice, potatoes, or grains such as quinoa, millet, or kasha. Fruit can be used as an additional side or as a dessert. This way, the majority of the meal is naturally gluten-free and delicious, and everyone can enjoy it.

- For more adventurous meals, try naturally gluten-free cuisines. Examples of these types of dishes include chickpea curry, chicken satay with peanut sauce, or rice noodles with stir-fry vegetables.

- Cheese sauces and gravies can be made with corn starch or gluten-free flours.

- For the members of the family who don't have celiac disease, traditional crackers, bread, pasta, or cookies can be served on a separate plate from the gluten-free items.

- Make sure similar gluten-free items (biscuits, bread, scones, or another treat) are always available.

- Friday night is often pizza night in many households. You can order delivery of a regular pizza for the non-celiac household members and prepare a gluten-free version for those with celiac disease. There are many gluten-free pizza crusts for creating your own masterpiece, or you can choose from the many frozen gluten-free pizza options.

Baking your own gluten-free food

As we discuss in this section, baking at home often presents the greatest challenge when it comes to cooking gluten-free. Preparing gluten-free baked goods has become easier over the years due to the increased availability of a wide variety of gluten-free mixes for everything from cookies to scones and quick breads. However, these mixes are often expensive.

TIP

You will likely find your baking challenges are, well, somewhat less challenging if you have at least one good cookbook on hand that is specifically written for people who, like yourself, want to prepare high-quality, tasty, gluten-free baked foods.

Learning how to bake gluten-free cakes, quick breads, muffins, cookies, piecrusts, and brownies is important for most families living with celiac disease. Mixes for various baked goods are available from both companies that specialize in gluten-free products, as well as many mainstream manufacturers.

Note that gluten-free mixes and purchased gluten-free baked goods, though often very welcome time-savers, are generally more expensive than made-from-scratch gluten-free foods and may not be as good as the homemade product.

Bread relies on glutenin (as we discuss in Chapter 2, glutenin is a component of gluten) to give it the texture and other qualities, such as elasticity, that we learn to characterize as belonging to bread. Gluten-free breads have gotten better over time but are often dry and crumbly and need to be toasted to make them more palatable.

Planning meals for the newly diagnosed

If you or a family member has just been diagnosed with celiac disease, you will likely find that getting started on a gluten-free diet can be a daunting task. Here are some strategies to help you get started with meal planning:

>> **Use naturally gluten-free foods as the building block for meals.** Try dishes from naturally gluten-free cuisines (for example, Indian, Thai, and Ethiopian).

>> **Shop the perimeter of the store.** That's where the good (and gluten-free) stuff is located!

>> **Keep things simple and organized.** After you've mastered the basics, allow yourself to move on to more complicated and varied gluten-free food shopping and meal preparation.

>> **Use the resources available to you.** Your dietitian, local support groups, gluten-free cookbooks, reputable websites, and books (like ours!) can help you learn about where to find gluten-free foods and how to prepare them.

>> **Plan meals and snacks ahead of time.** Make a shopping list before going to the store. Become familiar with stores that sell gluten-free items and learn to read labels.

>> **Start with a tried-and-true recipe.** When baking, start with a simple gluten-free recipe that other people you know have already mastered.

(We also included a two-week menu in Appendix A as a guide.)

If you are the parent of a child with celiac disease, once your child is old enough, be sure to involve them in the shopping and preparation of meals as we discuss in Chapter 14.

Eating Out Gluten-Free

Eating out of the home presents special challenges for people living with celiac disease. Whether it's going to a restaurant; attending a wedding, birthday party, or other family celebration; joining the gang at the annual office holiday party; or simply visiting friends or family, these situations create dilemmas and difficulties that you don't encounter at home. In the following sections, we look at these challenges and provide helpful tips to assist you when you're in these situations. (In Chapter 14, we discuss the special challenges that the childhood and teenage years present.)

Eating in restaurants

Eating gluten-free in restaurants, though not easy, is easier than it once was. The reason is that more and more national chain restaurants are offering gluten-free foods on their menus. Most restaurants, however, do not provide this information; so, just like when buying anything else, the old adage of "buyer beware" holds true here.

When it comes to successfully navigating restaurant foods, bear in mind the following:

» **Avoid fast food.** Fast food restaurants, which are often life-savers for busy families, are generally off limits for those with celiac disease. Sorry. The problem is that many of their staples — including hamburgers, chicken nuggets, seasoned French fries, pizza, hot dogs, and the like — contain gluten.

» **Pick the right restaurant.** In general, restaurants that are more expensive or are very small are more likely to be able to (and willing to) prepare custom meals from scratch that are free of gluten.

» **Look for high-quality cuts of meat or fish.** When navigating the menu, be aware that dishes prepared with high-quality cuts of meat or fish, and that use ingredients such as cream, butter, and wine, are more likely to be gluten-free.

» **Pay special attention to the side dishes.** Even if you've ordered a gluten-free food item, an accompaniment such as a bread roll may contain gluten, even if the waiter assures you it doesn't! (To be fair to restaurant staff, they may simply have insufficient training and, as a result, may not know what they don't know. As we said earlier, it's always best to follow the old adage about buyer — or, in this case, eater — beware.)

Here are some gluten-free foods to look for when scanning a restaurant menu for suitable foods (or about which you can ask knowledgeable wait staff):

>> Natural broths

>> Cornstarch-thickened gravies and sauces

>> Gluten-free soy sauce

>> Tortillas made from all-corn grain

>> Desserts such as crème brûlée, sorbet, and sherbet, as well as ice cream that has no gluten-containing ingredients

TIP

Some traditional specialties, such as gnocchi and matzoh balls, may be available in gluten-free forms, but you need to check with the restaurant to confirm they do not contain wheat or other gluten-containing flours.

Just like bringing crayons and the like makes dining out with little ones immeasurably easier, so too will following some "heads-up" tips make your gluten-free restaurant dining experience — with or without children — less stressful and, ultimately, more pleasant. When you're dining out, consider doing the following:

>> **Call ahead.** Call ahead to ask questions and let the restaurant know of your needs.

>> **Avoid busy dining times.** Avoid dining at the busiest times, especially on your first visit to a restaurant. That way, the wait staff will be able to provide you with the extra time you may need to discuss your food needs with them.

>> **Explain your dietary restrictions.** In the United States, because using the gluten-free diet has become trendy, we recommend framing your dietary needs as an allergy because many of the restaurant workers have allergy training. We recommend saying, "I have a severe food allergy to wheat, which means my food needs to be prepared with no bread, flour, bread crumbs, or malt." Although this statement may not be scientifically accurate, it communicates the medical necessity of your dietary needs. Explain your dietary restrictions to the staff. Some staff will be very knowledgeable (in which case the conversation will be brief), but others may need a more detailed explanation.

>> **Ask questions.** Ask about what gluten-free items or meals the restaurant has on its menu. Ask how meals are prepared and how gluten-free the kitchen and food preparation areas are. In Appendix C, we discuss online resources that address issues associated with dining out and having celiac disease.

>> **Check about cross-contact.** Check into situations of possible cross-contact, wherein non-gluten-containing foods become exposed to gluten-containing

products. (We discuss this topic in detail in the section, "Dealing with Cross-Contact," later in this chapter.)

>> **Use dining cards.** If you encounter a language barrier as you try to explain your dietary needs, show wait staff dining cards that provide information about celiac disease dietary restrictions in a wide variety of languages. Depending on the supplier of the cards, these are available in English, Thai, Chinese, Japanese, Indian, Spanish, French, German, Italian, Dutch, Portuguese, Greek, and even Swahili. These cards make it easier for you to order and eat a gluten-free meal in restaurants in many places around the world.

>> **Express appreciation.** Make sure the staff know you're appreciative when their extra effort has helped you have a good experience. This can be in the form of a generous tip, a thank-you note, or another token of appreciation. (We realize this point may seem kind of patronizing, but hey, the more that restaurant staff are rewarded for being gluten-savvy, the more likely that they will put in extra effort the next time a person with celiac disease comes to dine. And we think that would be great!)

>> **Offer repeat business.** Return to dining establishments where you have had an enjoyable gluten-free meal. Being a "frequent flyer" will likely help you get better service.

Traveling with celiac disease

Taking a flight presents its own special challenges. Airline meals (whether provided gratis or offered for sale) typically consist of a sandwich or other gluten-containing food. Even snacks can be off limits for those with celiac disease because fewer airlines pass out peanuts and instead offer gluten-containing pretzels, crackers, or cookies. For these reasons, we recommend you bring your own gluten-free food with you. Also, any of you who have flown in recent years know your own food will likely taste better and cost less than what you'd get onboard.

One way of getting around the onboard eating dilemma is to eat a meal before you leave home. Don't leave home with the expectation you'll be able to find gluten-free food at the airport because there are limited gluten-free meals or food options in most airports.

TIP

Good gluten-free snacks to bring with you on your flight include a dried fruit/nut mixture, pieces of fruit such as apples and oranges, peanut butter and gluten-free bread, hard-boiled eggs, and chunks of cheese and gluten-free crackers. Bear in mind that if you're traveling to another country, bringing in certain foods, such as fruit, will be off limits.

Traveling by train can also present challenges because, depending on the train you take, the food selection available may be very limited. It's always safer to bring along a few gluten-free items like those we just discussed.

Car travel allows far more options because you can pack items in a cooler for longer trips, and you can also stop to buy gluten-free food supplies along the way. Nonetheless, even here, some advanced planning is needed since the average rest stop will, naturally enough, not have the gluten-free selection of a full grocery store, and you may find yourself needing to take an unwanted detour off the highway to find a shopping area.

Visiting friends and family

If you were found to have celiac disease when you were very young, it's likely that your friends and loved ones have become at least somewhat familiar with your special dietary needs and have learned to make some accommodations for them (even if only to accept that you may opt to bring your own food to get-togethers). On the other hand, if you have only recently been diagnosed, your friends and relatives may not yet know this, and even if they do, like many people, they may have minimal knowledge of celiac disease and even less knowledge of its dietary requirements.

EXAMPLE

Thirty-year-old Mercedes visited her grandmother the day after she'd been diagnosed with celiac disease. Her grandmother had lovingly and painstakingly prepared her favorite casserole, a dish now off limits because it contained gluten. Try as she might, Mercedes was unsuccessful at explaining to her grandmother why she couldn't eat the food, and it was clear her grandmother felt hurt and disappointed. Over the next few months and after a number of further conversations, Mercedes' grandmother did ultimately come to a firm grasp of the condition and was able to come up with new favorites for her. A few years thereafter, when Mercedes's own daughter was diagnosed with celiac disease, Mercedes remembers marveling at the totally nonchalant way in which her grandmother greeted the news and whipped up an exquisite gluten-free dish in no time.

TIP

The best way of avoiding the potentially uncomfortable situation of having friends and family perplexed at your new eating needs is to inform them of your new dietary requirements *in advance* of a get-together. You may even want to share your copy of this book with them (but remember to ask for it back!). Depending on your comfort with this, you may elect to do as some folks with celiac disease have done and let friends and family know via the annual holiday letter of your or a family member's new need for a special diet.

You will likely discover that for smaller get-togethers, so long as you provide your host or hostess with some advance warning of your dietary requirements, they will be pleased to do their best to accommodate. However, for larger events such as a wedding, it may not be possible to make changes to a menu. In this situation, bring along snacks or even eat in advance of going to such a social event where you can't be assured of receiving gluten-free foods.

REMEMBER

Although you may feel it is impolite to refuse your aunt's famous trifle or your uncle's ultimate macaroni and cheese, if they contain gluten, you must refuse them. Always offer to bring a dish to a gathering of friends or family. That way, you'll know there is at least one safe gluten-free dish you can enjoy with everyone else. Hurt feelings are unpleasant; harming your health is worse. Just like Mercedes's grandmother in the preceding anecdote, your friends and loved ones will gradually learn to deal with your dietary needs and will ultimately be perfectly accepting of them. Why? Because they are your friends and loved ones.

Planning for Emergencies

In the wake of recent natural disasters, members of celiac support groups had renewed awareness of the need to be prepared for such situations. Everyone, whether they have celiac disease or not, should have an emergency prepared-ness plan that includes bottled water, flashlights, candles, matches, compasses, blankets, a can opener, butane lighter, pocket knife, something with which to boil water, and non-perishable foods.

If you have celiac disease, have the following (or similar) items available in the event that a hurricane, forest fire, floods, or other disaster forces you to leave your home:

>> **Staples:** Water, sugar, tea, coffee, and powdered milk or coffee creamer, powdered electrolyte mixes

>> **Protein sources:** Peanut or other nut butters, foil packets of tuna, chicken, canned salmon, tuna, chicken, dried meats, and jerky

>> **Instant foods:** Instant gluten-free mac 'n' cheese, gluten-free ramen, gluten-free oatmeal

>> **Snacks:** Gluten-free bars, gluten-free crackers, gluten-free pretzels and chips, dried fruits, nuts, tinned foods, dried packets of gluten-free soups

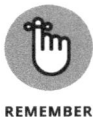

REMEMBER

Eat the items in your cache before they get too old and replenish these goods as they're used up, so if, heaven forbid, disaster strikes, you and your family are ready to make a hasty exit.

Dealing with Cross-Contact

Cross-contact, as it pertains to living gluten-free, refers to the process by which an item that should be gluten-free becomes exposed with gluten during the processing or preparation of the food. Cross-contamination can occur in manufacturing plants, grocery stores, restaurants, and in the home. Because having celiac disease means you must be strictly gluten-free, cross-contact is a very real concern.

These are examples of settings in which cross-contact may occur:

>> **During food processing in manufacturing plants:** As we discuss in Chapter 2, oats are often milled in plants where gluten-containing grains are also milled. This results in cross-contact of the oats and means you mustn't eat them. (If, however, the label says they are "certified gluten-free oats," then it is alright to eat them.) We list various sources of certified oats in Appendix A.

>> **In stores with bulk food bins:** It's is easy to imagine how a bit of the contents of, for example, the wheat flakes cereal bin makes its way into a bin of something that is supposed to be gluten-free, thanks to shared scoops, curious kids, and other things along those lines.

>> **When frying oil that was previously used to fry gluten-containing foods is used:** Breaded or battered meats, French fries dusted in spiced flour, or doughnuts can leave residue behind in the oil where they're fried. This can be an issue at restaurants and in the home.

>> **In shared spreads:** Have you ever looked at the butter in a butter dish? It always has an assortment of crumbs on it! Most families have found it easier to have separate containers for things like butter, margarine, peanut butter, jam — anything you would dip in and/or spread. Separating these items minimizes the risk of gluten-containing crumbs.

TIP

If you are making homemade gluten-free burgers, toast the gluten-free buns before the ones with gluten. This will reduce the risk of cross-contact.

>> **On grilling surfaces:** Grilling surfaces are likely to be used to prepare both gluten-containing and gluten-free foods. Therefore, after grilling a gluten-containing product, be sure to clean the grill before cooking gluten-free food. (Also, try to grill the gluten-free food first in any event.)

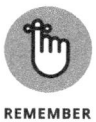

REMEMBER

Once a utensil or cutting board is properly washed, the risk of cross-contact with gluten disappears. Thus, there is no need for separate sets of dishes, cutlery, and other washable food preparation paraphernalia for different members of the family.

Sticking with a Gluten-Free Diet

If you have celiac disease, to maintain good health, it's essential that you follow a gluten-free diet. However, whether you are a kid at a birthday party or an adult in a fancy restaurant, it's human nature to want to taste a delicious (gluten-containing) cake or other treat that everyone else is oohing and aahing over. If you find yourself giving in to temptation (which, by the way, we recommend you *do not do*), don't beat yourself up over it or dwell on it. Instead, the best way to handle a little dietary indiscretion is to get back with the (gluten-free) program as soon as possible.

When it comes to voluntarily straying from living gluten-free, we don't like to call it *cheating.* Maybe it's just us, but we find the word *cheating* to sound patronizing. Besides, it tends to connote guilt, which isn't a particularly helpful feeling. (Well, maybe a tinge of guilt is helpful at times, but that's about it.) We prefer to call falling off the gluten-free wagon *straying* from the diet.

Unlike many others with a chronic illness, if you have celiac disease, you are able to fully take control of, or "own" your disease. You don't need medicines to control your celiac disease, you don't need fancy technologies, gadgets or wizardry; you just need *you.* And that involves finding the wherewithal to avoid any and all gluten. It also involves recognizing that to err is to be human.

TIP

Living gluten-free is often facilitated and, ultimately, more likely to succeed if one is a member of a support or advocacy group, and if there is regular follow-up with a dietitian. We recommend you do both. In Chapter 1, we discuss how to find a celiac disease support group.

Tracking Down Hidden Sources of Gluten

Through careful label reading and diligent homework, you will almost always be able to determine which foods are gluten-free (and hence okay for you to eat) and which contain gluten (and thus need to be avoided). There are, however, sources of gluten other than what is found in food. It is important that you be aware of these so-called hidden sources of gluten lest you inadvertently consume them and trigger your celiac disease. We look at hidden sources of gluten in this section.

Checking the ingredients of prescription medications

Always surprising is the number of different nonmedicinal ingredients present in their prescription drugs. Indeed, in addition to the actual medicine, drugs may contain one or more of many other ingredients, including (but not limited to) lubricants, coatings, preservatives, dyes, sweeteners, and, occasionally, gluten! (Gluten or corn starch can be used as a filler or as a vehicle to keep the active ingredient in suspension.)

You won't be able to tell from looking at a pill whether it contains gluten. If you've been provided with a package insert it may reveal this, but you'll likely only see this after you're home and long after you've already paid for the medicine. Your doctor is highly unlikely to know which company makes which drug with gluten. And your pharmacist may not know that you have celiac disease. We recommend that any time you are having a prescription filled at the drug store, tell the pharmacist you have celiac disease and ask them to check whether the particular drug contains gluten. The pharmacists can look this up on the computer or, if necessary, can call the manufacturer on your behalf. You can also check the website www.glutenfreedrugs.com, which lists both over-the-counter and prescription medications and indicates which have gluten as an ingredient, are manufactured on shared lines, or even if it has lactose as an ingredient.

Verifying the ingredients of over-the-counter medications

As with prescription medications, over-the-counter drugs may also contain gluten. Making things even more difficult is that if you simply pick the package up off the shelf and leave the store, you will not have had the opportunity to check with the pharmacist whether the product contains gluten. In these situations, the best thing to do is check www.glutenfreedrugs.com or contact the manufacturer to find out if the drug contains gluten.

TIP

Some celiac disease support groups maintain databases about the gluten content of common medications, but bear in mind these may not be fully reliable. As noted, there are websites such as www.glutenfreedrugs.com that are reliable sources.

Knowing other sources of gluten

Our patients with celiac disease commonly ask us whether it's hazardous for them to use gluten-containing shampoos, makeup, skin creams, and lotions. This misinformation is unfortunately commonly acquired from online sites. If you, too, have wondered about the safety of gluten-containing skin creams and lotions, then we can reassure you — as we do them — that using these products is perfectly safe. The only way gluten can cause intestinal damage is for it to be ingested; gluten applied to the skin or scalp, or hair, does not put you at risk. But please, no nibbling on your soap.

However, the following list is of some real and potential sources of gluten that aren't readily appreciated as problems:

» **Bakeries:** Occasionally, bakers who work with wheat flour may inadvertently ingest flour that has become airborne. If you work in a bakery, wearing a face mask may help minimize exposure.

» **Communion wafers and matzah:** Communion wafers and matzah typically contain gluten. Recognizing, however, that some individuals must avoid gluten, certain manufacturers have developed gluten-free communion wafers as well as matzah. We encourage you to have a conversation with your pastor or rabbi.

» **Play-dough and papier-mâché:** Young children who put things in their mouths are at risk of gluten if they consume play-dough made with wheat flour. Regardless of whether your child has celiac disease, it's advisable to avoid these items for many reasons (think of what makes them so colorful!!), unrelated to gluten. For older children, careful handwashing has been shown to eliminate the gluten residue from the child's hands.

IN THIS CHAPTER

» Delving into nutritional concerns related to the gluten-free diet

» Examining concerns about weight gain

» Exploring lactose intolerance

» Navigating vegetarian and vegan considerations on the gluten-free diet

» Investigating other important nutritional considerations

Chapter **11**

Exploring Other Nutritional Considerations

Years ago, before much was known about the disease, individuals with celiac disease often became increasingly malnourished. Today, with celiac disease being so much better understood and with increased availability of alternative gluten-free grains, products, and healthy gluten-free options, you can look forward to a healthy, active, full, productive, and long life.

As we discuss in Chapter 10 and throughout this book, the key to successfully living with celiac disease is following a gluten-free diet. In this chapter, we look at additional nutritional issues that need to be considered.

The Gluten-Free Diet and Adequate Nutrition

If you're like many people with celiac disease, once your condition is diagnosed and successfully treated, you'll probably look back and realize that your now-resolved symptoms had likely been with you for quite some time — perhaps years. Nonetheless, during those early years — even in the absence of symptoms — your damaged intestine was likely already interfering with your ability to properly absorb nutrients into your body. This, in turn, may have made you deficient in these nutrients.

In discussing the implications of nutritional deficiencies, it's helpful to first look at what are the types of nutrients that you need in the first place. This is the way in which most nutrients are categorized:

>> **Carbohydrates, fat, and protein** are the major components of your diet. Of their various roles, carbohydrates and fat provide energy (calories), and protein provides nutrients to maintain and repair the body.

>> **Fluids** are necessary to maintain hydration. (A human is 60 percent water after all.)

>> **Electrolytes** include sodium, potassium, and chloride and are vital for proper functioning of the body's cells, including those found in the nervous system, heart, and muscles.

>> **Minerals** include calcium, iron, magnesium, phosphorus, selenium, zinc, and other elements. Minerals play a variety of important roles. Calcium, for example, is necessary to build and maintain bone strength and mass. Iron is required to make red blood cells. (See Chapter 7 for more on calcium and iron.)

>> **Vitamins**, also discussed in Chapter 7, are typically divided into two categories:

- *Fat-soluble vitamins* are A, D, E, and K.

- *Water-soluble vitamins* are all the rest, including the large family of B vitamins and vitamin C.

Malnutrition in celiac disease

Malnutrition is a general term for the condition in which the body is lacking sufficient nourishment. Most people with celiac disease ingest what should be adequate quantities of nutrients in the form of food and liquid; the problem is that these nutrients are not sufficiently absorbed into the body — a condition called *malabsorption*. We discuss malabsorption in detail in Chapter 2.

If celiac disease is severe, it can lead to such marked damage to the small intestine that it results in profound malabsorption with dehydration, loss of muscle mass, and, in the case of children, failure to grow.

TIP

Although knowledge about celiac disease continues to grow in the medical community, it still isn't always considered as soon as it should be. For this reason, if you or someone you care about has symptoms or other health problems that we discuss in this book, and if celiac disease hasn't been considered, raise this possible diagnosis with your physician.

Some common nutritional challenges

As we discuss in Chapter 4, several forms of celiac disease exist, including the classical form in which the affected individual has, well, classical symptoms of this condition including diarrhea, abdominal pain, and, often, severe malnutrition. It is now known, however, that most people with celiac disease have the so-called atypical type in which symptoms are far less severe. Having less severe symptoms is, of course, good, but it can lead both patient and doctor alike to overlook nutrient deficiencies that can be present despite the small number of symptoms and a person's healthy appearance.

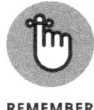

REMEMBER

Poor nutritional status is a concern for all people with celiac disease. Even following a gluten-free diet doesn't guarantee you are receiving all the nutrients you need.

Recent medical studies suggest that in treating celiac disease, too much emphasis has been placed on categorizing foods as "allowed" versus "not allowed," and too little emphasis placed on looking at the nutritional quality of a person's gluten-free diet. In particular, these studies have found evidence that many people with celiac disease who are following a gluten-free diet are not consuming enough of the following:

>> Calcium (see the later section "Consuming calcium" and Chapter 7)

>> Fiber (see the section "Figuring out fiber" and Chapter 13)

>> Iron (see the section "Ironing out iron deficiency" and Chapter 7)

>> Vitamin D (see Chapter 7)

Some studies have also suggested that people with celiac disease following a gluten-free diet tend to have too much of the following ingredients in their diets:

>> Sugar

>> Refined grains and carbohydrates

>> Fat

>> Salt

Part of the reason the gluten-free diet can lead to nutritional deficiencies is that gluten-free foods are rarely fortified with (that is, contain added) iron, calcium, and other nutrients. These dietary deficiencies of a gluten-free diet can make it difficult to correct the deficit in nutrients that were caused by the untreated celiac disease in the first place.

TIP

Make sure to meet with your dietitian regularly. As we discuss in Chapters 14 and 16, some families elect to have everyone in the household follow a gluten-free diet, even if only one person has the condition. If this is true of your situation, then be sure you ask your dietitian about whether the other members of your family are having their nutritional needs met. Children in particular have different requirements than adults.

Ironing out iron deficiency

As we discuss in Chapter 7, many people with active celiac disease have iron deficiency due to malabsorption of this mineral. Once you're on track with a gluten-free diet and your small intestine has healed, you will recover your ability to properly absorb iron into your body. Nonetheless, you may still find yourself being told by your doctor that your iron level (measured on a blood test) is low. The reason for this is that a gluten-free diet often contains insufficient iron. You need, therefore, to make a point of ensuring your diet is sufficiently rich in iron to meet your body's needs.

Foods that can supply iron in your gluten-free diet include

>> Red meat, chicken, and other poultry

>> Seafood (clams, oysters, mussels, sardines)

>> Legumes (lentils, kidney beans, chickpeas, soybeans)

>> Dark green leafy vegetables (spinach, kale, chard, collards, beet greens)

>> Tofu

>> Eggs

>> Molasses

>> Certain gluten-free grains (amaranth, buckwheat bran, quinoa, millet, teff)

>> Some types of dried fruits (apricots, figs, raisins, dates)

>> Seeds and nuts (cashews, almonds, walnuts, sunflower seeds, sesame seeds, pumpkin seeds)

Look for gluten-free baked goods made with enriched vitamins and minerals.

TIP

When you're looking to make sure you meet your nutritional iron needs, it's important to remember that iron from plant foods is less bioavailable (that is, less easily absorbed into the body) than is iron from animal sources. Certain plant compounds such as phytates found in legumes and grains can decrease iron absorption. However, to increase the amount of iron you absorb from plant sources you can do the following:

>> Add foods rich in vitamin C, such as citrus fruits (oranges, tomatoes), bell peppers, berries, kiwi, and broccoli. These enhance plant iron absorption.

>> Don't drink coffee or tea or take calcium or fiber supplements with these foods. These interfere with plant iron absorption.

REMEMBER

If, despite following a gluten-free diet, ingesting sufficient quantities of iron-rich foods, and, when necessary, taking iron supplements, your iron level doesn't return to normal, then your physician needs to ensure your celiac disease isn't still active (that is, still causing inflammation and damage to your small intestine). The first step in making this determination is typically to recheck your tissue transglutaminase IgA (TTG IgA) level. We discuss this test in detail in Chapter 3, and in Chapter 13, we look at the role of this test in monitoring your celiac disease.

Consuming calcium

Many people — regardless of whether they're following a gluten-free diet — don't consume sufficient amounts of calcium. This is especially challenging if you also follow a lactose-free diet (see "Lactose intolerance" later in this chapter) or a vegan diet because both these diets are intrinsically low in calcium.

These are the recommended daily amounts of calcium intake:

>> **For infants, children ages 1 to 3:** 500 mg

>> **For children ages 4 to 8:** 800 mg

>> **For pre-teens and adolescents ages 9 to 18:** 1,300 mg

>> **For adults ages 19 to 50:** 1,000 mg

>> **For adults over age 50:** 1,200 mg

>> **For pregnant and lactating women:** 1,000 to 1,300 mg

You can also include the following gluten-free, calcium-rich foods in your diet:

>> Milk products including milk, yogurt, ice cream, and certain cheeses

>> Tofu

>> Canned salmon or sardines containing bones

>> Dark green vegetables (kale, spinach, chard, collards), beans

Calcium is also often added to foods such as some brands of orange juice and rice, almond, and soy beverages.

If you have lactose intolerance (which we discuss later in this chapter), you can still ingest these calcium-rich dairy products because they are (intrinsically) lactose-free:

>> Yogurt

>> Kiefer

>> Other fermented milk products (sour milk, buttermilk)

>> Hard cheeses (Parmesan, cheddar, Swiss)

TIP

The best-absorbed source of calcium in the diet is found in dairy products. If you cannot consume any dairy products, getting enough calcium can be an extra challenge. There are, however, a number of nondairy sources of calcium that you can include in your diet:

>> Amaranth (75 mg, ¼ cup)

>> Blackstrap molasses (172 mg, 1 Tbsp)

>> Bok choy (Chinese cabbage) (~175 mg, 1 cup cooked)

>> Broccoli (79 mg, 1 cup cooked)

>> Collard greens (239 mg, 1 cup cooked)

>> Figs (137 mg, 5 figs)

>> Kale (99 mg, 1 cup cooked)

- » Mustard greens (109 mg, 1 cup cooked)

- » Orange juice with calcium (333 mg, 1 cup)

- » Salmon, pink with bones, canned (181 mg, 3 oz)

- » Sesame tahini (128 mg, 2 Tbsp)

- » Soybeans, green (edamame) (130 mg, ½ cup)

- » Soymilk, fortified (100–159 mg, 1 cup)

- » Teff (82 mg, ½ cup dry)

- » Tempeh (92 mg, ½ cup)

- » Tofu, firm, calcium-set (137–230 mg, ½ cup)

Figuring out fiber

Over the past few decades, much has been discovered about the importance of consuming sufficient fiber. Not only does a fiber-rich diet help "keep one regular" (that is, helps prevent constipation), there is also strong scientific evidence that eating lots of fiber reduces the risk of developing a variety of diseases, including heart disease and certain types of cancer.

Unfortunately, a standard gluten-free diet tends to have less fiber than you need. This is a result of the low fiber content of many gluten-free flours and other gluten-free products. There are several delicious ways to increase the fiber content of your gluten free diet. You can select gluten-free whole grains such as these:

- » Brown rice

- » Rice bran

- » Wild rice

- » Whole grain corn

- » Amaranth

- » Millet

- » Quinoa

- » Teff

Adding beans, nuts, seeds (chia flax meal), or even more fresh fruits and vegetables will help increase your daily fiber intake.

Deliciously gluten-free and healthy-eating tips

There are many other healthy ways you can add variety, fiber, and a whole host of nutrients, including vitamins and minerals, to your diet while at the same time avoiding gluten:

>> Eat fruits or vegetables with every meal.

>> Have a kiwi or two for an evening snack.

>> Sprinkle nuts and seeds (sesame, poppy, sunflower, pumpkin) on salads, stir-fry dishes, cooked vegetables, and other dishes.

>> Add dried fruits (raisins, currants, cranberries, cherries, apricots, apples), various fresh fruits, and berries of all kinds to cereal, salads, desserts, baking batter (pancakes, quick breads, muffins).

>> Add chia seeds or flax seed meal to foods to increase the fiber content.

>> Use brown rice or quinoa instead of white rice.

>> Add legumes (like pinto beans, navy beans, black-eyed peas, kidney beans), cabbage, and cruciferous vegetables (cauliflower and broccoli) to your diet.

Sorting out saturated fats

Saturated fat is the type of fat that comes from animal sources. Saturated fat is found in meat (for example, bacon or the marbling seen on steak), butter, and cream. *Unsaturated* fat comes vegetable sources such as olive oil, canola oil, and margarine.

The increased amounts of saturated fat in the diets of some people with celiac disease is explained by the tendency for individuals with this condition to eat relatively more meat and dairy products at meals because they cannot eat gluten-containing foods, such as bread or pasta.

EXAMPLE

An athletic young man with celiac disease found that while the rest of his family was filling up on a single hamburger (with bun), he needed to eat two or more gluten-free hamburger patties (sans bun) in order to feel satiated. Instead of a single sandwich for lunch, without benefit of having bread to fill him up, he found that he would eat slice after slice of cold meat and cheese. Breakfast out of the home could be eggs, bacon or sausage, and fried potatoes instead of including toast.

REMEMBER

A gluten-free diet doesn't have to be rich in saturated fats. As we discuss in Chapter 10, a gluten-free diet can be very healthful because eating fresh foods instead of processed, packaged, or prepared foods is the best way to avoid ingesting gluten. Adding the extra nutritious foods listed in the preceding section to every meal is one way to keep the gluten-free diet more varied and minimize the tendency to rely on fatty (and sugar-laden) foods.

Here are some other ways you can reduce the saturated fat in your diet:

>> Instead of bacon and eggs, serve gluten-free cereal or yogurt topped with fresh fruit, dried fruit, and/or nuts.

>> Replace processed meat-containing sandwiches for lunch with a salad with cheese, nuts, unprocessed meat, and lots of chopped vegetables. Include multigrain gluten-free breads, biscuits, or crackers.

>> Rather than meat at a meal, have a meatless meal once or twice a week with beans, gluten-free whole grains, nuts, seeds, and fruit or vegetables. Try a black bean and quinoa bowl or gluten free lentil pasta with roasted vegetables and tomato sauce.

Celiac Disease and Weight

More than half of the people with celiac disease living in the United States are overweight at the time their condition is diagnosed. Even overweight people, however, may still be malnourished due to the malabsorption of certain nutrients.

Historically, celiac disease was considered to be a childhood ailment. However, celiac disease is commonly diagnosed throughout the lifespan. Since many people gain weight as they age, this also applies to people with celiac disease.

Weight tends to go up with age due to multiple factors (sedentary jobs, less time for organized sport, or many other reasons). Every person, regardless of whether they have celiac disease, should strive to be at a healthy weight. In Chapter 3, we discuss how you can determine if you are overweight (or underweight), and in Chapter 13 we look at helpful measures you can follow to achieve and maintain a healthy body weight while living gluten-free.

Celiac Disease and Lactose Intolerance

Lactose intolerance, a situation in which one cannot digest lactose, the sugar found in milk, is a very, very common condition among all people. Although lactose intolerance is seldom a serious problem, it can cause additional difficulties for people with celiac disease. Also, symptoms of lactose intolerance are often confused with symptoms of celiac disease. In this section, we sort through these issues.

Lactose is a sugar (which is a form of carbohydrate) found in all mammalian milk (human, cow, sheep, goat, and so on). Lactose is also present in milk products such as ice cream, cheese, cream, and butter. Lactose is comprised of two smaller sugars (galactose and glucose) that are joined together. Lactose is not directly absorbed into the body; instead, it must first be broken down into these two smaller sugars. This is accomplished with the aid of a special enzyme called *lactase* that is found on the inner surface of the small intestine in an area called the *brush border.* (See Chapter 5 for more on the what the small intestine does.) If an individual lacks sufficient lactase, the result is that lactose is not properly broken down and absorbed into the body.

Who gets lactose intolerance?

It's hard to consider lactose intolerance a disease or an abnormal condition since most of the world has it. It affects the majority (over 85 percent) of people originating from Asia, Africa, the Mediterranean, as well as also native North and South Americans. Even in northern European populations, lactose intolerance affects about 30 percent of the healthy population.

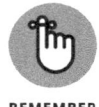

Almost everyone in the world is born with normal intestinal levels of lactase. This is of tremendous importance since ideally a newborn's nutrition comes from drinking breast milk, and without lactase, an infant isn't able to absorb the milk's lactose. As people grow up, the amount of lactase present in the intestine progressively declines, eventually leading, in many people, to lactose intolerance. The reason for the decline is not known for certain, but probably lies in the evolutionary fact that, in prehistoric times, a child who had outgrown drinking breast milk would have had no need for lactase because the only other milk products available for consumption would have been fermented milk products such as cheese and yogurt, in which bacteria did the work of digesting the lactose.

How lactose intolerance makes you feel

Symptoms of lactose intolerance include flatulence (that is, farting) and diarrhea. These arise because the lactose-intolerant person is unable to sufficiently break down (and absorb) lactose in the small intestine, so the lactose travels to the large intestine where bacteria find it a tasty snack and munch on it, thereby turning it into gas and diarrhea-promoting substances. Oh joy. Fortunately, these symptoms are rarely severe, and affected individuals typically learn to recognize which foods cause the problems and so avoid them.

Unlike celiac disease or a food allergy, it is important to note that lactose intolerance doesn't cause any lasting or even transient damage to the intestine.

Celiac disease and your lactase levels

As we mention earlier in this section, the amount of lactase in the small intestine normally falls as a person becomes an adult. Nonetheless, there is typically a sufficient level to keep most adults free or nearly free of symptoms of lactose intolerance. However, if you have celiac disease and your small intestine becomes damaged as a result, you're prone to having profoundly low levels of lactase. As a result, you may have symptoms not only from your celiac disease (see Chapter 2) but also from lactose intolerance.

If you continue to have symptoms of abdominal bloating, flatulence, and diarrhea even though you're following a gluten-free diet, let your doctor know. It could be that you have lactose intolerance. We discuss how to diagnose and treat this condition next.

Diagnosing lactose intolerance

Lactose intolerance in otherwise healthy individuals is typically easily recognized — both by people with the condition and by doctors — based on two findings:

>> The rapid development of abdominal cramping, bloating, and diarrhea soon after drinking milk or a milkshake, eating ice cream, or consuming other lactose-containing products.

>> Quick improvement in these symptoms once lactose-containing substances have been removed from the diet.

The diagnosis of lactose intolerance is often straightforward enough that an affected person can correctly identify it before they even consult with a doctor. When a person has the typical features of lactose intolerance that we just described, no special diagnostic tests are needed.

In some situations, the diagnosis of lactose intolerance is less apparent, and a doctor may request you have a special diagnostic procedure called a *breath test*. In this test, you drink a lactose-containing beverage, and your breath is then analyzed to see how much hydrogen gas it contains. If you have lactose intolerance, you have excess amounts of hydrogen gas. (As we discuss in the earlier section "How lactose intolerance makes you feel," lactose intolerance leads to excess gas being produced in the large intestine.) Some of this gas is absorbed from the colon into the body and is then present in the mouth where the breath test can measure it.

TIP

If you're asked to perform the breath test, be sure to hang out near a toilet for a few hours after the test. If you have lactose intolerance, the extra lactose you consume during the test can act as a laxative.

If you have celiac disease, the main reason to have a breath test would be if, despite following a gluten-free diet, you continue to have symptoms such as abdominal bloating, cramps, and diarrhea, and the cause is unclear.

Treating lactose intolerance

You can treat your lactose intolerance in three ways:

>> **Take a lactase enzyme supplement immediately before ingesting a lactose-containing food.** These are available as drops or pills that serve the same digestive role as naturally occurring lactase enzyme found in the healthy gut. This is the preferred option for most people.

>> **Avoid consuming any lactose-containing foods.** This option is effective, but it can be very restricting.

>> **Consume milk products which, prior to sale, have been treated so that they no longer contain lactose.** This is also an effective option; however, these products are more expensive than simply adding your own lactase drops to a jug of milk at home.

Despite what many people think, if you have lactose intolerance, there are some dairy products you can consume. Since almost all aged (hard) cheeses, yogurts, and buttermilk are naturally lactose free, you can safely consume these.

TIP

Many manufacturers label their lactose-free products as, well, "lactose-free." Also, the symbol "live and active culture" on yogurt denotes that the yogurt is lactose-free.

REMEMBER

If you have celiac disease, you must avoid any and all gluten because consuming even tiny amounts will damage your intestine. If, on the other hand, you have lactose intolerance or another form of milk intolerance, consuming milk products won't damage your gut, but it will make you feel unwell.

Gluten-Free Diet for Vegetarians and Vegans

A vegetarian diet that excludes animal flesh, whether it is meat, fowl, fish, or seafood, or a vegan diet that avoids all animal products, including eggs and dairy products, can still provide a nutritious (and yes, very delicious) gluten-free diet.

As people who follow a vegetarian diet invariably know, there are a number of health benefits to this diet (compared to a nonvegetarian diet) including these:

TIP

» Less consumption of saturated fat and cholesterol.

» Greater intake of fiber.

» Increased ingestion of the mineral magnesium.

» More ingestion of certain vitamins such as folic acid, vitamin C, and vitamin E.

» Greater intake of some antioxidants such as carotenoids.

   Antioxidants are substances that protect cells from damage caused by *free radicals* (compounds formed during the metabolism of oxygen in our bodies). *Carotenoids* are certain nutrients, like provitamin A and lycopene, that are found in yellow, orange, or red fruits and vegetables.

» Less likelihood of being overweight.

» Better blood cholesterol levels.

» Lower blood pressure.

» Less risk of heart disease.

Although there are health benefits to following a vegetarian diet, there are challenges as well:

» By avoiding meat, poultry, fish, and seafood, your diet is devoid of the major sources of protein, iron, zinc, omega-3 fatty acids, and vitamins A and B12.

» Eliminating eggs and milk products removes from your diet calcium and vitamin D in addition to other sources of dietary protein.

Despite these obstacles, with knowledge and care, a nutritious vegetarian or vegan gluten-free diet is possible.

TIP

Earlier in this chapter, we look at sources of calcium and iron, many of which can be consumed by people following a vegetarian diet. See the sections "Consuming calcium" and "Ironing out iron deficiency" for details.

WARNING

Getting sufficient protein can be a challenge for vegetarians, especially vegans, so make sure you eat a variety of alternative protein sources such as nuts, legumes, and various soy products like tofu. Many gluten-free grains such as amaranth, buckwheat, millet, quinoa, sorghum, teff, and wild rice contain higher levels of protein than wheat. Quinoa is probably the best grain in this regard because it's considered a *complete protein*; that is, it contains adequate levels of all essential amino acids, the building blocks of proteins.

Absorption of the mineral zinc is enhanced by ingesting animal protein and inhibited by consuming *phyates,* compounds found in legumes and whole grains. Because of this, it's recommended that vegetarians consume twice as much zinc as nonvegetarians. Nonanimal sources of foods that are high in zinc include nuts, seeds, legumes, and various grains, including wild rice.

Insufficient ingestion of vitamin B12 is only a problem for vegetarians who do not eat eggs or dairy products. Vegans must use either vitamin B12-fortified foods such as soymilk or take vitamin B12 supplements.

TIP

If you're following a vegetarian or vegan diet, it's important to meet with a dietitian on an ongoing basis to ensure you're getting all the nutrients you need. A gluten-free vegetarian and vegan menu plan is included in Appendix A.

Chapter **12**

Figuring Out What Comes Next

I f you have very recently been diagnosed with celiac disease and are now starting on your gluten-free diet, you're probably wondering how long it will take for you to feel better, what symptoms will go away the fastest, and how long it will take for you to feel 100 percent again. In this chapter, we look at these issues and also discuss what you should do if, despite following a gluten-free diet, things just aren't coming around the way you expect.

REMEMBER

To succeed with a gluten-free diet, you must know what a gluten-free diet is in the first place! We discuss this in detail in Chapter 10, but even if you've read and reread that chapter, we cannot emphasize strongly enough the importance of you meeting with a skilled, celiac disease-savvy dietitian to receive expert advice on how to live gluten-free.

Knowing Whether Your Gluten-Free Diet Is Working

There are several ways in which you and your healthcare team can determine whether your gluten-free diet is working. You can keep a lookout for symptoms, blood tests can be performed, and, in some cases, a repeat small intestine biopsy is performed. We look at these topics in this section.

REMEMBER

Speaking of blood tests to monitor your response to a gluten-free diet: It's important to realize that the blood tests we use to diagnose celiac disease are great for diagnosis, but not perfect for monitoring dietary adherence or healing of the small intestine.

Surveying your symptoms

The best and easiest way for you to tell whether your gluten-free diet is working is for you to simply ask yourself, "How am I feeling?" If you're like most people with celiac disease, within a matter of weeks of starting a gluten-free diet, you'll find yourself answering with a resounding, "A whole lot better."

TIP

If you had celiac disease for a long time before it was discovered, and especially if you've been quite ill from it, it may take a while for you to feel better.

Following are key symptoms you and your doctor can monitor to track your progress (we discuss these and other symptoms in detail in Chapter 2; in Chapter 13, we talk about monitoring celiac disease):

>> **Your general sense of well-being:** This is often one of the very first things to improve.

>> **Your energy level:** This tends to improve in tandem with your sense of well-being.

>> **Gastrointestinal symptoms:** Your indigestion, bloating, flatulence, and diarrhea will likely start to ease within a few weeks.

REMEMBER

Although monitoring how you're responding to your gluten-free diet by keeping tabs on these symptoms is very helpful, it's important to remember that these and other symptoms also can be present due to conditions totally unrelated to celiac disease. For this reason, although doctors put great emphasis on learning about and following your symptoms to help gauge your response to your diet, if your symptoms persist, neither you nor your doctor should automatically assume the problem is your celiac disease. It could, in fact, be that you have some other condition altogether. In this situation, your doctor will need to send you for other investigations to determine what is amiss.

Antibody blood tests

As we discuss in Chapter 3, the single most important blood test to help diagnose celiac disease is the tissue transglutaminase (TTG) IgA antibody. Because it can take a long time — years, for many adults — for the intestine to fully heal, following the TTG IgA antibody is a way to monitor your response to the gluten-free diet sooner, and more frequently, compared to a repeat biopsy. If checked a few months after you've been on your gluten-free diet, your TTG IgA antibody level should be lower in amount than before you started treatment.

If you are IgA-deficient (see Chapter 3 for more in-depth information), monitoring your response to your gluten-free diet by measuring your TTG IgA antibody level won't be helpful because your body can't make IgA in the first place. If this is the case, your doctor will use other means to monitor your progress, including other blood tests such as the IgG form of TTG antibody (although this is likely to come down even after adopting a strict gluten-free diet), a hemoglobin level to monitor for anemia (if you were anemic to begin with), or a vitamin D level if, prior to treatment, it was low. Sometimes, a follow-up endoscopy and small intestine biopsy are required (see Chapter 13).

Other blood tests

If, when you were diagnosed with celiac disease, your doctor discovered you had a low hemoglobin level (that is, you were anemic) or were deficient in iron, vitamin D, calcium, or other nutrients, your physician can monitor your progress by checking these levels in your blood from time to time. As you follow your gluten-free diet, your bowel should be healing and regaining its ability to absorb these nutrients into your body; hence, your levels should gradually return to normal.

Once your blood chemistry levels are back to normal, if your doctor had previously advised you to take supplements (such as iron), they may now tell you to discontinue them. If so, it's important to then have these levels rechecked a few months later to ensure they remain normal. If they've fallen again, it may indicate that your intestine has not yet sufficiently healed and is unable to sufficiently absorb nutrients into your body.

TIP

Vitamin D deficiency is so common in the general population (that is, in people without celiac disease or any other health problem) that some physicians and other health advocates recommend vitamin D supplements be taken routinely. This is especially so in middle-aged and older women who are also routinely advised to take supplemental calcium (to help preserve bone strength and mass). Therefore, if you're a woman in this age group and you have celiac disease and your doctor advises you that you can discontinue your vitamin D and calcium because your bowel has healed, ask if you should continue these nutrients anyway.

Another intestinal biopsy

Not everyone with celiac disease undergoes a second endoscopy and small intestine biopsy. Experts disagree about whether a second biopsy should be routinely done in everyone or should be reserved for those in certain circumstances. For example, if you have

>> Persisting gastrointestinal symptoms (like abdominal cramps and diarrhea) despite following a gluten-free diet.

>> Persisting, unexplained iron deficiency.

>> Persistent elevations in antibody levels, despite a dietitian's assessment that there is no identifiable source of accidental gluten exposure in your diet.

>> The return of gastrointestinal symptoms or anemia, yet no rise in your antibody levels. (If your antibody levels go up simultaneously with the redevelopment of symptoms or anemia, the first step would be to determine if gluten is inadvertently sneaking into your diet.)

>> The new development of weight loss, anemia, and/or severe diarrhea despite following a gluten-free diet. In this situation, an endoscopy and small intestine biopsy may help confirm these symptoms are due to celiac disease or may reveal some other, unrelated gastrointestinal disorder.

>> Celiac disease, but you never had antibodies (such as the tissue transglutaminase antibody) present that are typically seen with active celiac disease. In this case, your doctor cannot monitor your antibody levels to determine if your bowel is healing.

The persistently abnormal small intestine biopsy

If your repeat biopsy shows classical features of active celiac disease, such as *villus atrophy* (explained in Chapter 3), your celiac disease is still active. If the biopsy reveals mild inflammation, then your celiac disease may, nonetheless, be well controlled. It can take years for these mild inflammatory changes (particularly an increased number of intraepithelial lymphocytes; see Chapter 3) to resolve, and sometimes they never do. Studies suggest that people with mild inflammation on their follow-up biopsy have long-term health outcomes that are just as good as those with totally normalized biopsy results. On the one hand, people with persistent villous atrophy in the long term appear to have higher rates of complications of celiac disease, such as lymphoma and fractures. For that reason, the resolution of villus atrophy is seen as an important goal of the gluten-free diet.

REMEMBER

If ever you have a repeat biopsy performed and you're told it shows evidence of active celiac disease, it's important to compare the results of your first biopsy and discuss with your doctor what specific findings were found. If villus atrophy is still present, it may be due to a slow or gradual improvement compared to the initial biopsy. Some people — particularly older adults — may take three to five years or longer of strict avoidance of gluten to have fully regrown villi.

Although it is unknown why increased intraepithelial lymphocytes (a possible sign of ongoing inflammation) can still be found in biopsies of some patients who have been on a gluten-free diet for years, possible explanations include the following:

>> Accidental ingestion of minuscule amounts of gluten (which could maintain ongoing, mild inflammation in the gut).

>> A very slow-to-heal digestive system.

>> Having some other condition that causes biopsy findings similar to celiac disease but occurs unrelated to gluten ingestion. For example, increased intraepithelial lymphocytes in the small intestine can sometimes result from anti-inflammatory medications or infections (such as those caused by the *Helicobacter pylori* bacteria).

Exploring Why Your Gluten-Free Diet May Not Be Working

In most cases, it is readily apparent if a person is succeeding with their gluten-free diet. Usually, an individual with symptoms newly diagnosed with celiac disease is placed on a gluten-free diet and, within a matter of a few weeks, is feeling much better. Soon thereafter, his blood tests are improving, and they're on their way to restored good health. Simple as that. But what about the person who doesn't quickly feel better, or whose lab tests don't show improvement? It could be that they aren't responding to the gluten-free diet (that is, they have *nonresponsive celiac disease*). The single most important clue to you and your doctor that you're not sufficiently responding to your gluten-free diet is if, despite carefully following it, you're not feeling any better or, especially, if you're feeling worse. An additional, strong clue that your gluten-free diet isn't working the way it should is if your lab tests are not improving (refer to the preceding sections for information on follow-up tests). However, there could be other reasons that you do not feel better once you start the gluten-free diet, such as an increase in the amount of fat, less fiber, or other additives (gums) than in your regular diet. Other issues include small bacterial overgrowth (SIBO) and lactose intolerance, as we discuss later in this chapter in the "Conditions complicating celiac disease" section.

REMEMBER

It's important that you not wait months and months to get in touch with your doctor or dietitian if you feel that you're not responding the way you should to your gluten-free diet. Your healthcare providers will want to know if you don't feel better so that they can figure out why.

TIP

If you're not responding to your gluten-free diet the way you should, take heart. There's always a reason, and once the reason is discovered and corrected, you'll be back on the road to recovery.

Continued gluten exposure

The most common reason for someone to fail to get better on a gluten-free diet is that that person may not be completely gluten-free. This is typically due to one of three things:

>> You're unintentionally consuming gluten. Sometimes, despite your best efforts, you're still ingesting gluten-containing food. In this case, it's a matter of sitting down with your dietitian and identifying the potential sources. Other times, nonfood sources of gluten are being inadvertently consumed. In Chapter 10, we look at these nonfood sources of gluten, including (rarely) certain medications or play-dough.

>> You know you're consuming gluten and are aware that it can hurt you, but, for whatever reason, you elect to ignore medical advice (oh yes, this does indeed happen; perhaps more often than you might think) and to carry on with your old diet.

>> You (incorrectly) believe that "just a little bit of gluten won't hurt" and therefore continue to ingest it.

REMEMBER

If you aren't responding to your diet, it may be that some gluten is inadvertently getting into your diet. It's important to work with your dietitian to find the sources of unintentional gluten so you can remove those foods or products from your diet. The only way for your intestine to heal and for you to recover your health is to be completely gluten-free. Keeping a food diary will help identify the source of gluten exposure. A celiac disease-savvy dietitian may well discover sources of gluten that are not always easy to identify.

TIP

Don't be too hard on yourself if and when you inadvertently eat something with gluten or even when you decide to taste just a tiny piece of a homemade gluten-containing baked treat. Just climb back on that horse (the gluten-free horse that is) and keep fighting to stay gluten-free. We certainly don't advocate consuming *any* gluten at all, but we also recognize that nobody is perfect.

Conditions complicating celiac disease

Another relatively common reason why people with celiac disease may remain unwell despite following a gluten-free diet is if they have some other, additional gastrointestinal ailment that causes similar symptoms to their celiac disease. We look at these in this section.

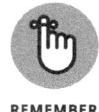

REMEMBER

Even if you are found to have one of the conditions we discuss here, the treatment is the gluten-free diet first, followed by other additional therapies you may need.

Lactose intolerance

As we discuss in detail in Chapter 11, lactose intolerance is a very, very common condition in which an individual lacks sufficient lactase enzyme to properly digest lactose (the sugar found in milk products). As a result, they may experience gastrointestinal (GI) symptoms such as abdominal cramps, flatulence, and diarrhea.

Because lactose intolerance is so common in most population groups, many people with celiac disease also have this condition. Indeed, it may well be that before you were diagnosed with celiac disease, you were already known to have lactose intolerance. In that case, after you've been diagnosed with celiac disease, you will need to continue with your lactose-free diet (with or without the use of lactase supplements). Otherwise, even if you're following a gluten-free diet, you might have GI symptoms.

Some individuals may develop temporary lactose intolerance due to the transient loss of normal levels of lactase with newly diagnosed celiac disease. As a result, you may have GI symptoms from both your celiac disease and your lactose intolerance. These may be indistinguishable from one another. Because temporary lactose intolerance is fairly common with newly diagnosed celiac disease, you may want to follow a lactose-free diet for a few weeks after you begin your gluten-free diet. At that point, although your bowel won't be completely healed, it will have sufficiently replenished its quantity of lactase that you can resume ingesting lactose-containing products.

Small intestinal bacterial overgrowth (SIBO)

Microorganisms (such as bacteria) — also known as microbes — live within much of your digestive tract. The number of microbes present increases as one moves (figuratively speaking) from the upper small intestine to the end of the large intestine. As many as 100 *trillion* microbes per 1 milliliter of fluid are within the lower part of the large intestine. How many is a trillion? Well, written out it's 100,000,000,000,000! Can you imagine that many bugs living in a space that is ⅕ of a teaspoon of liquid?

Although much remains to be discovered regarding the role (or roles) that gut bacteria play in maintaining human health, it is known that they are essential in helping normal digestion proceed. If there are excessive numbers of bacteria in the small intestine — a condition called *small intestinal bacterial overgrowth* (or SIBO for short) — the bacteria can interfere with the absorption of fat, protein, carbohydrates (including lactose), and other nutrients, which, in turn, causes symptoms such as diarrhea. (We discuss malabsorption in Chapter 7.)

SIBO is an area of tremendous uncertainty. Some experts believe that SIBO contributes to common symptoms that can cause frequent discomfort or distress, such as gassiness and bloating. On the other hand, studies have found that SIBO is often present in healthy people with no symptoms. In people who have previously undergone intestinal surgery, the link between SIBO and symptoms is stronger. But for everyone else, there is disagreement among doctors about whether SIBO is an important contributor to symptoms.

SIBO is diagnosed using tests, including those that measure the amounts of certain molecules in your breath. Some studies have shown that tests for SIBO are more likely to be positive in people with celiac disease compared to the general population. The treatment of SIBO typically consists of a 7- to 14-day course of an antibiotic. Often, your dietitian may recommend adding some probiotic-rich foods — such as yogurt — when you finish the antibiotics to increase the levels of more helpful bacteria, such as *lactobacillus*. Breath tests are imperfect and are subject to both false positive and false negative results. For that reason, some physicians prescribe a course of antibiotics for suspected SIBO without ordering a breath test.

Pancreatic insufficiency

As we discuss in Chapter 5, the pancreas is very important in digestion because it makes enzymes that travel down into the gut and assist with the breakdown of nutrients into small molecules that can then be absorbed into the body. This is called the pancreas's *exocrine* function. (The pancreas's other function, referred to as its *endocrine* function, is to make insulin and other hormones that help regulate blood glucose levels.)

When the pancreas's exocrine function becomes impaired (a condition called *pancreatic insufficiency*), the person develops malabsorption. Symptoms include bloating, flatulence, diarrhea, and weight loss. Because these symptoms are often also seen with celiac disease, your doctor may not necessarily consider pancreatic insufficiency as a cause of your symptoms . . . in which case we're thrilled you're reading this section! Because now that you've read this, should your GI symptoms not be responding to a carefully followed gluten-free diet, you can bring the possible diagnosis of pancreatic insufficiency to your doctor's attention.

Because there are no particularly good ways of testing for pancreatic insufficiency and because therapy is safe and simple, most physicians treat suspected cases on speculation (what doctors call *empirical therapy*). Treatment consists of taking, in pill form, the enzymes that the pancreas normally makes. We admit this isn't the most scientific process in the world, but sometimes a quick-and-dirty approach is the best.

EXAMPLE

Wendy had persistent complaints of loose stools and upper abdominal discomfort in spite of being on a strict gluten-free diet for two years. Her regular gastroenterologist suggested a lactose-free diet with lactase supplements. This helped, but not completely. The gastroenterologist ordered additional testing to find out why Wendy's symptoms weren't responding. The subsequent blood tests, including TTG IgA antibody (which had been mildly elevated to start with), were normal. The gastroenterologist organized an endoscopy and small bowel biopsy, and these were normal. The doctor prescribed pancreatic enzyme supplements and, lo and behold, just a few weeks later, Wendy reported that since starting the enzyme supplements, her symptoms had entirely gone away.

Microscopic colitis

Microscopic colitis is an autoimmune disease in which a special type of inflammatory cell — called a *lymphocyte* — accumulates within the lining of the large intestine (the colon). There are two types of microscopic colitis: *lymphocytic colitis* and *collagenous colitis*.

People with celiac disease, for unknown reasons, are more prone to microscopic colitis. The most common symptom is severe, watery diarrhea, typically far worse than the diarrhea that may occur with celiac disease alone. The condition is diagnosed by obtaining a biopsy of the colon (this is done when a colonoscopy is performed; in this procedure, a flexible tube is placed through the anus into the large bowel).

Intriguingly (well, at least to us), the large intestine biopsy in lymphocytic colitis shows increased numbers of *intraepithelial lymphocytes* (see Chapter 3), which is the same feature that is seen in small intestine biopsies in active celiac disease. This hints at some connection between the two conditions, but what, precisely, the connection may be is unknown.

In some individuals, ingesting gluten can sometimes promote or exacerbate the symptoms of microscopic colitis. Therefore, as you may expect, treatment includes following a gluten-free diet. This diet, of course, also treats celiac disease.

TIP

There is some scientific evidence that taking aspirin and non-steroidal anti-inflammatory drugs (such as ibuprofen or naproxen) or certain other medications either causes or, at least, aggravates microscopic colitis, so your doctor will likely advise you to withdraw these medications if possible.

If following a gluten-free diet and stopping any offending drugs aren't sufficient to control your microscopic colitis, you then need other therapy. Options include prescription drugs such as budesonide and over-the-counter bismuth-containing products like Pepto-Bismol.

Gastroparesis

Gastroparesis is a condition in which the stomach takes an overly long time to empty its contents into the small intestine. Although gastroparesis can affect people with celiac disease (hence the reason we discuss this condition), fortunately, this seldom happens.

The most common symptoms of gastroparesis are

>> Early satiety (that is, feeling full far sooner than normal during a meal)

>> Upper abdominal bloating or discomfort

>> Nausea

Because these symptoms can also be seen with celiac disease, on occasion, the two conditions may be confused.

Gastroparesis is diagnosed by a special nuclear medicine test called a *gastric emptying scan* in which you ingest a piece of food (usually an egg sandwich) into which a tiny amount of radioactivity has been placed. Pictures are then taken of your abdomen to see how long it takes for the food to pass from your stomach into your small intestine.

If you have gastroparesis due to celiac disease, following a gluten-free diet typically helps both conditions, and, indeed, your gastroparesis may entirely resolve. If, however, this doesn't happen, prescription medicines are available to help your stomach work better.

Conditions coexisting with celiac disease

Having celiac disease does not, of course, mean that you cannot have other, unrelated diseases, including other gastrointestinal (GI) disorders. Indeed, if you have celiac disease, you remain as prone to GI conditions unrelated to celiac disease as does anyone else. Therefore, if, despite carefully following a gluten-free diet, you find yourself having ongoing GI symptoms, you and your doctor should not automatically blame it all on your celiac disease. Rather, the two of you need to consider that you may also have another, coincidental GI problem.

These are the three most important coincidental GI ailments to be considered:

>> **Gastro-esophageal reflux disease (GERD)** is a condition in which stomach acid travels up into your esophagus and causes heartburn. We discuss this condition in Chapter 2.

>> **Functional dyspepsia (also called *non-ulcer dyspepsia*)** is a condition in which you experience persisting or recurring pain or discomfort centered in the upper abdomen despite the absence of "structural" (that is, physically apparent) diseases like ulcers of the stomach or duodenum, stomach inflammation (*gastritis*), stomach cancer, and so on. Symptoms may also include nausea, feeling full overly quickly as you eat, and/or feeling bloated after finishing a meal.

>> **Irritable bowel syndrome (IBS)** is a very common condition with variable features, but most commonly involving recurring abdominal pain or discomfort that improves with having a bowel movement. Affected people also typically notice a change in the frequency or the appearance of their bowel movements (for example, their stools may become long and skinny like licorice). Some people with IBS have problems with constipation and bloating, whereas others have diarrhea and urgency. IBS is not damaging to the body, but the symptoms can be physically and emotionally debilitating.

Because conditions like functional dyspepsia and IBS can cause symptoms similar to those seen with celiac disease, some people who have *not* been diagnosed with celiac disease mistakenly ascribe their symptoms *to* celiac disease and initiate a gluten-free diet without first having these other conditions looked for and without having been tested for celiac disease. As a result, individuals may be following a strict gluten-free diet without getting relief from symptoms and potentially unnecessarily restricting their nutrient intake.

Wrong diagnosis

You and your doctor should question the diagnosis of celiac disease when there is little or no improvement on your gluten-free diet. As we discuss in Chapter 3, it's not so rare that a diagnosis of celiac disease is made, for a variety of reasons, in someone in whom the condition isn't actually present.

Following are some of the most common conditions that are mistakenly diagnosed as celiac disease (when, in fact, they are entirely different ailments):

>> **Irritable bowel syndrome:** We discuss this condition in the preceding section.

>> **Functional dyspepsia:** We discuss this condition in the preceding section.

>> **Other functional gastrointestinal disorders (FGID):** This is a large group of conditions that include IBS, functional dyspepsia, and other problems that can either coexist with celiac disease or be mistakenly labeled as celiac disease. (For further information on FGID, see www.iffgd.org or https://theromefoundation.org.)

>> **Inflammatory bowel disease:** This includes *ulcerative colitis* and *Crohn's disease*. These are ailments of unknown cause, where the intestine becomes inflamed and people experience abdominal pain and diarrhea.

The number of other, less common or even rare conditions that can be misdiagnosed as celiac disease is lengthy and stretches from immune diseases (such as common variable immunodeficiency) to other forms of bowel disease (such as eosinophilic gastroenteritis) to other forms of food intolerance, and the list goes on (and on and on and . . .). There's no need, however, to look for these other, rare birds unless more common conditions, such as those in the preceding list, have first been excluded.

The overall approach if you are not responding to your gluten-free diet

If your celiac disease symptoms are not improving despite following a gluten-free diet for at least a few months, we recommend you follow this step-wise approach:

1. **Meet with your dietitian to review your diet in detail to ensure you are not inadvertently (or even intentionally) consuming gluten; if there's no evidence that you're ingesting gluten, move on to step 2.**

2. **Remove all lactose from your diet (if you haven't already done so). If this has not helped within a few weeks, then go to step 3.**

3. **Speak to your celiac disease specialist about the possibility that you may also have a complicating condition. If this isn't the case, proceed to step 4.**

   Complicating conditions include SIBO or pancreatic insufficiency. See the earlier section "Conditions complicating celiac disease" for a more complete list.

4. **Speak to your specialist about the possibility that you may also have an unrelated, coexisting condition. If this isn't the case, move to step 5.**

   Coexisting conditions include functional dyspepsia, irritable bowel syndrome, and others discussed in the earlier section "Conditions coexisting with celiac disease."

5. **Speak to your specialist about the possibility that the diagnosis of celiac disease is inaccurate and that you have some other ailment altogether.**

   There's no harm in raising this possibility at *any* time; you don't have to wait until this step to bring this up with your doctor.

TIP

If your doctor elects to treat you for conditions in the preceding list, we recommend that you be treated for only one condition at a time; otherwise, neither you nor your doctor will know which treatment was working for what condition.

When Your Celiac Disease Won't Settle Down

Though it's not at all likely, it's possible that you will not improve despite having gone through all of the steps we discuss earlier in this chapter. You've reviewed with your dietitian every morsel that enters your mouth, and nary a spec of gluten is to be found; you and your doctor have either excluded or have sufficiently treated any complicating or coexisting condition; the diagnosis of celiac disease has been convincingly made, but, well, you're just not feeling the way you should. What then? In this section, we look at two important causes of nonresponsive celiac disease that you and your doctor need to consider.

Refractory celiac disease

Refractory celiac disease (RCD) is a rare condition in which a person's celiac disease doesn't settle despite meticulously following a gluten-free diet for at least one year. The following two additional features need to be present for the diagnosis to be made:

>> Repeated small intestine biopsies must show persisting abnormalities of celiac disease. We discuss these in Chapter 3.

>> All other causes of persistent gastrointestinal symptoms, including gluten exposure, need to be excluded.

Some people have RCD from the get-go — that is, from the time they are first diagnosed with celiac disease. Other people who develop RCD had initially responded to treatment, but as time passed, they redeveloped symptoms that wouldn't go away.

TECHNICAL STUFF

The underlying mechanism involved with refractory celiac disease is not fully sorted out, but it is likely related to chronic stimulation of the immune system. It is as if the immune system has gotten so chronically overstimulated that it simply won't shut off. As part of this process, special types of white blood cells called *T lymphocytes* can transform so that they first become prone to developing cancer (that is, these lymphocytes become precancerous), then may subsequently become frankly cancerous. We discuss this rare type of cancer, a form of immune system malignancy (lymphoma) called EATCL, in the next section and, in more detail, in Chapter 9.

Who is at increased risk of refractory celiac disease?

Not every person with celiac disease is at equal risk for developing refractory celiac disease. Refractory celiac disease is most likely to occur in

>> The elderly

>> People in whom the diagnosis of celiac disease is very delayed

>> Individuals with known celiac disease who, nonetheless, elect to continue a gluten-containing diet year after year

>> Adults who were diagnosed with celiac disease when they were children but were subsequently told they had "outgrown it" and thus resumed consuming gluten (Sadly, often these patients present later in life with complications of untreated celiac disease.)

How is refractory celiac disease monitored?

If you have refractory celiac disease, your specialist will monitor you very closely. They will keep a special eye out for evidence of complications from the condition, including ulcers of the small intestine and enlarged lymph nodes (lymph glands), the latter being a possible sign of lymphoma.

You may also be sent for tests that allow for an examination of that long portion of the small intestine that lies beyond the reach of a regular endoscope. These tests include capsule endoscopy and enteroscopy. We review these tests in Chapter 9.

TECHNICAL STUFF

If you have refractory celiac disease, your doctor may mention to you that you have either the type I or type II variety. Cancer is rare with either, but of the two, cancer is more likely to occur with the type II variety. Hence, if you have this form, you will be especially closely monitored for the development of cancer.

How is refractory celiac disease treated?

There are many different treatment options for RCD, including using potent drugs like *corticosteroids* and other medications that suppress the immune system.

Despite these measures, people with refractory celiac disease remain at increased risk of death from infection, malnutrition, and certain types of cancer, especially EATCL (which we discuss next).

REMEMBER

Given the seriousness and rarity of refractory celiac disease, it's usually best managed by a specialist who has specific expertise in celiac disease and has access to highly sophisticated resources, such as is most commonly found in university-based teaching hospitals. We list such centers in Appendix D.

Lest we've created undue concern, before we leave this section, we'll reiterate that refractory celiac disease is a rare disease, so you'll be highly unlikely to ever get it. Far less than 1 percent of people with celiac disease are diagnosed with refractory celiac disease.

Enteropathy-associated T cell lymphoma

As we discuss in detail in Chapter 9, enteropathy-associated T cell lymphoma (EATCL) is a rare form of cancer that starts in the immune system cells located in the small intestine. EATCL is more likely to occur if you have refractory celiac disease (see the immediately preceding section). Symptoms of EATCL include malaise, loss of appetite, weight loss, worsening diarrhea, abdominal pain, and fevers.

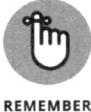

REMEMBER

If you have these symptoms, you must see your physician as soon as possible. When your doctor examines you for suspected EATCL, they may find enlarged lymph glands, a skin rash, an enlarged liver, or an abdominal mass. Investigations typically include special X-rays (such as CT or PET scans) of the chest and abdomen and upper endoscopy (see Chapter 3). Treatment may include chemotherapy, radiation therapy, and surgery.

4

The Long-Term: Living and Thriving with Celiac Disease

IN THIS CHAPTER

» Monitoring your condition

» Watching for ongoing nutrition issues

» Falling off your gluten-free diet

» Taking control of your celiac health

» Becoming your own best advocate

Chapter **13**

Ongoing Care of Celiac Disease

I f you've recently been diagnosed with celiac disease and have now started a gluten-free diet, you may be wondering what to expect next, both in the near term and over the long haul. Perhaps you've asked yourself questions such as "What do I need to keep an eye on?" or "What does *my doctor* need to keep an eye on?" In other words, what is the ongoing care of your celiac disease? It's also quite possible that these are questions that you may have even if you've had celiac disease for many years. In either case, you've come to the right place, because in this chapter, we answer these very questions.

Monitoring Your Celiac Disease

In medical school, doctors-to-be are taught rule after rule about how to manage a person's health (or illness). Indeed, by the time newly crowned med students walk up to get their diplomas, their heads are crammed with literally thousands upon thousands of "proper ways" to do things. What a shock it is when one actually starts to work as a doctor and immediately learns that, in fact, there are no rules! There are approaches, guidelines, recommendations, policies . . . yes. But as for rules, well, not so much. Or, looked at another way, there are as many unique situations as there are unique patients, which is everyone a doctor sees. Why this preamble? Simply this: You are a unique individual, so the monitoring you require and how often you require it depend on your specific situation. (And, lest any of our colleagues take offense, we admit there are *some* rules in medicine, but not very many.)

Determining how often you should see your healthcare providers

The factors that influence how often you need to be seen by your healthcare providers, including your primary care physician, your celiac disease specialist, and your dietitian, are based on a number of factors, such as these:

>> How you are feeling.

>> If you were diagnosed with celiac disease in the recent past, how sick were you when you were first diagnosed?

>> Whether you're having a hard time adhering to your gluten-free diet. We discuss the gluten-free diet in Chapter 10.

WHY NO RULES EXIST WHEN MONITORING PATIENTS WITH CELIAC DISEASE

In the world of medicine, the stronger the scientific proof of something, the stronger the recommendations that result from the scientific proof. For example, many thousands of studies show that smoking is harmful to one's health — enough studies that doctors can say with complete confidence and conviction to all their patients that they should not smoke and, if they do, they should do their utmost to quit. Unfortunately, in the world of medicine, things are seldom this cut and dried. Indeed, there is seldom scientific evidence of such overwhelming, incontrovertible, perfectly consistent, and universally applicable character that a doctor can reflexively recommend to a patient a single course of action. This reality is very much the case when it comes to monitoring a person who has celiac disease.

Because of the paucity of studies on this subject, guidelines for monitoring celiac disease vary considerably with regard to what tests to do when and how often. When healthcare providers find themselves in this situation, they end up choosing those recommendations that make the most sense to them, but they should also share with the patient the great uncertainty and variability about what is recommended.

>> Whether you're having complications from your diet, such as undue weight gain, weight loss, or constipation. We discuss these topics later in this chapter.

>> If you have complications from your celiac disease. We discuss this topic in Chapter 7.

>> If you have conditions associated with celiac disease. We discuss this topic in Chapter 8.

>> What laboratory test abnormalities did you have when you were diagnosed, how severe they were, and whether they're improving.

By way of extreme examples to make a point: If your celiac disease was only recently diagnosed, and if you were very unwell at the time with bad symptoms and markedly abnormal blood chemistry tests, you will need to be a frequent visitor to your celiac disease specialist. If you've had celiac disease for years, you've had no problems adhering to your gluten-free diet, you're feeling well, and you've had no complications, then your specialist may need to see you very seldom. As you may imagine, most people with celiac disease — likely including yourself — fall somewhere in between.

TIP

As a very rough rule of thumb, if you're pretty healthy overall when you're first diagnosed with celiac disease, you may expect to see your celiac disease specialist and your dietitian collectively no more than a handful of times in the six months after your diagnosis and less and less often as time goes by. Gastroenterologists or celiac disease specialists routinely see healthy, uncomplicated patients with celiac disease every year, but again, there are no rules.

Knowing who does the monitoring

The healthcare professional who is most responsible for monitoring your celiac disease varies depending on your specific circumstances and, in part, on the availability of a specialist. Although the diagnosis of celiac disease is almost always made by a specialist, and although the early monitoring is typically done by this same doctor and a dietitian, as time goes by, if you're doing well, your primary healthcare provider will likely have a central role in keeping tabs on your progress. Of course, if you are not responding to therapy as you should or if you have complications from your celiac disease, then the ongoing involvement of a specialist will be essential.

If you've been doing very well — and especially if there is limited availability of celiac disease specialists — the entirety of your celiac disease medical care may be handed back to your primary care doctor by the specialist. If that is the case, you should not take that to mean that you can't see a specialist again. Indeed, if ever you run into problems with your celiac disease — or if you or your primary care doctor even *thinks* you may have run into problems — you can be referred back to a specialist.

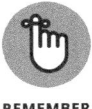

Registered dietitians are an invaluable resource when it comes to matters of nutrition. If your problem may relate to dietary issues, a dietitian is typically the best person to see.

Knowing what is discussed during a monitoring visit

When you see your doctor for a routine celiac disease monitoring appointment, your doctor will want to find out from you many details regarding how you've been feeling since your last appointment. We discuss these details in this section.

You may find reviewing this section helpful to prepare for an appointment with the healthcare providers assisting you with your celiac disease. You will be less likely to feel caught off-guard during the meeting or, even worse, leave the interview only to then say to yourself "Oh shoot, I forgot to tell/ask the doctor. . . ."

When you see your doctor for your appointment, that appointment is *your appointment,* and you should not feel constrained in what you bring up. You absolutely must share with your doctor anything at all that you feel may relate to your celiac disease. You never know when something that seems, at first blush, to be unimportant will in fact turn out to be highly significant.

How you're feeling in general

When discussing various health concerns, regardless of whether the issues are related to celiac disease, very often doctors and patients (appropriately) spend considerable time discussing specific issues such as, for example, chest pain, joint pain, diarrhea, and so on. What risks getting missed, however, is an overview of how you're feeling and managing with the gluten-free diet. This includes your overall sense of well-being and whether you find that celiac disease is impairing your quality of life.

What your energy level is like

If you lack energy and feel generally fatigued, listless, or tired, this can be an important clue to your physician that something is amiss with your health. The cause may be entirely unrelated to your celiac disease, but of the many possible causes for these symptoms, quite a few are known to be associated with celiac disease; therefore, they need to be considered by your healthcare provider. Possible causes include anemia, iron deficiency, thyroid disease, and depression, to name but a few. We discuss this topic in detail in Chapter 2.

How your bowel habits are and, in particular, whether you're having diarrhea or constipation

Although celiac disease can show itself in varied ways, the common denominator with this condition is inflammation of the bowel, and so keeping tabs on whether you have symptoms related to your intestines is important.

If you're having diarrhea, letting your doctor know is essential. A slew of possible causes of diarrhea exist, some serious, some not. As we discuss in detail in Chapter 12, possibilities include gluten remaining in the diet (that is, your diet isn't truly gluten-free), having a complication from celiac disease, having some other, possibly unrelated condition, and so on.

Constipation, as we discuss later in this chapter, is a common consequence of following a gluten-free diet. Be sure to let both your physician and your dietitian know if you've developed constipation so that they can assist you not only with determining the cause but also with helping relieve you of the problem.

Whether your weight is going up, down, or remaining steady

As we discuss further on in this chapter (see the section "Weighty issues"), treatment of celiac disease can lead to both weight loss and weight gain. A few pounds in either direction is seldom a cause for concern, but if your weight is changing in amounts beyond a few pounds, be sure to let your physician know. Your doctor will need to determine whether anything of concern is present. If no additional medical issue is responsible, then a visit to your dietitian will be in order.

For children, their pediatrician must make sure that they are on track on the growth curve — that is, gaining the appropriate amount of height and weight for their age. (You can find growth curves at www.cdc.gov/GrowthCharts.) Often, children are below the expected height and weight for their age when they are first diagnosed with celiac disease. Once they're on a gluten-free diet and their intestines start to heal, they regain the ability to properly absorb nutrients into their body, and they begin the process of catching up on height and weight. The amount they catch up will depend on the age of the child when they first begin treatment. We discuss this in detail in Chapter 2.

If you have any doubt whether your child is growing and developing normally, and if the physician doesn't happen to bring up this topic when you take your child in for a visit, be sure to raise your concerns with the doctor.

Whether you are on track with your gluten-free diet

As we mention literally dozens of times throughout this book, if you have celiac disease and continue to ingest gluten, you will experience ongoing inflammation in your small intestine and risk developing complications of this condition. How essential is following a gluten-free diet if you have celiac disease? In a word, *absolutely.*

Letting your doctor know whether you're on track — or whether you're not on track — with your gluten-free diet is essential. If you're not following the diet, your physician needs to spend time with you discussing what obstacles or barriers are limiting your adherence to your nutrition program. Your doctor may ask you about your last known or suspected gluten exposure, the circumstances surrounding it, the symptoms you experienced, and how often this occurs. The great majority of people coming in for follow-up have the experience of being *glutened* (that is, accidentally eating gluten), and reviewing these circumstances can help you and your team explore strategies for prevention going forward.

REMEMBER

Your doctor is not there to judge you. If you're not following your gluten-free diet, you must — this is crucial — let your doctor know. If you don't, your doctor may end up sending you for all sorts of unnecessary tests as they try to discover why you're not responding to your treatment program the way you should.

Several situations exist where additional testing becomes more important. Here are some examples:

>> **If, despite following a gluten-free diet, you continue to feel unwell:** In this case, you need to have further testing done to see whether evidence exists of ongoing intestinal damage.

>> **If you have complications from your celiac disease:** In this situation, you need to have testing done to ensure that the complications are resolving. Here are some examples of complications (we discuss these in detail in Chapter 7) that would require monitoring through further testing:

  ● *Iron deficiency anemia:* If you have this problem, your doctor needs to keep tabs on your blood count and iron storage levels.

  ● *Vitamin D deficiency:* In this case, your doctor needs to monitor your blood levels of this vitamin.

  ● *Osteoporosis:* If you have osteoporosis, your doctor needs to monitor your bone density with periodic bone mineral density (BMD) tests.

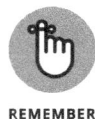

Although tests can be very important in monitoring your progress, testing is always of secondary importance compared to the crucial information your doctor will learn about you by simply hearing from you how you're feeling, how you're doing with your diet, if you're having symptoms, and so on.

Understanding the role of repeat blood antibody testing

As we discuss in Chapter 3, the IgA tissue transglutaminase antibody (TTG IgA) is a key blood test to help determine whether someone may have celiac disease. Almost all people with active celiac disease have this antibody. As you continue your gluten-free diet, your level of this antibody progressively falls and eventually becomes normal.

Monitoring your TTG IgA level is particularly helpful when you're not responding to your gluten-free diet. For example, if, despite having eliminated gluten, you continue to have symptoms (such as abdominal cramping or diarrhea), your doctor can then test your TTG IgA level. If your level hasn't significantly fallen since you started your nutrition program, your doctor and you will know that the odds are darned good that gluten is somehow continuing to make its way into your diet (and thus into your gut). At that point, solving the mystery is a matter of donning your Sherlock Holmes cap, determining the source of the gluten, and eliminating it.

When the TTG IgA is no longer elevated, most specialists recommend that this test be checked annually, even if you're well and all the laboratory studies are normal. The rationale for doing this is that the level unexpectedly going up is strong evidence that a person's celiac disease has again become active. No one has examined whether this type of laboratory monitoring practice is medically useful, but the tests are commonly done anyway. (In medicine, as all physicians would readily admit, there is both art and science.)

Though used less commonly, the deamidated gliadin peptide antibodies, which come in both IgA and IgG forms, can also be used together with the TTG IgA when monitoring for unintentional gluten exposure. Though this is a more sensitive way to look for gluten in the diet, there is also a greater likelihood of a false positive. For instance, if three antibodies are checked and only one is mildly elevated and the other two are normal, this is unlikely to be a sign of gluten exposure. But if all three are newly elevated after first normalizing, it's highly likely that a person is eating gluten.

Knowing the role of a repeat small intestine biopsy

As we discuss in Chapter 3, the diagnosis of celiac disease usually involves a biopsy of your small intestine. Although a repeat biopsy is not universally advocated for all people with celiac disease, doctors may recommend one in a number of circumstances, including these:

>> **Ongoing symptoms or evidence of malabsorption:** If you're having ongoing symptoms of celiac disease or if you have persistently low iron levels or other evidence of malabsorption despite following a gluten-free diet, your doctor may recommend proceeding with a repeat biopsy because only a biopsy provides definitive evidence of whether there's ongoing bowel damage.

>> **Failure of your antibodies to return to normal levels:** If your celiac disease antibodies (see the preceding section) don't normalize despite what appears to be complete abstinence from gluten, a repeat biopsy will help determine whether, despite your careful diet, there's ongoing evidence of small intestine injury. If present, it's once again a matter of playing detective and hunting down where the ingested gluten is coming from.

>> **Having had no evidence of celiac disease except on a biopsy specimen:** If when you were diagnosed with celiac disease you had no other features to suggest you had this condition except for a positive biopsy, the only way your doctor can know whether you still have active celiac disease is to once again perform a biopsy. (In other words, if you never had symptoms, never had abnormal antibodies, and never had other abnormal lab tests, then monitoring these parameters will not be of value in determining whether you do or don't have active disease; only a biopsy will tell the tale.)

>> **Involvement in a research study:** If you're enrolled in a research study looking at new therapies for celiac disease, the study protocol may involve having a follow-up biopsy. (If so, you'll be made aware of this at the time you sign on to participate in the study.)

>> **Checking to see if you're avoiding gluten strictly enough:** Even if you feel well and your antibody levels have normalized, unintentional gluten exposure can lead to internal intestinal inflammation and damage. For that reason, some celiac disease specialists, as a matter of routine practice, recommend to their patients that a repeat biopsy be performed two years after a gluten-free diet has been started. When it's done in this context (that is, if you're feeling better with normalized antibody levels), the result usually shows healed villi. This validates your current degree of precautions. If it doesn't show healed villi, circling back with an expert dietitian to identify sources of gluten exposure is the common next step.

In some situations, during monitoring of your celiac disease, the TTG IgA level is elevated and a repeat endoscopy and small intestine biopsy are performed, yet — lo and behold — the pathologist finds the biopsy to show nothing wrong at all. When this happens, it's a reassuring finding because a normalized biopsy is seen as a more reliable marker of long-term control of celiac disease.

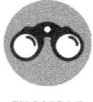

EXAMPLE

Here is a case where an abnormal repeat small intestine biopsy provided invaluable information. Shawn was a 37-year-old man who had been diagnosed with celiac disease three years earlier after an endoscopy and small intestine biopsy showed typical changes of the disease. He was treated with a gluten-free diet and did very well, but his symptoms had returned. Shawn had his blood tested and had a persistently elevated TTG IgA, despite his certainty that he was not consuming gluten. A subsequent small intestine biopsy nonetheless showed evidence of active damage from celiac disease. The mystery was solved when it was discovered that he had switched to a breakfast cereal that he thought was gluten-free but, unbeknownst to him, contained gluten. He stopped eating the cereal and soon thereafter started to feel much better.

Using capsule endoscopy

As we discuss in Chapter 3, capsule endoscopy is a procedure in which you swallow a pill-sized camera that then transmits pictures of your gastrointestinal system. Some studies have been done to determine whether this may be a better way to monitor the response of celiac disease to a gluten-free diet. At the present time, using capsule endoscopy is not a common practice. (Also, this test is not necessarily covered by health insurance, especially if you are doing well on your treatment.) However, if you're having ongoing difficulties and a regular endoscopy and biopsy can't sort out what's wrong, then a capsule study may be a good next test.

Managing Ongoing Nutrition Issues

If you felt unwell at the time you were diagnosed with celiac disease, you will almost certainly find that, soon after you've gotten on track with your gluten-free diet, you start to feel better. Previous symptoms you may have had — such as abdominal discomfort, diarrhea, bloating, gas, indigestion, or fatigue — quickly ease, and abnormal body chemistry such as anemia and low vitamin levels also start to correct. All of this, of course, is wonderful news. There are, however, a few possible downsides to following a gluten-free diet, including gaining or losing weight and developing constipation. We discuss these issues here.

Weighty issues

As we discuss in detail in Chapter 10, adopting a gluten-free diet isn't a simple matter. It requires much learning and requires great attention to pretty much everything that goes into your mouth.

Aside from water and a select few other beverages and foods, everything you eat contains energy in the form of calories. And everything a person does, from sleeping to walking to running a marathon, uses up calories. For most people, balancing calorie intake with calorie expenditure is a huge challenge; indeed, most Americans tip the balance (in a manner of speaking) in favor of excess ingested calories for their body's needs, and as a result, the majority of Americans are overweight. Having celiac disease and following a gluten-free diet can add to this challenge — at least for some people with this condition, it can be even harder to avoid weight gain. On the other hand, some people find that adopting a gluten-free diet results in losing weight. We look at both sides of this issue in this section.

The ideal weight ranges for height for adult men and women are known as *body mass index* (BMI), which we also discuss in Chapter 3. BMI has come to be criticized as too unrefined, because it does not distinguish between sources of weight (that is, muscle or fat). Thus, some people who are "big boned" may be classified as obese using the BMI when their weight is not necessarily unhealthy. Still, BMI is often useful, even if it is imperfect. You can calculate your BMI by using an online calculator. Many online calculators are available, including one you can find at www.cdc.gov/bmi/adult-calculator/index.html.

A normal BMI is 18.5 to 24.9. This range is most strongly associated with good health and, hence, is the target. These are the other categories:

>> Less than 18.5 is considered underweight.

>> 25.0 to 29.9 is called overweight.

>> 30.0 to 39.9 is termed obese.

>> 40.0 or more is considered morbidly obese.

Gaining weight

As we discuss in Chapter 6, some people with untreated celiac disease do not properly absorb nutrients into the body (a condition called *malabsorption*), and they consequently lose weight. When you follow a gluten-free diet, these nutrients — and the calories they contain — become properly used by the body, and you may gain weight. Another reason for gaining weight is that eating gluten-free foods can sometimes lead to an increase in fat in your diet. We discuss this and other nutritional issues associated with a gluten-free diet in Chapter 11.

If you found yourself gaining weight after you started your gluten-free diet, you're not alone. In one study from Ireland, more than 80 percent of people with celiac disease gained weight over the two years after starting on a gluten-free diet. (Only 15 percent lost weight.)

For some people, it can seem that each calorie seems to end up on the hips. This can be a shock for someone who was underweight and never watched — or needed to watch — what they ate. If you find yourself in this situation, you need to not only watch what you eat (to ensure that your diet is gluten-free) but also how much you eat (in terms of the number of calories you are consuming).

EXAMPLE

Maurice was a fit, 30-year-old personal support worker at a nursing home. His family doctor sent him to see a specialist after having been found, at the time of a routine physical, to be low in vitamin D. Investigations were undertaken, and it was determined that Maurice was malabsorbing nutrients — including vitamin D — because his small intestine was damaged from celiac disease. Maurice then met with a dietitian, a gluten-free diet was successfully instituted, a vitamin D supplement was begun, and in short order, Maurice's vitamin D level started to improve. Unfortunately, his weight also climbed. Maurice didn't feel that he was overeating, and he hadn't reduced his level of exercise, yet over the next two months, he gained 10 pounds. For the first time in his memory, he was overweight. Maurice met again with the dietitian, and it was determined that in attempts to increase his vitamin D levels, Maurice had been drinking an extra six glasses of vitamin D-fortified milk per day, each of which contained 120 calories. This was providing Maurice with an extra 720 calories per day! He was shocked by this discovery and, as he exclaimed at the time, "No wonder I'm gaining weight!" Maurice returned to his usual — perfectly sufficient — quantity of milk intake and, by following his gluten-free diet and taking a vitamin D supplement, his vitamin D level returned to normal while, at the same time, he lost the extra weight he'd gained.

Because gaining weight requires an excess of calorie intake compared to expenditure, if you're overweight, in addition to being careful about what you eat, increasing the number of calories you burn is also helpful. (That is, as long as you avoid the trap that so many fall into of eating extra heartily as a reward for the exercise you just did!)

TIP

If you're progressively gaining weight for no ready explanation, get in touch with your physician. Your doctor can check to see whether you have some other, additional health issue — such as thyroid underfunctioning (see Chapter 8). If not, then seeing your dietitian would be wise so that the person can review your nutrition program, including your calorie intake and expenditure, and help you come up with a plan to achieve and maintain a healthy weight.

WARNING

A person with celiac disease should *never, ever*, intentionally resume eating gluten to purposefully cause malabsorption of calories in attempts to control their weight. Doing so has the potential to lead to severe health problems, such as progressive, severe bowel damage, and even, potentially, cancer.

Losing weight

Although some people with celiac disease gain weight after they initiate a gluten-free diet, the opposite situation can also occur. If you've been eating pizza, pasta, and many other calorie-rich foods, once you go gluten-free, you may find yourself eating less of these and also being more circumspect in terms of food choices. As we discuss in Chapter 10, living gluten-free typically means avoiding junk food and also often means avoiding buffet meals or prepared foods (because many of the items contain gluten). As a result, many people with celiac disease end up eating a healthier diet that contains more natural foods and fewer processed foods. The net result can be a loss in weight in addition to other health benefits. Although we mention this "problem" here, we admit that we've not met too many people who complain to us about shedding excess weight they've been carrying around. And as for people who didn't need to lose weight, the pounds that are lost tend to be relatively few in number, and one's weight typically stabilizes within a few months.

EXAMPLE

Christine was a 22-year-old, somewhat overweight woman who, having just graduated from college, headed off to Europe to celebrate. While she was enjoying the sights and sounds of Paris, to her dismay, she developed abdominal cramping and diarrhea. She wondered if she'd "eaten something bad." Her symptoms persisted, forcing her to cut her trip short. Upon her return to the United States, her healthcare provider performed tests, including an upper endoscopy and small intestine biopsy (see Chapter 3). The results revealed that Christine had celiac disease. She began a gluten-free diet and eight weeks later, Christine was pleased to report that not only had her symptoms gone away, but to her pleasant surprise, she had noticed that — with her healthier eating style — the extra weight she had gained during her college years was disappearing. Later that year, Christine's weight had stabilized at a healthy level, she was carefully following her gluten-free diet, and she was feeling great. She celebrated by booking a flight to Paris!

WARNING

If, after starting a gluten-free diet, your weight progressively falls — especially if to the point that you're underweight — then you must see your healthcare provider to be assessed. The problem could be as simple as you not consuming sufficient calories (in which case you will then need to also see your dietitian) or as complicated as you having some other, undiagnosed, associated ailment (see Chapter 8).

Becoming constipated

If you have the classical form of celiac disease (which we discuss in Chapter 5), then you are well acquainted with the hassles of frequent trips to the bathroom with diarrhea. And we suspect you will be relieved to hear that following a gluten-free diet will correct this problem. Alas, although you will no longer have diarrhea, your new diet may lead to constipation. (Clearly, there is no justice here.) Indeed, regardless of what form of celiac disease you have, following a gluten-free diet can lead to this problem.

Constipation can be severe enough that your stools become hard and infrequent. The only good thing we can say about this is that it is a sure sign that you are on track with your gluten-free diet! Now, lest you think constipation is your new and ongoing destiny, let us reassure you that this is not the case. Here are some measures you can follow to, ahem, eliminate your constipation:

» **Drink more liquids:** Although the oft-cited advice to have at least eight (eight-ounce) glasses of liquid per day has been questioned, keeping hydrated is always a good idea. Also, be sure to ingest liquid-rich foods such as fruits. Be aware, however, that apart from water, diet soft drinks, and the like, liquids have calories, which you need to take into account.

» **Eat more (gluten-free) soluble and insoluble fiber:** *Soluble fiber* dissolves in water, and *insoluble fiber* does not dissolve in water. We discuss fiber in more detail in the next section.

» **Exercise more:** Exercise helps all aspects of one's physical and emotional health, including bowel regularity.

Treating constipation with soluble fiber

Ingesting soluble fiber, the kind that dissolves in water, not only helps ease constipation, but it can also help improve your cholesterol (and, if you have diabetes, can help lower your blood glucose levels). Soluble fiber is found in varying quantities in all plant foods. Here are some good sources of soluble fiber:

» Legumes, such as peas, soybeans, and other beans.

» Oats, including oat bran. (As we discuss in detail in Chapter 5, when purchasing oat-containing products, be sure you are getting "pure oats," not an oat product that is mixed in with other grains.)

>> Some fruits and fruit juices, including prune juice, plums, berries, bananas, and the insides of apples and pears.

>> Certain vegetables, such as broccoli, carrots, and Jerusalem artichokes.

>> Root vegetables, such as potatoes, sweet potatoes, and onions. (The skins of these vegetables, however, are sources of insoluble fiber, which we discuss in the next section.)

>> Psyllium is found in certain cereals and is widely available commercially in prepackaged containers.

Treating constipation with insoluble fiber

Insoluble fiber is also known as *bulk* or *roughage*. Unlike soluble fiber, insoluble fiber doesn't dissolve in water.

Here are good sources of insoluble fiber:

>> Whole grains — but only gluten-free grains, such as those listed in Chapter 11

>> Corn bran in gluten-free bran products (but no gluten-containing bran products such as wheat bran)

>> Nuts and seeds

>> Potato skins

>> Flaxseed

>> Vegetables such as green beans, cauliflower, zucchini, and celery

>> The skins of some fruits, including tomatoes

Four of the five most fiber-rich plant foods are gluten-free! These are

>> Legumes (including several types of beans, lentils, and peas)

>> Prunes

>> Asian pears

>> Quinoa

A complete list of gluten-free grains and other dietary sources of fiber are discussed in Chapter 11.

Treating constipation with commercial fiber supplements

If you find getting enough fiber in your diet difficult (for whatever reason, including simple aversion to fiber-rich foods), then eat gluten-free fiber supplements. At least 20 to 30 grams of fiber a day is recommended.

Here are some gluten-free commercial fiber supplements you can use (the type of fiber these supplements contain is noted in parentheses):

>> Benefiber (guar gum)

>> Citrucel (methylcellulose)

>> Konsyl, Metamucil (psyllium)

WARNING

Metamucil products are gluten-free with the exception of Metamucil Wafers; these contain gluten, so avoid this form of the product.

Generic versions of nearly all these and other brand-name fiber products are available, but you will need to check with the manufacturer to determine whether a particular product is gluten-free.

Treating constipation with laxatives

If you've followed the strategies we've just discussed, yet you continue to have problems with constipation, you may need to have tests done to make sure no other ailment is responsible. What tests, if any, you will need depends on a number of factors, including your age, how severe the problem is, whether you have other medical problems, whether you have previously had a colonoscopy, whether you have a family history of colon cancer, what medications you are taking (some can cause constipation), and so on.

If further investigations are either not necessary or are performed and found to be normal, it comes down to how best to treat your problem. This typically consists of stool softeners or laxatives, or both. Your doctor can advise you which of the following products is best for you to take for your particular situation:

>> **Osmotic laxatives:** Osmotic laxatives work by promoting the accumulation of water within the bowel. (This is termed an *osmotic effect*.) Polyethylene glycol (PEG) is a commonly used, highly effective osmotic laxative. These products contain smaller amounts of the same compounds used in the large volume clean-out preparations for colonoscopy. These are available over-the-counter (that is, without a prescription) and are very safe and effective.

>> **Stimulant laxatives:** These work by stimulating the intestine to contract and push materials along. Examples of these products are Ex-Lax, Senekot, Doxidan (*casanthranol*), and Dulcolax (*bisacodyl*). It's okay to use these on occasion, but they are not advised for long-term use because, if used in this way, the colon can become habituated to them.

>> **Stool softeners:** Stool softeners such as Colace contain a medicine called *docusate*. Stool softeners increase the water content of the stool, making it easier to pass. Their effect is mild, but some people find them very helpful.

WARNING

See your healthcare provider if, in spite of these measures, you have severe constipation (bowel movements once or twice a week or even less), if you develop rectal bleeding, if you have severe abdominal pain, or if it appears that you have become obstructed (nothing, not even gas, is coming out). These symptoms may signify that you have a serious medical problem that requires prompt attention.

Falling Off the Diet

As you continue your journey with gluten-free living, you may find yourself tempted, at times, to either abandon or, at the very least, not fully adhere to your gluten-free diet. If you feel this way, you're in very good company. Many other people with celiac disease feel the same way. Nevertheless, we strongly encourage you not to "give in to temptation" or, if you have, to as quickly as possible get back to being gluten-free again.

The problem with resuming the consumption of gluten is that it will lead to the redevelopment of damage to your intestine, can cause symptoms of celiac disease to reappear, and may lead to the serious condition called *refractory celiac disease* (which we discuss in Chapter 11) that causes dreadful symptoms and increases your risk of cancer (specifically, a form of immune system cancer called EATCL, which we discuss in detail in Chapter 9). For all these reasons — and at the risk of sounding redundant — we strongly advise against resuming *any* gluten ingestion.

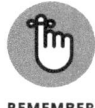

REMEMBER

Don't fall victim to the illusion — which we recognize can so easily happen — of believing that, if you've resumed consuming gluten yet you feel well, that everything therefore must be alright. This simply isn't the case. You may feel perfectly fine (at least initially, anyway) all the while your small intestine and, potentially, other parts of your body, are being progressively damaged.

We recognize that all this may sound pretty scary. We also recognize that the simple fact of human nature remains that following a gluten-free diet (or, for that matter, many other forms of restricted diet) can be very tough and that, people being people, you may find yourself at times not only tempted to fall off the gluten-free wagon, but actually doing just that. Many people with celiac disease do indeed have periods of time where this occurs. To put it succinctly, life happens.

If you find yourself in this situation, then we have two things to share. One, what you need to do is pick yourself up, dust yourself off, and start living gluten-free all over again. And two, not that we'd *ever* counsel people with celiac disease to even fleetingly resume eating gluten (because we don't and never would), but, having said that, so long as you get back on track right away and so long as the period of time for which you were consuming gluten was very brief, you'll likely be fine.

TIP

People with celiac disease are less likely to fall off their gluten-free diet if they have the support of others — not just family but also membership in a celiac disease support group. We suggest you consider joining such a group. For many people, joining a group is hugely helpful. Your celiac disease specialist or dietitian may be able to tell you of a group local to you. Another option is to join an online discussion group. In Appendixes C and D, we list some organizations for people living with celiac disease.

Taking Charge of Your Celiac Health

As we emphasize throughout this book, we want you to have control over your health and, in particular, control over your celiac disease. We bet you feel the same way, or you wouldn't be reading this book right now! In this section, we share with you some tips on how you can empower yourself by ensuring you get the best possible care from your celiac disease healthcare providers. We also discuss being an advocate for you or your loved one with celiac disease in matters that extend beyond routine healthcare.

Preparing for your appointment with your celiac disease specialist

Just like the Boy Scouts motto, when it comes to your forthcoming appointment with your celiac disease specialist — especially if it's your first visit — be prepared. Being prepared helps ensure you — and your doctor for that matter — get the most out of your visit and sets the stage for future good care.

Here are some ways you can help make your visit to the doctor a success:

>> **Bring your records.** Bring records of your prior medical history, including previous test results. If you were diagnosed with celiac disease prior to this visit, bring the test results that established the diagnosis, including blood test and biopsy reports. Some offices ask you to send these records in advance for review. (This is only necessary for your first visit to the doctor.)

>> **Bring your medications.** Bring a list of all your prescription and nonprescription drugs with you.

>> **Bring someone with you.** Bring a loved one or trusted friend with you to act as a second set of ears. (See the next section for more information.)

>> **Bring questions.** Write down questions you have prior to the visit. That way, you won't forget your questions when you're at your appointment. (Also, make notes during the visit and write down questions as you think of them.)

>> **Arrive sufficiently early.** Arrive ahead of time for your appointment, but understand that the doctor may be running late. Often this is due to the fact that the physician is spending extra time with sick patients, and you can be confident they will do the same with you.

REMEMBER

Before you leave the appointment, be sure to also prepare for what comes next. Are you going to the lab for blood tests? Are you supposed to call the office to report on your progress? Are you planning to book a return visit with the doctor? Knowing what you are to do is essential; trust us, you don't want to risk being "lost in the shuffle." Your doctor or their staff will likely spontaneously bring up the answers to these questions before you leave. If that doesn't happen, however, be sure to bring them up yourself.

Knowing what to ask your doctor

Asking questions when you visit your doctor is always a good idea. And, of course, your questions will only help you if they get proper answers! If what you're told is confusing or doesn't make sense, ask for clarification. It's your health after all, and you deserve to have sufficiently clear answers given to you.

Here are some questions to consider asking your doctor (if they didn't happen to get discussed routinely when you spoke with your physician):

>> Is my diagnosis of celiac disease certain, or is there an element of doubt? If an element of doubt exists, how is this going to be sorted out?

>> What kinds of tests will I need to have done to monitor my celiac disease? How often will these need to be done?

>> When do I need to see you again? How often, if at all, will I need to be seen by you on an ongoing basis?

>> What symptoms should I look out for? What should I do if they develop? Whom should I contact if they occur, and how?

TIP

We are strong believers in having two sets of ears present during your first visits to your celiac disease specialist. During these early appointments, a great deal of information is being shared, and questions like those just listed are most likely to come up. At this time in the process, people are most likely to be nervous and thus least likely to retain information. Bring a loved one or trusted friend with you to your doctor's appointment; you'll be glad you did.

Becoming an expert on your condition

We hope that you find this book to be a helpful resource to allow you to master your celiac disease (or to allow you to help a loved one master his condition). Indeed, we'd be disappointed if you don't. We also hope that you will avail yourself of the myriad resources available to you online. Online resources are a great storehouse of information on celiac disease (and every other topic under the sun). However, some sources provide misinformation, so you must tread with care and not be taken in by "experts" who are out to take you for a financial ride by offering some (useless) "miracle therapy" for celiac disease. It's also very important to take with a very large grain of salt those online sources that offer expertise (or even just plain opinion) without providing any scientific references or background to support their statements.

To help you find reputable information online, have a look at Chapter 2, as well as Appendix D, where we list celiac disease organizations and centers you may want to contact.

Being an Advocate for Your Celiac Health

Celiac disease is a condition in which you, the person living with the condition, are largely in charge of your own treatment. You should also feel empowered to advocate for yourself to make sure you receive the care that you (or a loved one who cannot advocate for themselves) deserves.

The first step to being an effective advocate is being knowledgeable about your condition, so we're glad you're reading this book. Making sure that you get the medical care you need is also critical. In the previous few sections, we look at how to help ensure productive sessions with your doctor. In the following sections, we discuss some other situations you may encounter and how you can effectively advocate for yourself.

Having your doctor help you advocate for yourself

Your doctor can arm you with information that will help you advocate for yourself. Most often, this information is in the form of a letter that spells out important details such as the following:

>> Your diagnosis

>> Your treatment plan

>> How long you've been under their care

>> Your treatment costs, including

- The extra costs of buying gluten-free foods

- The need for extra travel (for example, to and from appointments with the doctor)

>> The doctor's invitation (with your permission, of course) to speak to relevant third parties (such as a potential insurer) on your behalf

This letter should be printed on the doctor's letterhead and signed by the doctor. Make a digital copy to use as you need.

TIP

Remember to ask your doctor to update the letter periodically, especially if you will need it for tax purposes or for travel out of the country.

Handling hospitalizations

As a well-informed patient, you know how to look after your celiac disease. Indeed, often a person with celiac disease knows more than the average health-care provider, including those working in hospitals. For this reason, if you are in the hospital, you need to work especially hard at being your own best advocate. Here are some ways you can advocate for yourself from within a hospital:

>> Tell all your healthcare providers, including doctors, nurses, dietitians, and so forth, that you have celiac disease.

>> Before you eat anything that is brought to you, ensure the tag on the food tray states that the food is gluten-free.

>> Tell the clerk who admits you to the hospital that you need to eat a gluten-free diet. You may find it helps to tell them you are "allergic" to gluten, wheat, rye, and barley products.

>> Bring to the hospital copies of an information sheet on celiac disease. (Many of the celiac societies and organizations — see Appendix D — have these for their members.) You can then hand these out to the members of the health-care team who are looking after you.

>> Ask for a dietitian to visit with you. The dietitian will help ensure you get a gluten-free diet while you're in hospital.

>> If the admission is not an emergency, you may want to bring some gluten-free supplies with you, including crackers, cereals, and breakfast bars. However, before you eat any food you've brought, make sure to ask the doctor or nurse whether it is okay for you to eat. Sometimes tests, health issues, or other reasons require you to not eat anything at all for a period of time.

IN THIS CHAPTER

» **Getting pregnant and having celiac disease**

» **Dealing with celiac disease in infancy**

» **Diagnosing celiac disease in children**

» **Knowing how celiac disease can affect your child**

» **Helping a child manage a gluten-free diet**

Chapter **14**

Celiac Disease and Pregnancy, Children, and Beyond

Although everyone living with celiac disease shares certain things in common — such as the need to avoid consuming gluten — children face additional, special challenges that adults do not. And, if you are the parent of a child with celiac disease, you likely have already discovered that you, too, have challenges that other parents may not have to contend with.

If you have celiac disease and are trying to have a child, you may face certain hurdles. Undiagnosed (and untreated) celiac disease can cause infertility and, once you're pregnant, it can increase the risk of certain obstetrical complications, including miscarriages.

In this chapter, we look at these important issues. As always, we encourage you to bear in mind that, although having undiagnosed celiac disease increases your risk of fertility and obstetrical difficulties, after diagnosis, the great majority of people living with celiac disease are able to conceive, deliver, and raise healthy children successfully.

Pregnancy and Celiac Disease

Celiac disease can interfere with a woman's reproductive function. This fact is unknown to most healthcare providers and, less surprisingly, is also unknown to most people living with celiac disease. Reproductive difficulties range from infertility to miscarriages to delivering a small baby. We discuss these important topics in this section.

REMEMBER

Like so very many other complications of celiac disease, these reproductive difficulties apply to *active* celiac disease. When you're on track with your gluten-free diet, these problems typically resolve.

Female infertility and celiac disease

Infertility is typically defined as the inability to conceive (that is, to become pregnant) despite a year or more of regular intercourse without contraception. Active celiac disease in women can cause infertility for a number of reasons.

In order for a woman to get pregnant, she must be able to ovulate. *Ovulation* is the process wherein an *ovum* (an "egg") is released from an ovary. After leaving the ovary, the ovum makes its way down the fallopian tube where, if one has had recent intercourse, it can then meet up with a sperm and the ovum can then be fertilized.

In the absence of ovulation, pregnancy cannot occur (except through in vitro fertilization — IVF — but that's a subject for a different book). Women with untreated or insufficiently treated celiac disease have fewer years in which they ovulate and, hence, fewer opportunities to become pregnant. This can occur on either side of the fertile age spectrum; in other words, women with active celiac disease may experience the following:

>> First start ovulating (and therefore, first begin having periods) later than normal.

>> Stop ovulating (and hence, develop menopause) earlier than normal.

>> Have times where ovulation — and, hence, periods — stop. (This is referred to in medical jargon as *secondary amenorrhea*.)

It is not known with certainty why some women with active celiac disease have these problems with ovulation, but possible factors may be

>> **Malabsorption of nutrients:** Celiac disease can result in malabsorption of important nutrients required to allow for normal female hormone production

that regulates ovulation and the menstrual cycle. The poor nutrition that results from malabsorption is especially likely to play a role if untreated celiac disease has led to a lower-than-normal body weight. We discuss malabsorption in detail in Chapter 2.

>> **Endocrine dysfunction:** Having celiac disease increases the probability of a person also having certain endocrine (that is, hormonal) disorders, such as thyroid disease, which in their own right can disrupt ovarian function. We discuss this issue further in Chapter 8.

The preceding discussion applies to women with active celiac disease. If you follow a strict gluten-free diet, your celiac disease will be *in*active, and you will likely have normal ovulation and normal ability to conceive. Nonetheless, and for reasons that are not fully understood, even when having normal ovulation and menstrual cycles, occasionally a woman with celiac disease may still be at increased risk (compared to women without celiac disease) of having difficulty conceiving.

TIP

Infertility (or recurring miscarriages, which we discuss in the section, "Miscarriages") may be the only manifestation of celiac disease and can be the very first clue that you have this condition. If you're having unexplained problems with infertility or recurring miscarriages, ask your doctor about the possibility that you have (undiscovered) celiac disease.

One final observation before we leave this section: IVF aside, unless you're having intercourse, pregnancy ain't gonna happen. One scientific study found that couples in which one of the partners had celiac disease had sex less often than couples in which celiac disease wasn't present. The reason? Probably that the person with celiac disease didn't feel well and as a result was less interested in having intercourse. Makes sense. So too, does it make sense that, once the affected person started a gluten-free diet, the frequency with which they were having sex — and their satisfaction with their sex life — both returned to normal. The moral of the story? Forget about the oysters, dark chocolate, and the like; the newest aphrodisiac on the block is clearly following a gluten-free diet! (Well, at least if you have celiac disease.)

Complications of pregnancy

Most women with celiac disease have uneventful pregnancies; however, some evidence exists that women with undiagnosed and untreated celiac disease are at increased risk of pregnancy-related complications. (Reassuringly, studies suggest that even among women with incompletely treated celiac disease, the risk of these complications is not greater than what you may expect in individuals without celiac disease.)

Miscarriages

A *miscarriage* is the spontaneous end of a pregnancy at a stage where the embryo or fetus is incapable of surviving, generally defined in humans as being prior to 20 weeks of pregnancy (*gestation*). Women with active celiac disease have an increased risk of miscarrying a pregnancy. Indeed, as we mention in the preceding section, miscarriage may be the only clue that a person has (as yet undiagnosed) celiac disease.

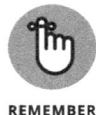

REMEMBER

If you have a miscarriage, lest you automatically attribute it to your celiac disease or, even worse, blame yourself for not being careful enough with your gluten-free diet, bear in mind that miscarriages are common among all women. Indeed, 25 percent or more of pregnancies result in a miscarriage within a few weeks of conceiving. Miscarriages are not only common, but they can also occur for many different reasons. Therefore, if you have celiac disease and you have a miscarriage, it may well be unrelated to your celiac disease. Having said all that, it always remains terribly important — especially if you are pregnant — to follow a healthy, nutritious, gluten-free diet. We discuss the gluten-free diet in Chapter 10.

Small babies, intrauterine growth restriction, and premature delivery

A fetus that is smaller than expected for the length of time a woman has been pregnant is referred to as being *small for gestational age*. Being small for gestational age occurs as a consequence of *intrauterine growth restriction* (IUGR); IUGR is a condition in which the fetus grows and develops more slowly than normal and is typically underweight at birth.

Many causes exist for IUGR, including a fetus having a genetic defect or infection, or the pregnant woman having diabetes or a malfunctioning placenta. An additional cause of IUGR may be celiac disease, which, in some studies, has been associated with as much as a threefold increased risk. This finding, however, has not been corroborated in other medical studies, which, in fact, suggested there was no increased risk.

Another reason for delivering a small baby is an early delivery called a *pre-term* or *premature* delivery. Here, too, the evidence that celiac disease may be responsible is contradictory.

If celiac disease does contribute to an increased risk of a fetus being small, having IUGR, or being delivered prematurely, the cause remains to be determined.

Helping avoid pregnancy complications due to celiac disease

Although no woman with celiac disease can ever be guaranteed that she can avoid pregnancy-related complications, women with celiac disease can follow certain precautions to make what are good odds of a healthy outcome even better odds.

We recommend that if you are a woman with celiac disease and you are contemplating pregnancy, do the following *before* you try to get pregnant:

» Make sure you're following your gluten-free diet.

» Ensure your celiac disease symptoms, such as diarrhea, abdominal discomfort, and fatigue, are improving. (We discuss symptoms of celiac disease in Chapter 2.)

» If you've had problems with anemia, iron deficiency, or other abnormal blood chemistry tests, review these with your family doctor or celiac disease specialist to make sure they're being treated. (We discuss anemia and iron deficiency in Chapter 7.)

» Check with your celiac disease specialist that your celiac antibody tests (such as your IgA tissue transglutaminase antibody level) are coming down. (We discuss antibody tests in Chapter 3.)

» Speak to your obstetrician/gynecologist to determine that you are in suitable gynecologic health to attempt to conceive.

TESTING INFERTILE WOMEN AND WOMEN WITH RECURRING MISCARRIAGES FOR CELIAC DISEASE

So, should women with infertility and recurring miscarriages be tested for celiac disease? Well, given that

● Some women with celiac disease are infertile due — often in unknown ways — to their celiac disease, and

● Treating celiac disease can, in many such women, restore fertility, and

● Testing for celiac disease is *relatively* straightforward.

We believe that if you have infertility (or recurring miscarriages), your doctor should check you for celiac disease. Unfortunately, this is not always done, even by infertility experts.

Timing of Gluten Introduction in Infancy

Growing interest exists among people living with celiac disease who are about to become (or are new) parents regarding when to introduce gluten into the diet of their infant child. Because celiac disease is more common among close family members, these parents recognize that their child is, therefore, at increased risk of developing celiac disease and, of course, like any loving parent, they want to lessen the likelihood of this happening.

Some medical studies suggested that the risk to a child of later developing celiac disease is reduced if the child has gluten introduced into their diet at a very early stage (before they are four months of age). But subsequent studies failed to prove that. In fact, no strategy has been definitively shown to reduce the chances of a child developing celiac disease. The latest studies suggest that even though early introduction (before 4 months) does not reduce the risk of celiac disease, delaying the introduction of gluten for a long time (beyond one year) could actually *increase* the risk of developing celiac disease.

How is a parent to know what to do? Pending further studies, the current consensus among most celiac disease experts is that gluten can be introduced at any time between 4 and 12 months of age.

Breastfeeding has not been consistently shown to reduce the risk of celiac disease. Still, breastfeeding carries many benefits, including a reduced risk of various childhood infections and other autoimmune conditions later in life, even if celiac disease risk is not affected.

Detecting Celiac Disease in Children

Until not too long ago, celiac disease was thought to be a pediatric condition and was seldom first detected in people beyond young adulthood. Today, however, we know that celiac disease is not exclusively a pediatric condition. In fact — and you may find this surprising — it's most commonly diagnosed in people in their thirties and older.

As we discuss in Chapter 4, there are several forms of celiac disease. In the past, most children diagnosed with celiac disease had the classical form with the main symptoms being gastrointestinal in nature. These children would have diarrhea and abdominal discomfort (and, because of malnutrition, would often have failed to properly grow, develop, and thrive).

Today, increasing numbers of children are diagnosed with non-classical celiac disease with few or no gastrointestinal symptoms; instead, the main or only features are impaired development or growth.

Thankfully, studies suggest that the time to make a diagnosis is shorter in children than in adults, where a diagnosis can be delayed by more than ten years. Also, increasing numbers of children are being diagnosed through screening (we discuss screening in detail later in this chapter), which means they are able to be successfully treated for their condition long before it has had time to cause them to fall ill.

Diagnosing children with celiac disease

As we discuss in Chapter 3, the first step that must occur when a doctor diagnoses an illness is that she must think of the possibility that the illness is present. For celiac disease in a child, certain observations — as we discuss in the following sections — may lead a physician to consider this ailment.

We think that you should be aware of these features, too; this way, if you have a child without known celiac disease who develops these symptoms, you can mention, when you see the doctor, that you are wondering whether your child has this condition. Who knows? Perhaps you will have helped make an otherwise overlooked diagnosis. (As we say elsewhere in this book, unless you are concerned that your doctor will admonish you for telling them their business, feel free to take this book with you and blame us for putting you up to the task!)

Looking at symptoms

TIP

Unlike in adults, where the doctor gets the story directly from the patient, when it comes to children — especially young children — the doctor needs to rely on you, the parent, to provide your observations. It will, therefore, be helpful for you to mull over the information we discuss in this section *before* you take your child to the doctor so that you have collected as much information as possible to share with the physician.

These symptoms can be present in a child with celiac disease (note that these symptoms can also occur with other conditions and thus are not unique to celiac disease):

>> **Abdominal discomfort.** Cramping and distention.

>> **Abnormal bowel habits.** Loose or watery stools, frequent large stools, and very smelly stools. Sometimes, however, constipation is the main problem.

>> **Behavior problems.** Irritability, restlessness, and the inability to remain attentive or focused.

As we discuss in detail in Chapter 8, there is some evidence that certain neurological and behavior problems, such as ADHD and autism, are more likely to occur in children who have celiac disease. Nonetheless, the great majority of children with ADHD and autism do not have celiac disease, and conversely, the great majority of children with celiac disease do not have ADHD, autism, or other neurological or behavioral difficulties.

>> **Dermatitis herpetiformis.** A very itchy skin rash with little blisters over the elbows, shoulders, and buttocks. (We discuss this condition in Chapter 8.)

>> **Insufficient growth and development.** Failure to grow and develop normally (called *failure to thrive*), lack of normal weight gain, and, especially, the development of weight loss. The child may be shorter than others of the same age and may also be shorter than their siblings were at a comparable age.

Some children, because of malabsorption of calcium and vitamin D, develop a condition called *rickets* in which the bones have impaired growth and strength. We discuss rickets in detail in Chapter 7.

>> **Other nonspecific symptoms.** Generalized, nonspecific symptoms such as pale skin, lack of energy, malaise, and fatigue.

TIP

If your unwell child is still in diapers, pay special attention to your infant's stools because your doctor will find it helpful to hear from you regarding how often diapers need to be changed and the consistency of your infant's stools.

Another set of important observations you should make before you see the doctor is to note your child's mood, energy, and level of physical activity. Does your child appear sullen and withdrawn, or happy and energetic? Does your child appear listless, or is your child crawling, walking, or running around all day? A child who is fatigued, sullen, and listless may have these symptoms for a host of different reasons, one of which is celiac disease.

We recommend that you also share with the doctor when your child reaches various developmental milestones (such as sitting, crawling, standing, walking, and talking) and whether your child is smaller or shorter than your other children. A child who is slow to reach milestones and is shorter than their siblings were at that age does not necessarily have celiac disease, but it's certainly something that needs to be considered.

All these pieces of information will help your doctor fit the puzzle together.

Undergoing a physical examination

When a doctor examines any sick child, there are many features they are seeking. However, specifically in terms of whether the child may have celiac disease, the doctor will be checking for the following:

» **Abnormal behavior:** Evidence of abnormal behavior, failure to achieve developmental milestones, and reduced energy level.

» **Anemia:** Pale skin, which might indicate anemia.

» **Dermatitis herpetiformis:** Skin rash with characteristics suggesting dermatitis herpetiformis. (See the previous section.)

» **Insufficient growth and development:** One way the doctor determines this is by comparing the child's weight and height to the child's peer group average, as well as the child's prior measurements.

» **Malnourishment:** Evidence of malnourishment can reflect the presence of malabsorption.

Testing for celiac disease

If, after talking to you and assessing your child, the doctor suspects celiac disease may be present, investigations will be required:

» **Stool samples:** These are most often analyzed to look for other ailments — such as a bowel infection — that may be masquerading as, or mimicking, celiac disease.

» Blood tests may be requested to look for a variety of different abnormalities, including the following:

- Anemia

- Vitamin deficiencies

- Abnormal body chemistry

- Celiac disease antibodies, including the tissue transglutaminase (TTG) IgA antibody and total IgA level. We discuss these tests in detail in Chapter 3.

» **Endoscopy and small intestine biopsy:** As we discuss in Chapter 3, an endoscopy and small intestine biopsy is — regardless of the age of the patient — the definitive way to diagnose celiac disease. For this reason, if the doctor has a strong suspicion that your child has celiac disease, she may recommend proceeding directly with this test rather than first doing much, if any, other preliminary testing.

TIP

If your child's doctor sends your child directly for a small intestine biopsy and it confirms celiac disease, the doctor will still likely ask for the TTG IgA antibody test to be done because the result will be helpful to monitor your child's progress. For more info on this topic, have a look at Chapter 15.

Doing an endoscopy in kids is not too much different from how it is for adults. In very young children, different sedative medications are used, and kid-sized endoscopes may be used as well. Typically, a parent comes into the endoscopy room to provide support until the child is sedated and is then again present when the child awakens in the recovery area of the endoscopy unit.

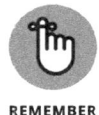

REMEMBER

An endoscopy and small intestine biopsy are usually necessary before a diagnosis of celiac disease can be made with certainty. Although there are select cases where a biopsy is sometimes justifiably skipped (see Chapter 3), that is an exception to the rule. Celiac disease is a serious, lifelong condition, and following a gluten-free diet is no mean feat. Saddling a child with the diagnosis and treatment without first being certain of the diagnosis is simply neither fair nor appropriate. (Also, lest you think that a child who feels better on a gluten-free diet must surely have celiac disease and that other, confirmatory testing is unnecessary, we will note that lots of kids — and adults, too — feel better on a gluten-free diet whether or not they have celiac disease.)

Screening children for celiac disease

As we discuss in Chapter 6, screening for a disease is testing a person for it even if that person has no symptoms or other manifestations of the condition being looked for.

Several specific situations exist in which a doctor should consider screening a child for celiac disease, including when the following situations apply to a child:

>> **The child has an immediate family member (or members) who is known to have celiac disease.** If one person in the family has celiac disease, other immediate family members are at increased risk of also having the condition.

>> **The child has type 1 diabetes.** As we discuss in Chapter 8, type 1 diabetes is an autoimmune disease often onsetting in childhood and associated with an approximately 5 percent likelihood of the child also having celiac disease. Quite commonly, such children do not have any symptoms of celiac disease, and celiac disease wouldn't have been detected if they hadn't been screened for it.

For children who are being screened for celiac disease because they have an immediate family member with this condition, the best initial screening test is to see whether the child has the HLA DQ2 and/or DQ8 genes. If these genes are not present, the risk of the child having or later developing celiac disease is so low that further screening for celiac disease is unnecessary.

Knowing these genetic screening results — whether positive or negative — can be a huge help, as we describe here:

>> If your child does *not* have the HLA DQ2 or DQ8 genes, you can feel greatly reassured that the child will almost certainly never develop celiac disease and, as mentioned, repeat screening is not be required.

>> If your child does have either of these genes, you will be armed with the important knowledge that further action needs to be taken. Specifically, the next step is to check for TTG IgA and total IgA (see the immediately preceding section, "Testing for celiac disease," and the following discussion).

In the event that your child has the HLA DQ2 or DQ8 genes, testing for celiac disease antibodies should first be performed when your child is around 3 years of age. If these antibodies are normal (that is, depending on the laboratory's testing methods, either completely absent or, at least, in the so-called "normal range"), most pediatric celiac disease specialists suggest repeating the antibody tests every 2 to 3 years until the child reaches age 18. At that point, if the antibody tests have remained negative, they're typically no longer tested for. However, if at any point your child later develops symptoms that suggest celiac disease and they are known to be genetically at risk, then a TTG IgA antibody test should again be performed, regardless of what age your child is (indeed, even if your "child" is now an adult). If the antibody tests are increased at any point, an endoscopy and small intestine biopsy should be performed to determine if celiac disease is present.

TIP

If your child has type 1 diabetes, an elevated TTG IgA is not as reliable as it is in other circumstances. It could indicate celiac disease, but it could also be a false positive. The intestinal biopsy in this case is critical.

REMEMBER

If your child has the HLA DQ2 or DQ8 genes, or has TTG IgA or AGA IgA antibodies, that does not mean they necessarily have celiac disease. (In fact, most people with a DQ2 or DQ8 gene never go on to develop celiac disease.) It does, however, mean that your child may have the condition and that further investigations could be warranted, including an endoscopy and small intestine biopsy. Only the presence of a confirmatory small intestine biopsy allows the diagnosis of celiac disease to be made.

Starting Your Child on a Gluten-Free Diet

After your child has been diagnosed with celiac disease, they should begin a gluten-free diet. Chapter 10 covers in detail the reality of following a gluten-free diet; this section revisits some tips from that chapter.

TIP

Living gluten-free can pose quite a few challenges, especially for children. Here are some tips — some admittedly harder to follow than others — that parents of children with celiac disease have shared with us that helped them deal with these challenges:

>> Base the family's diet around naturally gluten-free foods such as fruits, vegetables, nuts, gluten-free grains and carbohydrates, meats, fish, and dairy products.

>> Keep on hand (a limited number of) gluten-free treats that the whole family can enjoy. These can include gluten-free packaged and prepared foods like rice crackers or rice snacks, popcorn, ice creams, sorbets, and candies.

>> When buying items such as cookies, cereals, and certain baked goods (scones, loaves), purchase both gluten-free and gluten-containing versions. Of course, the gluten-containing version should be given only to those family members who do not have celiac disease.

>> When baking, prepare gluten-free and gluten-containing versions. Placing similar foods on everyone's plate helps the child with celiac disease not feel left out.

As you embark on creating a healthy, gluten-free diet for your child, you may wonder if life would be easier if your entire family were also eating gluten-free. Many parents tell us that doing this simplifies shopping and preparing food, and also makes keeping the child with celiac disease on track with the diet easier. (Less temptation is present if everyone in the family is eating the same way and if no "off limits" foods are nearby.)

There are, however, challenges to having the entire family eat gluten-free, including the difficulty of finding sufficient quantities of gluten-free foods each time you shop, incurring additional expense (as we discuss in Chapter 10, gluten-free foods often cost more than other foods), and asking the entire family to take on what are otherwise unnecessary dietary restrictions.

Some parents of children with celiac disease say teaching young children to eat gluten-free is best. They feel that having the rest of the family eat normally allows the child to develop the "right attitude" and learn boundaries at home. Other parents have very different and equally strongly held opinions. Needless to say, this topic is hotly debated among families and members of celiac support groups.

Shopping and Cooking with Your Child Who Has Celiac Disease

Your child with celiac disease, at the appropriate age, needs to learn how to recognize gluten-free foods and where to find them, not only at home, but also in stores and online. Of course, educating your child in these ways is a gradual process that evolves as your child grows up.

Even more important is to encourage your child to develop an interest in cooking and baking gluten-free. Cooking and baking gluten-free are skills that will help throughout the rest of your child's life.

In Chapter 10, we look in detail at shopping and cooking gluten-free.

Growing Up Gluten-Free

As any parent knows (or eventually finds out), parenting a child presents different challenges that depend on the age of the offspring. In this section, we look at some of these age-dependent challenges as they pertain to celiac disease.

Dealing with the preschool years

One of the most challenging aspects of keeping a preschooler gluten-free is when the child is away from home and, especially, when they are out of your supervision. Whether attending daycare or preschool, going to a friend's house, or attending a birthday party, your child will be constantly at risk of being exposed to gluten. Children like to share their food and try others' food.

The best way to deal with this issue is to educate the people (teachers, other parents, babysitters, and so on) who will be interacting with your child about celiac disease. Make them aware of what a gluten-free diet is and the importance of not deviating from it.

Working with others on this issue will require diligence on your part because some people are not particularly conversant with celiac disease and may mistakenly believe that "just a little bit" of gluten couldn't possibly hurt. If they feel this way, make sure you correct them on this potentially dangerous misconception! (If you're concerned that you will be met with skepticism — or worse — consider showing them this book; as always, we're happy to be the heavies here.)

You may find that providing your child with gluten-free snacks and treats to take with them when they're attending celebrations or even simply visiting a friend's house is often helpful — not only for you and your child, but also for the parent(s) of the child that they're visiting.

Helping your child through the elementary school years

As your child goes through the elementary school years, a main challenge will be living gluten-free while eating in cafeterias or at sleepovers, camp, and other such away-from-home activities. Fortunately, at this age, your child can be actively involved in their care by letting those people (and their supervisors) with whom they're spending time know about the need to follow a gluten-free diet and, depending on your child's age and level of maturity, telling others what that diet consists of.

We recommend that, when appropriate, you speak to the people who will be supervising your child when outside of the home to inform them about the basics regarding celiac disease and gluten-free eating. Again, feel free to let them borrow this book; perhaps with you having tagged key pages for them to read.

Anytime your child will be away from home overnight, whether for a one-night sleepover or a summer-long stay at camp, they will be at increased risk of eating gluten. It's important to remind your child not to be lulled into thinking that eating gluten must be okay just because they don't feel immediately unwell after consuming it. You may well find their friends and camp-mates pressuring them into consuming gluten. Feel free to both forewarn your child of this and to prepare them with ammunition to resist such temptation by saying — even if not completely accurately — that they're allergic to gluten. Nowadays, with so many children having dangerous allergies to things like nuts, using the term "allergic" is more likely to convey a sense of importance than would be an attempt at explaining the true (and complex) immune nature of celiac disease (which, by the way, we describe in Chapter 5).

Grasping teenage challenges

As any parent of a teenager — regardless of whether the teen has celiac disease — knows, the teenage years pose their own special set of parental challenges. (We speak from experience in case you're wondering.) These years represent a time when your child wants to exercise his or her independence, and this often entails a certain amount of rebelling against things that are imposed by authority, including parents.

If your child has celiac disease, you may find that even if he was previously very good at sticking to a gluten-free diet, he may now go out with his friends to have regular pizza, burgers, and other gluten-containing fast foods. Sometimes, this experimenting leads to symptoms of indigestion, abdominal pain, and diarrhea, in which case the teen typically quickly gets back on track with gluten-free eating. If, however, your teenage child doesn't develop symptoms, he may be less inclined to resume living gluten-free. This, in turn, may put him at risk of developing complications of celiac disease (as we describe in Chapter 7).

Giving your teen control of their own gluten-free diet is important. You should start to let go even in the preteen or early teen years, depending on the maturity of your child. Here are some suggestions for you as a parent of a teenager with celiac disease:

>> **Don't punish:** Realize that gluten-ingestion "accidents" happen and don't punish them for this.

>> **Educate your teen:** Facilitate your teen's learning and allow them to develop an understanding of their own health issues. Talk to them about the gluten-free diet and celiac disease as you would or should for other health issues like texting while driving, alcohol, drugs, smoking, and sexual activities. Speaking in an open, educational, and non-threatening manner is often the best way of doing this.

>> **Involve your teen in the shopping and cooking:** Learning the ropes of how to identify food products that are gluten-free and where to find them is an important skill to acquire before leaving home. Similarly, being able to prepare gluten-free foods at home is another helpful skill to learn early in life.

>> **Have your teen check on gluten-free food availability:** Let your teen check out what foods will be available at parties, restaurants, school trips, and other activities. That way, they'll either be reassured that gluten-free foods are going to be available or, if not, can make alternative preparations.

>> **Encourage your teen to build a supportive peer group:** Just like friends don't let friends drink and drive, your child will want to have friends who support their efforts to stay gluten-free. Finding friends who won't make fun of him for his special diet or encourage him to stray from the diet is important in teenage years and beyond.

>> **Task your teen with exploring menu options at prospective colleges:** In addition to finding out about the expected educational and social experiences, determine what eating options are available. Once your teen knows where they'll be going to college, your child can then arrange to meet with the kitchen manager, cook, dietitian, or other relevant personnel at the college cafeteria to discuss your child's gluten-free needs.

We recognize that there are no easy solutions to dealing with a teenage child with celiac disease who elects not to follow a gluten-free diet. Each teenager is different, each situation is different, and what works for one family may not work for another. Letting your teenage child know that your concerns are born of love and caring is essential. You may also choose to enlist the support of others (family, friends, and so forth) who love and care about your child. If necessary, ask your doctor for help, either directly by speaking to your child or by referring your teenager to another appropriate healthcare professional, such as a social worker. Ultimately, however, it will be your child's responsibility to regain control of their health by returning to a gluten-free diet.

Sending your child off to college

By the time a child with celiac disease has reached young adulthood, they've typically become accustomed to living gluten-free. Nonetheless, new challenges emerge when it's time to leave home for college. In addition to the usual trials and tribulations (adjusting to campus life, dealing with courses that are typically harder than those in high school, exploring a new social life, and so on), your young adult will face the additional hurdle of trying to live gluten-free while eating at cafeterias and with meal-plans that typically center around gluten-containing foods such as pizza, pasta, burgers, subs, breaded meats, and breads. You probably aren't surprised to find that more than a few college students with celiac disease end up at the health services department with a flare of the disease.

Here are some food venues your teenage child must explore to stay gluten-free during the college years:

>> **Cafeteria or dining hall:** Meet with the chef or cook at the dining facility where your child will be eating. Your child can share their dietary needs with the chef or cook. In particular, your child can explain the importance of having gluten-free foods available. (Lest your child feel they're imposing by making special dietary requests, they can rest assured that celiac disease is common enough that many other students will likely share the same needs. Also, this is a health priority; nothing to be hesitant about here!)

>> **Living situation:** Choose a living situation that doesn't mandate use of the school or fraternity, or sorority meal plan. That way, your teenage child can buy and prepare their own food. (See the example that follows this list.)

>> **Nearby stores and online grocery providers:** Specialty food stores are often located in areas around colleges and universities. These shops and even some chains of grocery stores carry gluten-free foods. Identify these ahead of time, and if none are available, seek other options as listed below.

>> **Restaurants:** Locate local restaurants that have gluten-free offerings on their menus.

>> **Snacks:** Eat a gluten-free meal or snack before going out with friends. (This isn't usually necessary, but if your child isn't sure the gang will be heading out to a place that has gluten-free food offerings, it can be helpful.)

EXAMPLE

Melissa was diagnosed with celiac disease during her sophomore year of college. She did very well on her gluten-free diet (available to her at the school cafeteria) and remained symptom-free. As the year was coming to a close, Melissa confided to her doctor that her sorority required that she live in the sorority house for her third year, and this concerned her because many of the meals provided at the sorority consisted of gluten-laden items such as lasagna and other pasta dishes. At Melissa's request, her doctor wrote a letter to the head of the local sorority chapter explaining the need for Melissa to live gluten-free. As a result of this letter, Melissa was granted an exemption by the sorority and allowed to remain a member but live outside of the sorority house. This enabled Melissa to continue to live gluten-free, and she remained in good health. Did this put her at odds with her sorority? Apparently not; she was subsequently elected chapter treasurer!

TIP

Because gluten-free foods are often more expensive than gluten-containing foods, your young adult child's food budget may be higher than that of other students. As we discuss in Chapter 10, in some settings, these extra costs may qualify for a tax benefit.

IN THIS CHAPTER

» **Developing better ways of determining the risk of getting celiac disease**

» **Improving the tests used to diagnose celiac disease**

» **Discovering new treatments for celiac disease**

» **Preventing celiac disease**

» **Increasing awareness of celiac disease**

» **Furthering the research of celiac disease**

Chapter **15**

What the Future May Hold

So much has happened in recent decades to advance the scientific understanding of celiac disease, its diagnosis, how commonly it occurs, the different ways it presents, and perhaps most importantly of all, the greater availability of more and better-quality gluten-free foods. It's clear that if things continue to advance at the rate they have, the future for people living with celiac disease will be brighter and brighter.

In this chapter, we look at what this bright future may hold. Now we're the first to admit that predicting the future is, at the best of times, a fanciful thing to do. And we wouldn't want for one moment to suggest that *all* the things we discuss in this chapter are going to happen or even predict when any of them will happen. But we also wouldn't want to leave the impression that the status quo will persist indefinitely. It won't. Indeed, in one form or another, better and better ways of managing celiac disease will emerge. Doctors don't typically guarantee much, but this, indeed, we will guarantee.

In this chapter, we mention a number of different research studies that are underway. If you would like to keep abreast of these and other celiac disease studies, check out www.clinicaltrials.gov. This excellent website contains a huge inventory of medical studies on all manner of subjects, so to narrow your search to just those studies on celiac disease, enter that term into the site's search engine.

Devising Better Ways of Determining Your Risk of Getting Celiac Disease

As we discuss in Chapter 5, the genes a person is born with (conceived with, actually) predict many things about that person's future, including skin color, eye color, and, most relevant to this discussion, much of their risk for getting certain diseases, including celiac disease. Celiac disease is triggered by exposure to gluten, but this only happens if you are susceptible to celiac disease in the first place, and this susceptibility is directly related to your genetic makeup.

One of the most robust and exciting areas of medical research these days is the field of genetics. With each passing day, more and more discoveries are being made. In terms of celiac disease, over the past few years, scientists have discovered an increasing number of genes that are linked to the risk of a person getting this condition. It's only a matter of time before this stream of discoveries leads to the ability to more precisely identify who is and who is not at risk for celiac disease. And, armed with this information, a person with a very high (or near-certain) risk of getting celiac disease has a whole range of options available to help them avoid running into problems related to celiac disease, including being able to

>> Avoid gluten from day one. No gluten exposure, no risk of developing gluten-induced damage to the body.

>> Monitor for evidence that celiac disease has developed so that it can be picked up early before it has a chance to take a toll on the person who has it.

>> Intervene with other novel therapies, so as to prevent the development of celiac disease. (If you knew, based on your genes, it was a certainty you were going to develop celiac disease, would you submit to experimental therapy to prevent it before it happens? Perhaps yes, perhaps no; either way, this type of genetic knowledge would give you the ability to at least consider the option.)

Finding Out Why Genetically Susceptible People Get Celiac Disease

As we discuss in Chapter 5, people with certain genes, most notably the HLA DQ2 and DQ8 genes, are at increased risk for developing celiac disease. If you have neither of these genes, you have virtually no risk of developing celiac disease. The converse, however, is not true; that is, if you have these genes, you will not necessarily develop celiac disease.

Why does having certain genes make a person more susceptible to celiac disease (and why does the absence of these genes seemingly protect against getting it)? The quick answer is no one knows for sure. The more complex answer is that certain genes in people with celiac disease likely influence the behavior of their white blood cells (actually a particular type of white blood cell called a T cell), leading these cells, when they come across gluten protein, to think they've come across a foreign invader (like a bacteria) rather than recognizing gluten for what it is: a nutrient. The T cells' "intruder alert, intruder alert" announcement triggers an immune response, and the small intestine becomes damaged as a result. So that's the bad news.

The good news is that scientists are learning more and more about how the immune system of a person with celiac disease responds to gluten exposure. Armed with this knowledge, doctors can use novel therapies to target the immune problem seen with celiac disease, thereby preventing gluten from triggering the condition. ("Ah," a naysayer may say, "why mess around with the immune system when all you have to do is avoid eating gluten?" To which we would respond, you're right . . . except that millions of people with celiac disease either don't follow this advice or, try as they might, still inadvertently ingest gluten and become ill as a result; therefore, we need to find better treatment strategies.)

Improving Ways to Diagnose and Monitor Celiac Disease

As medical science and medical technology continue their rapid advance, newer and better ways of diagnosing and monitoring celiac disease are evolving. We discuss these here.

Better ways to diagnose celiac disease

As we discuss in Chapter 3, an endoscopy and small intestine biopsy is the *definitive* way to diagnose celiac disease. Blood tests that are currently available, though very helpful, are simply not sufficiently accurate to do away with the need for these other procedures.

There is ongoing research looking for more accurate antibody blood tests to help diagnose celiac disease. Although an endoscopy and small intestine biopsy aren't by any means particularly unpleasant procedures, they do require you to give up some time to visit a clinic, and it would certainly be far better if a simple blood test could instead be done.

It may turn out that highly elevated levels of antibodies to tissue transglutaminase (TTG IgA; see Chapter 3) when combined with other available information (for instance, the patient's age and/or other blood test results) may prove to be sufficiently accurate to allow for a definitive diagnosis without the need for a small intestine biopsy. Even if not, with time, other precise diagnostic tests will undoubtedly become available.

Better ways to monitor celiac disease that isn't responding to a gluten-free diet

When it comes to monitoring celiac disease, if you have ongoing or recurring unexplained gastrointestinal symptoms, your doctor may recommend an endoscopy so that they can directly visualize what is the state of affairs in your stomach and small intestine. An endoscopy (see Chapter 3) may not be particularly unpleasant, but, curious medical students aside, we don't know too many people who would line up to swallow a four-foot-long rubber hose if an easier alternative were available. At the present time, no other equivalent or better option exists to routinely provide the type of images that are seen with an endoscope, but newer ways are now playing a role in select situations, including refractory celiac disease (see Chapter 12) and cancer of the intestine (Chapter 9).

As time goes by, these emerging procedures will become increasingly sophisticated and increasingly used. Further studies are needed to assess how best to use the new technologies in monitoring celiac disease and to determine whether the endoscopic findings using a technique known as *confocal microscopy* may one day be able to replace the need for a biopsy. One limitation of the more advanced scoping procedures, such as *double-balloon enteroscopy*, is that they are time-consuming. Fortunately, technology is continually improving, and in the future, better instruments and techniques, including better capsule endoscopy (see Chapter 3), will become available.

Developing New Treatments for Celiac Disease

The proven, highly effective way to treat celiac disease is to follow a gluten-free diet. There are millions upon millions of people — likely including yourself — who know this and do this. But we suspect that, given the choice, most of these people would happily return to consuming a full diet if they could safely do so. If you also feel that way, we're happy to tell you that there is a bit of light at the end of the gluten-free tunnel. In this section, we look at current research efforts being made toward finding celiac disease therapies that would allow you to once again consume gluten.

Breaking down gluten in the gastrointestinal tract

Have you ever seen a parent bird regurgitate some food and then drop it into the waiting mouth of its offspring? Well, maybe we can learn something from them. While we wouldn't want to suggest that human moms and dads should pre-digest food — yuck! — for their kids with celiac disease, if we could achieve this same effect by use of digestive enzymes, this could allow affected individuals to ingest gluten. In what is clearly a great bit of lateral thinking, scientists are looking at just this trick; that is, rather than avoiding gluten, one would ingest special enzymes that would do the work of digestion for you, and by the time the gluten hit your gut, it would have been transformed into smaller proteins that wouldn't trigger the immune response (and subsequent bowel damage) that is seen with celiac disease.

Even if it turns out that this type of therapy isn't able to completely and routinely replace your gluten-free diet, it could still be a great help in a pinch. Let's say, for example, that you're in a restaurant or at a party and you have some doubts about whether the food is totally gluten-free, despite assurances by the wait staff or host. All you'd need to do is reach into your pocket or purse, pull out your enzyme supplement, and swallow it (before eating). (If you're familiar with the treatment of lactose intolerance — which we discuss in Chapter 11 — you may note some similarities. Lactose intolerance is a condition in which one lacks an enzyme called lactase. One form of therapy for this condition is to swallow an oral enzyme supplement when you're consuming lactose.)

TECHNICAL STUFF

The enzymes that are currently being tested are called endopeptidases, which are found in nature in plants and microorganisms and can also be engineered in a laboratory. Two such products are currently being tested in clinical studies: Latiglutenase from ImmunogenX and TAK-062 from Takeda Pharmaceuticals. The research that led to ALV-003 was the work of Dr. Chaitan Khosla at Stanford University, an accomplished professor who turned his attention to celiac disease research after his son and wife were found to have celiac disease. Sometimes, necessity truly is the mother of invention!

We're very excited about the potential of this form of therapy. Although it wouldn't be a cure, it could make living with celiac disease immeasurably easier.

Decreasing gluten uptake by the intestinal wall

If you have celiac disease, greater than normal quantities of gluten can be taken up through the leakier intestine present with active celiac disease. The taking up of more gluten stimulates the immune system and results in damage to the lining of the small intestine, which in turn can cause symptoms such as diarrhea. As we discuss in Chapter 8, the specific component of gluten that is responsible for triggering the abnormal immune response is *gliadin*. Scientists suspect that a breakdown in the gut wall causes it to allow more gluten to get into the intestinal tissues, where it can cause activation of the immune system, which in turn leads to intestinal damage.

This theory has led to the development of a medication called *larazotide* that enhances the tightness of the gut lining. Preliminary clinical studies with larazotide showed favorable results in terms of reducing gastrointestinal symptoms during a *gluten challenge,* the intentional eating of gluten under experimental conditions. A larger study, testing whether larazotide helps people with celiac disease feel better (as compared to a placebo) was designed, but not completed because when the researchers looked at their results so far, larazotide did not appear to be having the beneficial effect they had hoped for. Is this the end of larazotide as a possible treatment for celiac disease? Not necessarily; sometimes it's a matter of testing the right dose under the right conditions. Stay tuned.

CHANGING THE IMMUNE RESPONSE TO GLUTEN

Because celiac disease is related to a problem with the immune system (see Chapter 8), one theoretical way of handling this condition would be to get the immune system to stop malfunctioning when exposed to gluten. If immune system therapy were to be helpful, there are several places this system could be targeted, including these:

- **Blocking tissue transglutaminase enzyme:** Doing so would make gliadin (gliadin is a component of gluten; see Chapter 8) less likely to stimulate the immune system; hence, there would be less small intestine injury. Preliminary studies have shown that TAK-227, a drug that blocks tissue transglutaminase, reduces symptoms and intestinal damage in people with celiac disease undergoing a gluten challenge. Further studies are in progress.

- **Blocking the action of proteins made by the HLA DQ2 or DQ8 genes:** Doing so would reduce the T cell immune response to gluten and result in less damage to the intestine. DONQ52 is a drug that specifically targets the DQ2 molecule when it's attached to gliadin. This drug is being tested in people with celiac disease who have the DQ2 gene.

- **Promoting a different T cell response to gliadin:** People with celiac disease have gluten-specific T cells that recognize gluten as foreign and dangerous. Could reintroducing gluten in a new way lead to a newly tolerant immune system? That is the thought behind TAK-101 and KAN-101, two medications that are in clinical testing. These drugs consist of fragments of gluten that are encased in such a way that they hone to the liver and spleen, which promote the generation of regulatory T cells, a type of T cell that tells the immune system to chillax and see gluten as nonthreatening. So far, early studies suggest that giving these medications by intravenous infusion is safe and leads to a decrease in the gluten-specific T cells that are thought to be the main instigators of gut damage in celiac disease. Further studies are in progress. If this route turns out to be successful, this could one day open a path to allow people with celiac disease to ditch the gluten-free diet entirely, but it's too early to know if that will come to pass.

- **Modulate the way in which specific cytokines, which are part of the immune response to gluten (as discussed in Chapter 2), act on the intestinal lining:** Certain cytokines, particularly interleukin 15 (IL-15) are thought to be key parts of the immune response to gluten in people with celiac disease. Several drugs blocking IL-15 are being tested. The hope is that this will diminish the intestinal damage that arises in patients with celiac disease.

(continued)

(continued)

Modifying the immune response to gluten is attractive in concept, and testing in people with celiac disease has shown some promising early results. But, because it isn't known how one could selectively change the immune system only within the gut, there are concerns that the immune system in the rest of the body would be adversely affected by this form of treatment. Further studies are designed to test whether these medications are both effective and safe.

Preventing Celiac Disease: When to Introduce Gluten in a Child's Diet

It's not known whether celiac disease can be avoided by specifically timing when first to introduce gluten-containing foods into a child's diet. Some studies suggested that early exposure to gluten decreases the risk of celiac disease, but other studies refuted that. Studies suggest that delaying the introduction of gluten for a long time (beyond one year) could actually *increase* the risk of celiac disease, so we advise not delaying gluten introduction beyond one year.

We discuss this topic in detail in Chapter 14.

Increasing Public Awareness

Not so very long ago, when celiac disease was thought to be a rare disease, relatively little attention was paid to it (by lay and professional people alike). Nowadays, however, armed with evidence that far more people are affected by celiac disease than was formerly thought, there is heightened awareness of the condition not only by the public, but also by the medical and scientific communities and, importantly, the press, too. In this section, we look at some of the implications of this.

Public awareness and public policy

For better or worse, it's a simple fact of life that if a disease garners lots of public attention, there's an increased likelihood that politicians and other healthcare and research funders will also pay attention and provide more robust financial support for researching and treating the condition. In terms of celiac disease, its increasing prominence in the public eye has enhanced the relative importance given to it by governments and other bodies that determine priorities for how research dollars are spent and medical care monies used. All this attention can only help lead to better ways to prevent, diagnose, treat, and, hopefully, one day cure celiac disease — to which we simply say, "Thank goodness!"

TIP

Do you want to get involved in the push to increase awareness and advances in the diagnosis and treatment of celiac disease? If you're not a member of a support group or another celiac disease organization (we list a number of these in Appendix D), you may want to consider joining one.

Grassroots organizations, advocacy groups, education, patience, and persistence have all contributed to bringing a once little-known condition to the attention of healthcare providers, politicians, and the public.

Public awareness, information, and misinformation

There has been a virtual explosion in the number of websites and organizations (see Appendix D for a listing of some of these) that focus on celiac disease. This is wonderful in so many ways (knowledge is power, after all), but as with any explosion, there can be untoward consequences.

The trouble with websites

The greater the number of websites and online discussion groups, the more likely it is that misinformation will creep in and potentially mislead people living with celiac disease. For example, some sites say one thing about what constitutes a gluten-free diet, and other sites say very different things. We see no solution to this — the Internet is a place of great freedom for the delivery of information — except to advise caution to always question not only the information one reads on the Internet, but the *source* of the information.

The difficulty with organizations and groups

Different celiac disease organizations sometimes offer very different and conflicting advice to their members on topics such as whether a person with celiac disease can safely consume buckwheat (you can) or vinegar (again, you can, so long as it's not *malt* vinegar).

Different celiac disease support groups sometimes offer discrepant information regarding the inclusion of oats into the diet. (Oats are almost always okay for a person with celiac disease to consume, as long as they are not contaminated with other grains; in other words, they need to be "pure oats.") Another unfortunate discrepancy is in regard to whether it is safe to use gluten-containing topical products, such as some lotions, shampoos, and soaps. (It most certainly is as long as you don't drink the stuff!) This misinformation can still be found in printed and online information of some support groups, but we hope this will be changed soon.

As you can likely imagine (or perhaps have already experienced), getting conflicting information or advice can be terribly frustrating and leave you not knowing what to do.

There can be a number of reasons behind well-intentioned organizations and groups providing less than fully accurate information. One thing's for certain: It isn't the result of malicious intent. Here are a few reasons why people and groups who are trying to be helpful sometimes get things wrong:

>> As most people have done themselves in other contexts, when one feels strongly about something, opinion sometimes manages to get in the way of the facts.

>> Even when one has the facts straight, they can, at times, be interpreted in different ways.

>> Scientific discoveries typically occur in research laboratories and are generally of a "basic science" nature, meaning that what has been found is something to do with molecules, genes, cells, and so on, not flesh and blood people. These discoveries can take ten or more years to lead to clinical applications (that is, therapy you can actually use). Unfortunately, what so often happens is that these very early, very preliminary discoveries, which are of uncertain ultimate value, are interpreted by the press and then by the world at large as being far more definitive and having far greater implications than they often actually do.

Making sense of new information

This is what we recommend you do when you read about some new "discovery" in the world of celiac disease. (Or, as so often happens, when it's a loved one or concerned friend who shares the news with you. "Hey Jim, did you see the news? There's a cure for celiac disease." "Thanks, Bob; yup, that's the tenth cure I've heard about this month."):

1. **Be skeptical — optimistic, but skeptical.**

2. **Check out the details.**

   Is it really a new discovery or just another article rehashing old data?

3. **Assess the validity of the source of the information.**

   Is it, for example, an article in the *New York Times* (a good sign that it's reliable) or was it on an anonymous online blog (in which case its reliability would be far more suspect)?

4. **Discuss the findings with your celiac disease specialist.**

   They'll almost certainly be aware of the information and can shed further light on it. Nonetheless, in this information age, you may have found something before they have, so be sure to bring a copy of the information you found and show it to the doctor.

Identifying Areas for Further Investigation

Huge strides have been made in the field of celiac disease in the past number of years. Indeed, a mind-boggling array of discoveries has been made, including in (but certainly not limited to) the following fields:

» **Genetics:** For example, the discovery of the role of the HLA DQ2 and DQ8 genes.

» **Immunology:** For example, the discovery of the tissue transglutaminase antibody.

» **Epidemiology (the study of diseases within population groups):** For example, the discovery that celiac disease is much more prevalent than was formerly thought.

» **Pathogenesis (the study of how diseases develop):** For example, the determination of the role of transglutaminase in making gliadin stimulate the immune system.

Armed with this new information, doctors are now better able to diagnose, screen for, and treat celiac disease.

In spite of all these exciting developments, there are lots of things that remain unknown. Fortunately, there are many, many scientists and clinical researchers busily working on filling in the numerous gaps that exist.

Though many areas of celiac disease research are needed, and at the risk — egads — of offending some of our colleagues and friends whose areas of study aren't included, in the rest of this section, we look at those topics that we feel are in special need of attention.

Discovering more about who gets celiac disease and why

Much is yet to be discovered in the realm of who gets celiac disease and why they get it. We suspect you've asked yourself these very questions after you or your loved one was diagnosed. Here are some areas in this domain that are in need of further research:

>> **Understanding more about the pathogenesis of celiac disease:** One example is learning what role, if any, the TTG antibodies play in causing intestinal injury. That is, are they directly damaging to the intestine or just innocent bystanders? We discuss celiac disease antibodies in Chapter 3.

>> **Finding those additional genes that predispose someone to acquiring celiac disease:** Much is now known about the importance of the HLA DQ2 and DQ8 genes, but other as yet largely undefined genes are also known to play a role. We discuss the genetics of celiac disease in Chapter 3.

>> **Discovering factors that lead to the development of celiac disease:** At present, we have *lots* of theories, but no certainty. (Is it a virus that leads to celiac disease? Improved hygiene in developed countries? We look at these and other possible factors in Chapter 5.)

>> **Finding out why celiac disease has increased in prevalence over time:** Studies by Dr. Joseph Murray and his colleagues at the Mayo Clinic using tissue transglutaminase IgA (TTG IgA) testing of stored blood samples show that celiac disease was far *less* common half a century ago.

>> **Knowing why the clinical presentation of celiac disease has changed over time:** For example, most cases are now diagnosed in adulthood, and most are of the non-classical type (whereas in the past, most new diagnoses were in children who had the classical form). This remains an area wide open for investigation. We discuss the classification of celiac disease in Chapter 4.

Preventing and screening for celiac disease

Although consuming a gluten-free diet is a very effective therapy for celiac disease, following this diet is not an easy task. Far better would be preventing celiac disease in the first place. Figuring out how to prevent celiac disease is an important area of research, and ongoing research studies are currently being conducted in this field.

Screening for celiac disease is designed to discover it before it has had a chance to make someone ill. Knowing who, exactly, should be screened for celiac disease is, however, both controversial and uncertain. (Naturally enough, uncertainty breeds controversy.)

As we discuss in Chapter 6, celiac disease is more common in some regions of the world than in others. In those countries with populations who are at significant risk of getting celiac disease, the prevalence of celiac disease is estimated to be approximately 1 percent. In the United States and many European countries, it's estimated that less than 50 percent of these individuals have actually been diagnosed. Finland is one country in which at least 50 percent have been diagnosed. This much higher rate of diagnosis was the result of increased awareness and testing rates. Large-scale screening of the entire population of Italy is being planned, which aims to bring the proportion of those diagnosed close to 100 percent.

To better know who should be screened among the general population, it would be a huge help to know the natural history of the silent and latent forms of celiac disease (we discuss the forms of celiac disease in Chapter 4). Because silent celiac disease has only been relatively recently recognized, there isn't all that much known about how it will affect people as time goes by. This isn't a moot point because if it turns out that, on the one hand, silent celiac disease only rarely causes damage to the body, then screening for it wouldn't likely be necessary because treatment wouldn't be warranted. On the other hand, if it's determined that, if left untreated, it often leads to a whole host of problems, then screening for silent celiac disease would be invaluable because treatment could then be undertaken before complications arise.

We discuss screening for celiac disease in detail in Chapter 6.

Finding better ways to make the diagnosis of celiac disease

At present, celiac disease can only be diagnosed by having an endoscopy and a small intestine biopsy. Other tests, such as blood tests and the like, are helpful but are never definitive. As we discuss elsewhere in this chapter and in Chapter 3, an endoscopy (and small intestine biopsy) may not be particularly unpleasant, but we have yet to encounter a single patient who wouldn't prefer, all things being equal, to take a pass on these tests if there were only a simple blood test that could establish the diagnosis. Finding better ways to diagnose celiac disease is an area of active research.

Finding out what happens to people with celiac disease as time goes by

As we discuss in Chapter 1, celiac disease was first described centuries ago. It was, however, only the classical form of celiac disease that was known to exist until fairly recently, when the other types (non-classical and silent) were discovered.

Whereas it's abundantly clear that people with the classical and non-classical forms of celiac disease must be treated because otherwise the disease will lead to progressively worsening damage to one's body, there is less known about the long-term implications of having silent celiac disease. These are huge gaps in knowledge about a condition that affects millions of people. More scientific research is needed to fill in these blanks.

Improving treatment

The treatment of celiac disease must be made literally and figuratively more palatable for people living with this condition. Meeting this need is essential.

Earlier in this chapter, in the section "Changing the immune response to gluten," we discuss current research that is looking at innovative ways of getting around the current need to avoid all gluten-containing foods. While the fruits of this research are awaited, what is needed in the here and now is better availability, nutritional quality, palatability (there's that word again), and affordability of gluten-free foods.

A need also exists for

>> Better labeling of gluten-containing foods

>> Easier methods to avoid cross-contact during food preparation (see Chapter 10)

>> Reducing the costs of living gluten-free, including how governments assist people in offsetting the costs

Finding better ways of managing refractory celiac disease

Another area of needed research relates to the therapy of refractory celiac disease (RCD). As we discuss in Chapter 12, this is a rare but serious complication of celiac disease in which severe intestinal inflammation is present. There are several treatment options to manage RCD, but none is clearly the best option and, accordingly, none is ideal.

One area of promising research relates to a type of medication called *JAK inhibitors,* which may reduce the inflammation seen in RCD. Blockers of IL-15, which are being studied to treat celiac disease (see the "Changing the Immune Response to Gluten" sidebar earlier in this chapter), may also be effective in treating RCD.

Discovering more about non-celiac gluten sensitivity

As we discuss in Chapter 5, some people react adversely to ingesting gluten, but for reasons not necessarily related to the immune system or to celiac disease. The reason or reasons for this are unknown and require further scientific investigation.

Knowing whether tolerance to gluten occurs

Gluten "tolerance" refers to the theoretical development of immunity to the damaging effects of gluten on the intestine of a person with celiac disease. Most celiac disease specialists doubt this exists, but could they be wrong?

There have been rare reports of adults with celiac disease who can resume eating gluten without apparent ill effects. This is obviously an intriguing prospect, but one that needs much more research before anyone with celiac disease — including you! — abandons a gluten-free diet.

Increasing public awareness of celiac disease

We feel passionately that the knowledge we're sharing in this book can be used to great effect by people living with celiac disease and by healthcare providers and researchers alike to advocate for causes related to celiac disease. Indeed, as a result of people advocating for celiac disease, there's now better funding of labs making innovative and potentially life-altering discoveries, a quickly expanding array of gluten-free foods available on grocery store shelves and in restaurants, and the availability of tax deductions for certain expenses related to living gluten-free, to name but a few success stories.

The work is, of course, not yet done, and it will require ongoing and concerted efforts at increasing public awareness of celiac disease if the recent, wonderful strides that have been made are to continue (which, by the way, we feel confident will indeed happen).

5
The Part of Tens

Chapter **16**

Ten Frequently Asked Questions

Over our combined 50-plus years in practice (how lucky that we started medical school at the age of 9!), our patients have collectively asked us hundreds of different questions regarding their celiac disease. Queries have ranged from the easily answered ("Can I catch celiac disease?" No, you can't.) to the almost-impossible-to-answer ("When will there be a cure for celiac disease?" Alas, we just don't know.). Some questions — whether easily answered or not — come up much more often than others. In this chapter, we've compiled the 10 most frequently asked questions (FAQs).

Do I Need to Have a Small Intestine Biopsy to Diagnose Celiac Disease?

Most likely yes.

This question is often raised — not only by lay people but also by healthcare professionals. Like much else in the world of medicine, people argue both for and against requiring a small intestine biopsy in order to diagnose celiac disease.

We'll start with the argument against requiring a small intestine biopsy to make the diagnosis. People in this camp argue that if someone has symptoms of celiac disease (see Chapter 2) and has antibodies that are typically present when someone has celiac disease (see Chapter 3), then the probability of celiac disease is high enough that there's no reason to burden the person with an endoscopy (and small intestine biopsy). Instead, the diagnosis can be made on these grounds alone, and treatment with a gluten-free diet can begin. In addition, even if the diagnosis is wrong, the person wouldn't come to harm by unnecessarily following a gluten-free diet, and if the diet wasn't helping because, in fact, the person didn't have celiac disease, they'd seek medical attention, and the correct diagnosis would ultimately surface anyhow. Fair enough.

Now, take a look at the other side of the argument: Those people who argue that a small intestine biopsy should always be done prior to diagnosing celiac disease say that symptoms of celiac disease are never specific and that similar symptoms can be seen with many other ailments, too. Further, they point out that the antibodies found in a person with celiac disease can be falsely positive. They may also add, given the great importance of knowing whether one has celiac disease (in terms of the risk of other family members having it, the need to adhere lifelong to a special — and costly — diet, the potential health complications arising from celiac disease, and so on), that it doesn't make sense to risk uncertainty regarding diagnosis when a simple, safe, fast, and very accurate endoscopy and small intestine biopsy can almost always provide definitive evidence one way or the other. Finally, they may point out that once someone starts the gluten-free diet, it becomes harder to figure out with certainty whether the person has celiac disease because these markers (antibody tests and biopsy findings) become normal over time in people with celiac disease.

These are pretty darn good arguments on either side. But we don't think it's a toss-up. In our opinion, the implications of having celiac disease are so great that, in most cases, the diagnosis should only be made if a small intestine biopsy has been performed and found to show appropriate abnormalities.

TIP

Now, we say "in most cases" because there are certain scenarios in which there are real safety concerns about doing a biopsy, such as for someone with a rare bleeding disorder or someone who has already started a gluten-free diet and develops severe symptoms when they eat gluten, making a gluten challenge impractical. In these scenarios, a highly (tenfold) elevated TTG IgA (not just any elevated celiac disease antibody level) could be used to make a diagnosis of likely celiac disease (see Chapter 3). But this is the exception to the rule.

EXAMPLE

Miguel was a 35-year-old man who was referred to a gastroenterologist because his family doctor thought he likely had celiac disease. This was a perfectly reasonable supposition because he had irregular bowel habits (constipation alternating with diarrhea) and a mildly elevated TTG IgA (this antibody is almost always found if someone has celiac disease). Miguel's gastroenterologist advised him that he thought Miguel's family doctor was likely correct, but still recommended that an endoscopy and small intestine biopsy be performed to be sure. With some reluctance, Miguel agreed to the procedure. As it turned out, Miguel's small intestine biopsy was normal, and further tests revealed that his symptoms were actually related to irritable bowel syndrome, which improved after fiber supplementation and avoidance of trigger foods such as broccoli and cauliflower. Miguel continued to eat gluten, and on repeat testing, his mildly elevated TTG IgA became normal. If Miguel hadn't been biopsied, a wrong diagnosis would have been made, unhelpful therapy (a gluten-free diet) administered, his correct diagnosis delayed, and proper therapy given only belatedly.

Can I Protect My Child from Getting Celiac Disease?

We are often asked by parents who have celiac disease whether they can do anything to lessen the risk that their child will also get celiac disease. This, of course, begs the question as to whether anybody can be protected from getting celiac disease.

The quick answer is no. There is no proven way to prevent your loved one — or anyone else, for that matter — from getting celiac disease. Medical researchers, however, are exploring several hypotheses about how to reduce the risk of getting celiac disease. One hypothesis, as we discuss in Chapter 14, is that the risk is reduced if you delay exposing an infant to gluten. Another theory, however, is opposed and suggests that giving infants small amounts of gluten early in infancy is the better thing to do to lower their risk. Geesh, how confusing is that?! Until this debate is resolved, we recommend you follow the current consensus among most celiac disease experts that it's best to first introduce gluten to infants who are genetically at risk of celiac disease between 4 and 12 months of age.

Strategies for preventing celiac disease are the subject of a number of ongoing research studies. Though some research has suggested that breastfeeding an infant reduces a child's risk of developing celiac disease, this has not been consistently shown to be the case. So, although there are many proven benefits to breastfeeding, we can't claim that prevention of celiac disease is one of them.

TIP

If being involved in medical research may interest you and your family, consider contacting a nearby university-based teaching hospital to find out whether that institution is performing any celiac disease prevention studies. If so, you may consider enrolling your child in one of these studies.

Should I Have My Child Tested for Celiac Disease?

If your child has symptoms of celiac disease (we discuss these in Chapter 2), your child's doctor should test to see whether celiac disease is present, unless there is some other apparent cause. If, on the other hand, your child is perfectly well, they don't need to be tested for celiac disease unless some other reason to do so exists. In other words, it isn't currently recommended to test all healthy children for this ailment. There are, however, two important circumstances for which you and your child's doctor should consider (there are no hard and fast rules here) when deciding to have your child tested for celiac disease:

>> If your child has a first-degree relative (mother, father, brother, or sister) who has celiac disease. (We discuss this further in the later section "If I Have Celiac Disease, Will My Child or Sibling Also Have It?")

>> If your child is known to have a health condition that puts them at increased risk of also having celiac disease. Most commonly, this other condition would be an autoimmune disease such as type 1 diabetes. (Having type 1 diabetes, for example, is associated with a 6 percent lifetime risk of also having celiac disease.) In Chapter 8, we discuss a number of different conditions — including autoimmune diseases — that are associated with celiac disease.

REMEMBER

We've worded this FAQ specifically as "should I have my child tested for celiac disease?" because, well, that is the frequently asked question we hear. Nonetheless, our answer would be the same if the question had been asked by any person who has a first-degree relative with celiac disease. (Assuming, of course, the first-degree relative was a biological first-degree relative, not an adopted relative; the increased risk is due to shared genes, not a shared environment.)

Testing for a disease in the absence of symptoms or other evidence that it is present is called *screening*. We discuss this topic in detail in Chapter 6.

Can You Outgrow Celiac Disease?

You likely recall how much better you felt soon after starting a gluten-free diet. And the odds are darn good that as you continued your diet, all your previous symptoms gradually resolved and you remained well thereafter. It could be — human beings being human after all — that at some point you inadvertently (or maybe even intentionally) resumed consuming gluten. It's likely that in short order, your old symptoms came back to haunt you, reminding you that you had not been cured of your celiac disease, but rather, that you still had it and needed to look after it. But what if you had resumed eating gluten and your symptoms didn't return? Or perhaps you have a child with celiac disease and, after being entirely well for years while on a gluten-free diet, you are now wondering whether your child needs to continue it? Could it be that you or your child has "outgrown" celiac disease?

So, then, with that preamble under our belt, can you, in fact, outgrow celiac disease? Alas, although you will outgrow your booster seat, your first bike, adolescence (thank goodness), your wedding-day tuxedo (sigh), and a million other things, you will *not* outgrow your celiac disease. Similarly, if you have a child with celiac disease, your child won't outgrow it either.

If you are a middle-aged person and were diagnosed in your youth with celiac disease, you may recall long ago being told by a doctor that you could — or would — outgrow your celiac disease. At one time, this possibility was entertained by some healthcare providers. Nowadays, we know this is incorrect.

So, what might happen if you feel completely well and you decide to resume eating gluten-containing foods? The answer is, one or more of the following problems could happen:

>> Your symptoms (see Chapter 2) may return, possibly becoming severe and exceptionally difficult to settle (see Chapter 12 for information on refractory celiac disease).

>> You may develop complications of celiac disease (such as iron deficiency anemia or osteoporosis); see Chapter 7.

>> You may expose yourself to an increased risk of several types of cancer, as outlined in Chapter 9.

The bottom line: As much as we wish it were otherwise, you cannot, in fact, outgrow celiac disease, and it's potentially dangerous to resume eating gluten, even if, having done so, you feel perfectly well.

Of course, all of this advice assumes that your initial diagnosis was accurate. For some people, the question isn't, "Do I still have celiac disease?" but rather "Did I *ever* have celiac disease?" If the initial diagnosis wasn't based on an intestinal biopsy, or if the full details of the diagnosis aren't retrievable in the long-lost archives of a shuttered doctor's office, then revisiting this question may be worthwhile (see Chapter 3).

If I Have Celiac Disease, Will My Child or Sibling Also Have It?

As we discuss in Chapter 6, celiac disease tends to run in families. The reason for this is that members of a family share many genes — including those for celiac disease — in common.

If you have celiac disease, your first-degree relatives (that is, your mother, father, brother, sister, or child) have a risk of around 11 percent of also having celiac disease. The risk varies by relative; for instance, it's higher in daughters and sisters and lower in sons and brothers. But for all of these groups, it's higher when compared to the risk of celiac disease in the general population (around 1 percent).

Because the risk of celiac disease is so much higher in first-degree relatives of an affected person, these relatives are often screened for the condition. We discuss this further in Chapter 6.

How Much Gluten Can I Safely Consume If I Have Celiac Disease?

We begin our answer to this question by being dogmatic: If you have celiac disease, you should consume *no gluten at all.* Celiac disease is an immune system disease, and even a minute stimulus can trigger the immune system, so don't play with fire and don't ingest gluten. Period.

Okay, so much for dogma; now let's look at practical realities.

Following a gluten-free diet doesn't mean that you will never ingest a single molecule of gluten. The U.S. Food and Drug Administration (FDA) defines gluten-free food as having fewer than 20 parts per million of gluten. This is based on studies that show that eating food that contains this minuscule amount of gluten would be unlikely to cause intestinal damage. In other words, although gluten-free doesn't mean zero gluten, it's so close that it can be considered the same.

As we say throughout this book, if you have celiac disease, it isn't only unwise, it's also unsafe to consume gluten. Having said that, we recognize that even the most conscientious person is likely to ingest gluten — accidentally or otherwise — at some time. Will this be a disaster-in-the-making, or will you be okay if this happens to you? Well, so long as it seldom happens, and so long as the amount consumed is very small, you will likely be fine.

Can I Skip the Diet and Just Take an Iron Supplement to Treat My Low Iron?

As we discuss in Chapter 4, many people with celiac disease have no — or virtually no — symptoms, and the condition is discovered only after a blood test, typically done for routine purposes, reveals iron deficiency, often with anemia present. Iron deficiency in celiac disease occurs because the damaged first part of the small intestine, the *duodenum*, is unable to properly absorb ingested iron into the body.

Given that a person who has celiac disease discovered in this incidental way typically feels healthy, it's not surprising that they may ask whether it's really necessary to follow a gluten-free diet and whether they can simply take an iron supplement instead. Our reply (which you may predict if you've read this chapter from the beginning) is that, regrettably, taking iron alone is not sufficient, and you must also follow a gluten-free diet.

Here are three important reasons why you can't simply consume iron and forego the gluten-free diet:

>> Even if you have no gastrointestinal symptoms, your gut is damaged and will remain so if you continue to ingest gluten. This damage prevents you from sufficiently absorbing into your body the iron you're ingesting and, as a result, despite taking iron supplements, you'll continue to be iron-deficient.

>> You may feel fine now, but if you continue to consume gluten, there's a good chance that you will eventually feel ill. Even if you don't, your celiac disease may still be taking a silent toll on your body (for example, by causing osteoporosis, which we discuss in Chapter 7).

>> Ongoing ingestion of gluten may increase your risk of developing certain types of cancer. See Chapter 9 for more on this risk.

Another question about treating iron deficiency that comes up fairly frequently is whether you can get around the problem of malabsorption of oral iron by taking iron by infusion. As we discuss in detail in Chapter 7, this is sometimes necessary in special circumstances, but it does not take away the need to adopt a strict gluten-free diet.

Should My Whole Family Eat Gluten-Free If Only One Member Has Celiac Disease?

If a person has celiac disease, there is a significantly increased risk that a close family member will be similarly affected. For this reason, we're often asked whether it's wise — or, at least, easier or simpler — to put everyone in the family on a gluten-free diet. (Following a gluten-free diet is the mainstay of treating celiac disease. We discuss this diet in detail in Chapter 10.) Like most things in the world of medicine, there are some good things about doing this, and there are — you guessed it — some bad things about doing this.

Here are some advantages of having the whole family eat gluten-free:

>> The person who is known to have celiac disease won't feel singled out for dietary restriction because everyone in the family is eating similarly.

>> Food shopping becomes more straightforward if everyone in the family is eating the same types of foods.

>> If another family member has — but has not yet been diagnosed with — celiac disease, they will be on track with therapy.

>> If a family member has been screened for celiac disease and it wasn't detected, that doesn't guarantee that it won't later develop. Starting a gluten-free diet early in the game introduces a diet that that person is going to end up requiring later anyhow.

And here are some disadvantages to having the whole family eat gluten-free:

>> Family members who don't need to follow a gluten-free diet will be eating an unnecessarily restricted diet.

>> Following a gluten-free diet typically entails greater grocery costs than a conventional diet. If you are buying additional gluten-free foods (as you would if your whole family is following this diet), then you'll end up spending more money than you would have otherwise.

>> A gluten-free diet is not an intrinsically healthy diet, and if adopted without the guidance of a dietitian (which may be the case in a non-celiac family member) could be imbalanced, with low amounts of fiber and high amounts of fat and calories.

>> If a person who is not known to have celiac disease is following a gluten-free diet, when they're tested for the condition, it will be more difficult to determine whether they have it. We discuss this further in Chapter 3.

>> The family member with celiac disease may not adjust as well to learning how to deal with staying gluten-free once they leave the home environment, as compared to someone who learns to live gluten-free while living at home. (We discuss this in Chapter 14.)

Although the final decision always rests with the family dealing with this issue, we advocate great caution before having an entire family follow a gluten-free diet when the whole family doesn't actually have to follow such a diet. Celiac disease is a lifelong and important disorder. We feel it best that one commit to the often-challenging gluten-free diet only if one has been definitively proven to have the ailment.

Is It All Right for Me to Eat Oats?

The short answer is, yes, but carefully.

The great majority of people with celiac disease can consume oat-based products so long as "pure" oats are being ingested.

As we discuss in Chapter 5, the misperception about oats triggering celiac disease likely arose because the oats that were typically available (and, therefore, consumed) were mixed in with other, gluten-containing products. In other words, the oats weren't triggering the celiac disease; the other products were. *Pure* oats (that is, oats not contaminated by other gluten-containing products) are now available and are fine for you to consume. Bon appétit!

As much as we'd love to end the discussion with the preceding paragraph, alas, in the interests of being entirely scientifically accurate, there is one qualifier we need to add to this discussion. There is a minority of individuals with celiac disease whose condition is triggered by oats. So, if you eat oats (or oatmeal) and develop gastrointestinal symptoms, it would be wise to have yourself checked out by your doctor to see what's causing you to be unwell.

Does Avoiding Gluten Protect Me from Getting Other Autoimmune Diseases?

As we discover in Chapter 8, if you have celiac disease (which is an autoimmune disease, a condition in which your body's immune system mistakenly attacks part of your own body), you're at increased risk of also having other autoimmune diseases like type 1 diabetes and certain forms of thyroid disease.

A unique feature of celiac disease, in contrast to other autoimmune diseases, is that the trigger (gluten) for this condition is known, whereas for other autoimmune diseases, it remains a mystery. We're often asked if this mystery is not so mysterious after all. Could it be that gluten exposure not only triggers celiac disease but is also responsible for causing these other autoimmune diseases (at least, in those people who already have celiac disease)?

In case you're wondering, we've saved this FAQ for last for a very good reason: It's the hardest to answer! It's known with absolute certainty that if you have celiac disease, you must not consume gluten because doing so perpetuates injury to your intestine and potentially leads to other celiac disease complications. What isn't as clear is whether avoiding gluten — if you have celiac disease — has the additional benefit of reducing your risk of acquiring other autoimmune diseases or, if they're present, helping to keep these other conditions in check.

This is a very important question for scientists to figure out. If avoiding gluten does actually help protect people with celiac disease from developing other autoimmune diseases, this knowledge will contribute to our understanding not only of the particular disease in question but also of how the immune system malfunctions in the first place. Regardless of the answer, following a gluten-free diet is an absolute necessity for everyone with celiac disease in order to protect them from complications of this disease. If it also helps prevent other autoimmune diseases from developing, that will be a true blessing. If it doesn't, well, the diet remains essential for maintaining good health anyhow.

Chapter **17**

Ten Tips for Living Successfully with Celiac Disease

As with any other health condition, when it comes to having celiac disease, the goal isn't just to avoid being ill; the goal is to be able to lead a full, active, and healthy existence. In other words, to live successfully.

In this chapter, we share ten key tips to help you climb the hills, traverse the valleys, and swim the seas of daily life with celiac disease. Now, just before — or just after, if you prefer — you do all that climbing, traversing, and swimming, in this chapter, we also share tips about dealing with workmates and friends, eating out, and otherwise navigating life with celiac disease.

Be Healthy and Gluten-Free: It's All About What to Add

"Living successfully" isn't, of course, being obliged to live the same routine day to day (although you're perfectly welcome to if that's what you prefer). For most people, living successfully also involves constantly reevaluating how you live life: looking at how you eat, what exercise you do (or are hoping to do), what bad habits, if any, you feel you should abandon, what good habits you want to adopt, and so forth.

If you're living with celiac disease, one of the things you've had to reevaluate is your diet as you've faced the challenges of living gluten-free. But as you have already discovered, or if celiac disease is a new diagnosis to you, you will soon discover, striving to be healthy by making the necessary dietary changes involves making healthy changes. Disruptive? Sure. Good for you? You bet.

Eating gluten-free isn't about adopting a stance of avoidance. Instead, it's about landing on a balanced diet based on fresh fruits and vegetables, a variety of carbohydrates, and different sources of protein, fats, minerals, and vitamins. A person lives gluten-free not only to *feel* well but to *be* well, and the necessary dietary changes make this all the more likely to happen.

We suspect that you know many people without celiac disease who are also striving to be healthy by making their own dietary changes. Perhaps they've cut down on their saturated fat intake or are trying to eat more vegetables, get more fiber, reduce how often they consume fast food, and so on. These people without celiac disease are looking at making many of the healthy eating changes that you with celiac disease already have. Bet it feels nice to know that you're ahead of the (healthy eating) curve!

For a detailed discussion on gluten-free eating, see Chapter 10.

Keep Informed About Your Disease

As a physician and dietitian at a major celiac disease center, we're constantly reading about new research findings, attending medical conferences, and doing our best to ensure we're current in our scientific knowledge. As a healthcare consumer, you, too, would be well served by ensuring you remain abreast of important aspects of living with your celiac disease.

Keeping informed provides you with ways to help you live successfully. Whether it's highly practical information, like what new gluten-free foods have recently made their way onto the shelves of your grocery store, or more academic information about new discoveries, knowledge is power.

You can remain informed in a number of ways:

» Your celiac disease specialist will be able to answer questions specific to you and your celiac disease. They're also a source of general information about what's new in the world of celiac disease.

» Your dietitian — especially if affiliated with a celiac disease clinic — is an invaluable resource when it comes to providing you with current information regarding gluten-free eating.

» You can avail yourself of up-to-date information provided by a number of very helpful organizations specifically charged with meeting the needs of people living with celiac disease. Here you find both practical information as well as scientific information that's geared toward a lay (but interested) audience. We list a number of these organizations in Appendix D.

» Reading informed publications keeps you abreast of what's new in the world of celiac disease. Remember, though, particularly when it comes to press releases and links on social media groups, you need to always consider the source of the information. Anyone with an Internet connection can post materials, however inaccurate, to websites. In Appendix D, we list websites that have a reputation for reliability and accuracy.

Live a Full Life While Avoiding Gluten

Gluten is everywhere, and people living with celiac disease inevitably discover this. No matter how well-meaning the wait-staff is, there is always the possibility of a slip-up. Whether it was the lone crouton buried in your garden salad or the wrong batch of pasta that made its way into your stomach, the experience can be frustrating, frightening, and sometimes painful. Since gluten is lurking around the corner like a horror movie villain, one potential reaction is to *avoid*: avoid restaurants, avoid traveling, and avoid that dinner party. (Small talk is exhausting anyway, right?)

We recommend that you take a different approach. The challenges are real. Speaking up for yourself to a stranger at a restaurant isn't easy, and no one wants to be a difficult guest at a dinner party. But some social discomfort and, yes, taking some degree of reasonable risk, can lead to rich experiences. You didn't choose to have celiac disease, but you can choose to learn to advocate for yourself and live a fuller life.

Prepare for Your Child's Visit to Friends

Being a parent of any child has all sorts of challenges. Oh, we'd be the first to say there are many, many, many joys, but we'd also volunteer that there are challenges, too. And if you're the parent of a child with celiac disease, you likely have already had to deal with some of the extra challenges that are present, including what to do when your child wants to eat "normally, just like the other kids." This perfectly natural and completely understandable desire to want to fit in with friends at school, in the playground, in the home, and so on, can at times be one of the biggest hurdles for both parent and child to surmount.

The most important thing about having your child cope with these situations is to have clear direction from you. And that direction must include a lovingly delivered but firm stance on the importance of your child not consuming gluten-containing foods. However difficult this may be, you must not yield. You love your child dearly, and born of this love is your desire for your child to be healthy. Consuming gluten if you have celiac disease is not healthy. Period.

As we discuss in Chapter 14, there are a few ways in which you can make the difficult task of keeping your child gluten-free:

>> **Teach your child, as early as is age-appropriate, about what foods contain gluten and the need to avoid them.** Again, as age-appropriate, take your child shopping with you at the grocery store and teach them how to tell the difference between foods that include gluten and those that don't, including knowing what to look for on food labels. Increase the sophistication of the explanation you provide as your child ages.

>> **Speak to the parents of your children's friends and explain to them about celiac disease and how it's treated.** You may find them surprisingly willing to do their best to accommodate your child's needs when your child is visiting their house.

>> **When going to a birthday party or other celebration, have your child take some gluten-free treats with them.** For example, if cupcakes are being served for Johnnie's birthday, send along a few gluten-free cupcakes so your child doesn't feel left out. If hot dogs or pizza are going to be served, preparing a gluten-free version to drop off with your child at a party or an end-of-the-season sports team celebration will be appreciated by the host or coach.

For more tips, have a look at the section "Growing Up Gluten-Free" in Chapter 14.

Eat Out without Standing Out

Unless you are on the flamboyant side, you likely prefer not to stand out when eating out. Oh sure, you want good service and you surely want good food, but you probably don't want the fact of your celiac disease to become an issue (even if it's as much the restaurant's issue as it is your own).

There are a number of ways you can have an enjoyable, stress- and gluten-free dining experience when at a restaurant:

>> **Pick the restaurant.** In a perfect world, knowledge of the gluten-free diet is uniform and widespread among food preparers, and all restaurants are equally excellent regarding the precautions they take. In reality, there's a good deal of variability and a lot of room for improvement. Some places just "get it," whereas others don't. As you learn the lay of the land, consider offering to pick the place to eat. This isn't always possible, but when it is, this is something you can control.

>> **Call the restaurant before you go and ask if gluten-free foods are on the menu.** If so, ask what ones. If not, feel free to suggest that the restaurant consider revisiting this and, in the future, include gluten-free items. The restaurant business is the most competitive one out there, and your suggestion may well be appreciated, especially if it helps to draw in more customers.

>> **Order "off" the menu.** If you're with friends or family at a pizza restaurant (where gluten-free menu items are not available), for example, feel free to ask the waiter to have the cook whip together a plate of fresh mozzarella, a couple of tomato slices, some basil, artichokes, and olives all drizzled with a little olive oil for a heartier salad. They'll likely be happy to do this. You might also ask if the owner is around (if it's a small restaurant, your waiter and the owner may be one and the same); small restaurant owners are, intrinsically, hosts and want to please their guests, so they are often very accommodating and will likely do their best to honor your needs and requests.

>> **Consider having a light meal or snack at home before you go out.** It's easier to retain your gluten-avoidance willpower if you aren't starving as someone offers you a tasty, but off-limits, gluten-containing morsel.

You can find more tips on eating gluten-free when out of the house in Chapter 10.

Save On Your Food Purchases

As you probably discovered when you went on your inaugural gluten-free grocery shopping trip, living gluten-free means incurring additional expenses. In a sense, wheat is the "great extender" in that it takes up a significant portion of the volume of many prepared foods. Replacing wheat-based components with alternative products means the manufacturer incurs increased food production costs, which, not surprisingly, are passed on to you. (There are multiple other cost factors also at play here, including the absence of the same economy of scale that's present with regular food production.)

Here are some ways that you can save some money on your gluten-free food grocery purchases:

>> **Apply for tax rebates that reimburse you for your additional food purchasing costs.** As we discuss in Chapter 10, this isn't always straightforward to do.

>> **Learn how to do your own gluten-free cooking and baking.** In addition to being a great hobby, it also helps you save money because cooking for yourself is typically less expensive than eating out or buying gluten-free prepared foods.

>> **Fill up your always-hungry teenager by having them eat rice, beans, corn (polenta), and potatoes to complement their other nutritious foods.** These foods are more filling than calorie-dense processed foods.

>> **Find suitable restaurants.** Because the less-expensive, fast-food types of restaurants typically don't provide much in the way of gluten-free food offerings (and are generally not very nutritious places), you may feel that you're limited to fancier, more expensive restaurants, which often are more likely to have gluten-free options. Another option is to find small, family-run restaurants where the owners are on site and typically do the food buying, preparing, and serving themselves. These types of establishments are likely to charge less than the fancy place down the street. More important, when it comes to you and your celiac disease, although they may not know much about celiac disease, they sure as shootin' know what ingredients are used in their recipes, and you can chat with them to make sure you make appropriate gluten-free selections.

We look in more detail at these and other money-saving food purchasing tips in Chapter 10.

Be Prepared for Blank Looks (or Worse)

You've likely had experiences where, when you told acquaintances, friends, or workmates that you have celiac disease, you got looks ranging from, at best, a blank stare to, at worst, one that says you may as well have told them you had the plague. Although things are changing, most people still know very little about celiac disease. And in any event, even when they do, discussing the details about a digestive disease hardly seems like a smooth beginning to a "normal" conversation and hardly an effective pickup line.

Many people may give you a blank look if you say "celiac disease," but be more familiar with the term *gluten-free*. Depending on how comfortable you are telling people you have celiac disease, the people to whom you're speaking, the specific situation, and so forth, you may find it helpful to have different comments or responses prepared in the event that the topic of your having celiac disease comes up. Most people with celiac disease find the simplest thing to do when chatting to people with whom they're not particularly close is to describe their celiac disease as a food intolerance or a food allergy. This brief description, even if not quite accurate, is usually effective at dispensing with the subject and moving the conversation on to other topics.

Have a Good Answer to the Inevitable Question — "What Happens When You Eat Wheat?"

As we mention in the preceding section, although people may be surprised to hear you have celiac disease, they usually drop the subject once you've explained it in a few words (assuming, that is, you elect to say anything at all) or, conversely, opt to provide a more detailed explanation.

Some people, however, out of either curiosity or caring — or, at times, even prying — may press you for more details than you're comfortable providing. Chief among these is typically a question along the lines of "What happens if you eat wheat?"

If you know the person well and want to provide a full answer, then, of course, go for it. If you're comfortable telling them, "I get diarrhea," or "I throw up," that is a matter-of-fact way to answer the question. If you'd rather not get too graphic, you can tone it down ("I get an upset stomach"). Or, if you don't develop symptoms when you eat gluten, you could tell them that gluten causes silent-but-significant inflammation internally that is bad for you in the long term. (You are also entitled to answer, "That's none of your business." We're offering polite responses, but sometimes there are situations where you don't have to be polite!)

Pack Your Bags, We're Going To . . .

Eating is one of the greatest pleasures on a trip, but also one of the biggest challenges or sources of anxiety for someone on a gluten-free diet. Even more daunting is the situation when traveling to a country where you don't speak the language. This is another example of how a little preparation can go a long way to making the trip go more smoothly.

Before you go, try to learn about the foods likely to be available and served in the place to which you'll be traveling. You can research online to find out what the regional dishes and local recipes are in pretty much any neck of the woods. Also, in many countries, food isn't as mass-produced and processed as in the United States, so dishes containing gluten aren't as prevalent.

Most countries have some spectacular gluten-free dishes that you may even want to introduce into your regular menu. Can't eat quiche? Try a frittata. Enjoy the Swiss *raclette,* which is melted cheese on potatoes. And fresh berries in *crème fraiche* with a drizzle of excellent balsamic vinegar puts most baking to shame. In Italy, you'll find that there are many alternatives to pasta, including corn-based polenta and risotto. Italy also has many food shops that cater to people who are living gluten-free. In France, try a *charcuterie* (a type of delicatessen specializing in meats and other prepared foods) for many gluten-free options for a great picnic. In Japan, rice is nice. Also, "spring rain" noodles are made from rice. And miso soup is gluten-free. In Scotland, they use a lot of wheat and bread crumbs, so eating gluten-free has some challenges. On the plus side, the whisky is gluten-free (due to the distillation process).

TIP

It's very helpful to learn a few key words of the local language. Learn how to say you're allergic to wheat and to ask whether something is made with wheat flour in the local language. Sometimes, however, nothing works quite as effectively (and succinctly) as pointing to a dish you recognize from your homework as likely to be gluten-free.

Bon voyage!

Deal with the Slip-Ups

Being aware of the importance of avoiding gluten in order to maintain good health, most people living with celiac disease strive, as they should, to be as careful as they can with their diet. But life happens, and the odds are darn good that at one point or another (or multiple points for that matter) you — and everyone else living with celiac disease — will either intentionally or inadvertently consume gluten-containing food.

If and when this happens, the first thing to do is to take a deep breath and reassure yourself that you haven't just swallowed plutonium and you're not about to die! In the next breath, tell yourself that your slip-up doesn't make you a weak person, it doesn't make you a dumb person, and it certainly doesn't make you a bad person. Following a strict diet of any type for even a few days or weeks can be tough; following a strict diet for the rest of your life can be that much more formidable a challenge.

In the third and with every subsequent breath, do your darndest to never refer to your gluten-consuming misadventure as *cheating*. Cheating is something devious or immoral. Eating gluten isn't those things. Eating gluten represents a break in willpower or an accident, or, for children, simply part of growing up and experimentation. The term *cheating* is patronizing at best, insulting at worst, and should never be uttered in the same sentence as the words *celiac disease* or *gluten*. Wow, we feel so much better now that we got that off our chests.

So, take pride in your usual success following your gluten-free diet, get quickly back on track, let any guilt you might be feeling pass quickly, for it won't serve you much good in the long run.

Chapter **18**

Ten Myths, Misperceptions, and Falsehoods about Celiac Disease

In some ways, celiac disease is a very straightforward condition: The bowel gets damaged from exposure to gluten, and if the person avoids gluten, all will likely be well. And in other ways, celiac disease is incredibly complex: Why does one person get celiac disease, yet someone else does not? Why does one person get a whole host of symptoms and someone else no symptoms at all? Why does one person run into other autoimmune diseases and someone else has no other health issues? The questions go on.

We think it's this mixture of the readily explained plus the complex and confusing that leads to so many of the myths, misperceptions, and, at times, downright falsehoods that surround this often puzzling condition. In this chapter, we look at ten common myths that come up.

Heavy People Can't Have Celiac Disease

As we discuss in Chapters 2 and 7, celiac disease causes malabsorption, meaning that nutrients you ingest are not properly absorbed into your body. These nutrients have to go somewhere, so if they are not being absorbed *into* your body, they then go *out of* your body (with your stool). Also, as the nutrients are lost from your body, so are the calories they contain. It makes sense, therefore, to conclude that losing calories from your body would lead to weight loss. Indeed, this is exactly what happens to many people with active celiac disease.

The thing is, however, when it comes to malabsorption due to celiac disease, it's not an all-or-none issue. The substantial majority of people with active celiac disease successfully absorb most of the nutrients (and thus, calories) they consume. They often do have some malabsorption; it's just that it's selective in terms of which nutrients are malabsorbed and limited in the degree to which they malabsorb. So if most nutrients — and the calories they contain — are being absorbed into the body, it comes down to how many calories are being ingested versus how many are being lost. For many people with celiac disease, just like for most people in general, the calories eaten exceed the calories used up, leaving the person with a net surplus of calories that ends up in excess weight.

Here are a couple of other reasons why people with celiac disease can be overweight:

>> Perhaps the person was considerably overweight before developing celiac disease. When they then acquired this condition, it could be they lost weight, perhaps even substantial weight, but depending on their size before they became ill, they may still carry around extra pounds at the time he was diagnosed.

>> Once you follow a strict gluten-free diet, any problems you previously had with malabsorption will resolve. At that point you will, just like everyone else, be at the mercy of that notorious and sometimes oh-so-frustrating balance between calorie intake and calorie expenditure.

Eat Gluten and You Feel Immediately Ill

If you have celiac disease, you should consume no gluten; it's the consumption of gluten that leads to damage to your gut and the symptoms (see Chapter 2) that then arise. Having said that, it's a myth that all people with celiac disease immediately develop symptoms after ingesting gluten. Here are some important reasons for this:

>> **Not everyone with celiac disease has symptoms.** You may well be one of the many people who were diagnosed either through screening (Chapter 6) or after an unexpected, abnormal test result was found (Chapter 3). So if you felt fine when you were consuming gluten *before* you were diagnosed with celiac disease, it's quite possible that you will continue to feel well when you consume gluten *after* you were diagnosed. (*Note:* This is not a reason to resume ingesting gluten! If you have celiac disease, you should consume no gluten at all! Hmm, we think we've said that before.)

>> **Although ingesting gluten triggers your immune system and leads to damage to your intestine, this isn't instantaneous.** For most people with celiac disease, it takes days, weeks, or even months before the damage becomes visible on an intestinal biopsy, so it's not unusual for it to also take time for gluten to cause symptoms in some people. This is unlike the immune problem seen if you have a peanut or bee sting allergy, in which case you have an immediate reaction upon exposure to these agents.

After reading the preceding list, you may have come to the conclusion that ingesting gluten will *not* make you feel immediately unwell. Excellent; we're glad we convinced you. But — well, yeah, there's a but — some people with celiac disease do start to feel unwell with symptoms of bloating, abdominal discomfort, and diarrhea developing soon after ingesting gluten. Some people experience nausea and vomiting, particularly after a large accidental exposure (such as eating at a restaurant where they were accidentally served a bowl of gluten-containing pasta).

So, is it a myth that if you consume gluten you will feel immediately unwell? For most people, yes, it's a myth. But for some people it's a reality.

You Can Have Only a Little Bit of Celiac Disease

We never take exception when a person advises us that they or a loved one has "a little bit" of celiac disease. Oh, sure, it's a myth, and one can no more have a little bit of celiac disease than one can be a little bit pregnant, but the person with this misperception got it from somewhere, and that somewhere is typically a well-meaning but misinformed friend, relative or — more commonly in years gone by — doctor. Like pregnancy, when it comes to celiac disease, you either have it or you don't. And speaking of the myth of borderline celiac disease, as we discuss in Chapter 16, it's also a myth that you can "outgrow" celiac disease.

If ever you have been told you had "a little bit of" celiac disease, or borderline celiac disease, this could be for a number of reasons. Perhaps the intestinal biopsy showed partially (as opposed to totally) flattened *villi*, the finger-like projections emanating from your intestinal wall. Or perhaps you had a biopsy showing celiac disease only in the first part of the duodenum (referred to as the *bulb*) and not anywhere else. Or perhaps you had clear-cut evidence of celiac disease on your biopsy despite having minimal symptoms or no symptoms whatsoever.

All of the above scenarios *are* celiac disease, and the treatment is a gluten-free diet. There's nothing "borderline" about it.

But there are other reasons you might be told of having "a little bit of" celiac disease. Perhaps you had an elevated tissue transglutaminase IgA level and a biopsy that was normal or showed only mild inflammation with no flattening of the villi. This is a case of *potential celiac disease* (see Chapter 4), a condition that is sometimes treated with a gluten-free diet but is usually monitored without eliminating gluten because some people with this condition have their antibodies normalize and never go on to develop celiac disease.

Because celiac disease is so important a condition, with so many health implications, if you've been diagnosed with "a little bit of" celiac disease, we encourage you to speak to your physician to find out on what basis this determination was made. If you had a small intestine biopsy, ask your physician what it showed and compare these findings to those we discuss in Chapter 3. If you didn't have a biopsy, ask what, if any, antibody studies were done and compare your results to those we also discuss in Chapter 3.

TIP

If you were told long ago that you had borderline celiac disease, it may (or may not) be worth your while to be retested for celiac disease beginning with having appropriate antibody or genetic testing done. (Often a genetic test is a particularly good way to start because, as we discuss in Chapter 3, if you don't have certain genes, you almost certainly cannot have had, or ever get, celiac disease.) Be sure to speak to your current doctor about this.

You Cannot Eat Buckwheat

You can't spell "Buckwheat" without W-H-E-A-T, so it must contain gluten, right? Nope. Buckwheat doesn't contain gluten; in fact, it isn't even closely related to the wheat family. This grain is a healthy, nutritious addition to your diet, regardless of whether you have celiac disease. Among other uses, buckwheat can be used as an ingredient in pancakes or added to salads and soups.

REMEMBER

There is, however, one important precaution: Some products contain both buckwheat *and* other, gluten-containing grains, so read labels carefully to make sure you purchase pure buckwheat or buckwheat mixed only with other gluten-free ingredients.

You Must Avoid All Products with Gluten

Sometimes it seems to us that gluten is about as ubiquitous as the air we all breathe. As we discuss in Chapter 9, gluten can be found not only in foods, but also in some shampoos, creams, and lotions. A commonly held myth is that if you have celiac disease or dermatitis herpetiformis (DH), using such gluten-containing products can trigger your celiac disease or your DH. In a word (well, two actually), it can't.

The only way that your celiac disease will be triggered is by you ingesting gluten. So long as your shampoo, cream, lotion, and so forth stay on your skin and out of your mouth, they won't come in contact with your small intestine and thus, will be unable to cause your disease to flare. This is also true of DH which, as we discuss in detail in Chapter 8, is a skin disease very closely linked with celiac disease. So even if you have DH, it's safe for you to use gluten-containing topical products.

Lipstick may also contain gluten, but so long as your lipstick does as its name says it should — that is, stick to your lips — your insides will remain a stranger to your lipstick's gluten and thus, your use of lipstick won't pose a risk.

TIP

For the sake of completeness, we'll add one qualifier here: Albeit very rare, it's possible that some speck of gluten-containing lipstick will, indeed, find its way into your insides and lead to problems. So if you're strictly avoiding gluten in your diet yet you continue to have gastrointestinal symptoms, make sure your lipstick is gluten-free. You'll need to check ingredients or contact the lipstick manufacturer to find this out.

Vinegar Is Forbidden

One commonly held myth about celiac disease is that if you have this condition, vinegar is off-limits. Well, if you, too, have this understanding, then we're pleased to say it ain't so. As it turns out, apart from malt vinegar, vinegar is perfectly fine for you to consume if you have celiac disease.

The reason for the exclusion of malt vinegar from the "vinegar is safe" policy is because it is made by malting barley and, as we discuss in Chapter 5, barley contains gluten. For this reason, if you have celiac disease, you should not consume malt vinegar.

Feeling Fine Means No Celiac Disease

People with celiac disease can have nausea, vomiting, bloating, abdominal cramps, diarrhea, weight loss and, as we look at in Chapter 2, many other symptoms. And people with celiac disease can have no symptoms at all. When someone with lots of symptoms gets a diagnosis of celiac disease as the cause of their problem, this is typically greeted with mixed emotions: relief at knowing that a cause has been found and that treatment will relieve their symptoms; and upset at finding out they have a chronic disease to contend with.

On the other hand, when someone who is entirely free of symptoms is diagnosed with celiac disease (for instance, due to screening, see Chapter 6), this can result in disbelief. "How can I have celiac disease? Celiac disease makes you feel lousy, and I feel fine," are common reactions.

As it is, however, you can feel perfectly well yet not only have celiac disease but actually have or later develop complications from it such as osteoporosis and anemia. Although in some ways, that you may feel perfectly well yet have celiac disease is good — who wants to feel unwell after all? — it can actually be a challenge because it understandably makes it harder for many people to accept the diagnosis and to follow a gluten-free diet.

WARNING

If your celiac disease was discovered during investigations to find out why you had some other health problem such as iron deficiency or osteoporosis, but, because you have no symptoms, you don't believe you actually have the condition and therefore haven't adopted a gluten-free diet, we strongly recommend you speak to your celiac disease specialist (or primary care provider) and share your thoughts with them. That person can then review with you on what basis the diagnosis was made and, if it turns out the diagnosis is uncertain, further evaluation would be in order. Otherwise, if the evidence is incontrovertible, we hope you come to accept that you have celiac disease and follow a gluten-free diet. It's your health after all, and you need to protect it.

If, however, you have potential celiac disease (see Chapter 4) without intestinal damage and with no apparent health problems, you and your physician need to decide together whether you should be treated.

You Are More Likely to Have Food Allergies and Food Intolerance

One common misunderstanding surrounding celiac disease is the impression that having this particular food-related condition makes you more likely to have *other* food-related conditions such as food allergies or intolerance. We can certainly see where this concern arises because all these conditions are related to the ingestion of food, but, in fact, with the exception of lactose intolerance (which we discuss in detail in Chapter 11) that's pretty well where the similarities end.

As we discuss in Chapter 5, there are major differences between celiac disease, food allergies, and food intolerance, including the time between when you eat something and when you start to react to it, the symptoms that occur, and the underlying immune problem, if any. Given the disparate nature to these conditions, discussing them in the same breath is, in keeping with our food theme, like comparing apples to oranges.

You Can't Share Cooking Implements

As we mention repeatedly in this book, having celiac disease means you must avoid any and all gluten. So you might reasonably conclude that would mean you should not share a toaster or cooking utensils with family members who are not on a gluten-free diet, lest these items become "contaminated" with gluten that might then be ingested.

Well, as it turns out, when it comes to sharing a toaster, this isn't quite as black and white as it might at first appear. It depends on the type of toaster you use:

>> **Toasters with removable racks:** If you use a toaster with racks, so long as you clean the racks (soap and water will do) before you use them, you'll be fine, and you don't require a separate toaster.

>> **Upright toasters:** If your family shares an upright toaster (which typically does not have removable racks), then it's very difficult to avoid having your bread pick up someone else's crumbs. Therefore, you may be better off using your own toaster.

As for sharing cooking utensils, again, so long as you wash them before you use them to prepare your own, gluten-free foods, you'll be fine.

For more information on these and other issues about cross-contamination have a look at Chapter 10.

If Your Old Symptoms Return, It's Likely Due to Celiac Disease

If you have celiac disease and you're meticulously following a gluten-free diet, you probably feel just fine. But, perhaps you can recall a time prior to your diagnosis, a time when — if you're like many people with celiac disease — you had gastrointestinal (GI) symptoms such as nausea or cramps or bloating or diarrhea or one of the many other celiac disease symptoms that we describe in detail in Chapter 2. Having this recollection, it would be perfectly understandable, should you happen to redevelop these symptoms, if you were to say to yourself "before I was diagnosed with celiac disease, I had these symptoms, and now they're back, so my celiac disease is likely responsible."

Well, although we agree that this line of thought would be perfectly reasonable, it may not actually be accurate. Indeed, if you're being really careful with your gluten-free diet, there's a darn good chance that your recurrent symptoms are unrelated to your celiac disease and may be due to something else altogether. In other words, having excellently controlled celiac disease doesn't protect you from getting the other health problems that anyone else can get. Also, as we discuss in Chapter 8, having celiac disease does increase your risk of developing certain other ailments.

Here are just a few examples of symptoms that may mislead you (and, by the way, your healthcare provider) into prematurely concluding your celiac disease is flaring:

>> **Abdominal cramps and diarrhea:** Sure, these symptoms could reflect a flare of your celiac disease. On the other hand, they could actually mean you've come down with a gastrointestinal infection (like stomach flu or food poisoning for example).

>> **Nausea:** Perhaps this is due not to your celiac disease but has occurred as a side effect from a new medication you're taking.

>> **Fatigue:** Type "fatigue" into a search engine and you'll get millions of hits. Type "fatigue" and "celiac disease" into that same search engine and you'll get several hundred thousand hits. In other words, there are tons of causes of fatigue unrelated to celiac disease.

>> **Weight loss:** Although active celiac disease causes malabsorption and this in turn can lead to weight loss, many other conditions also cause weight loss, including hyperthyroidism (thyroid overfunctioning) which occurs with increased frequency among people with celiac disease — regardless whether the celiac disease is under control.

Having said all this, you shouldn't discount the possibility that your symptoms are indeed indicative of your celiac disease flaring. What to do? We recommend, if you redevelop GI problems or other of your previous symptoms and they don't promptly settle, that you check carefully to see whether you are inadvertently ingesting gluten (see Chapter 10 for a discussion on what foods contain gluten and on hidden sources of gluten).

If you're accidentally consuming gluten, of course you need to eliminate it. If you're not, then, as we discuss in detail in Chapter 12, there remain a number of other possible causes that may account for your symptoms and for which you and your healthcare provider can explore.

Appendixes

Appendix **A**

Resources to Supplement the Gluten-Free Diet

The gluten-free diet is about more than just what foods to avoid. It's also about enjoying your new diet and being healthy. In this appendix, we provide resources that the dietitian covers beyond the basics of identifying and avoiding gluten. This includes having a diverse diet that includes gluten-free whole grains, and guidelines on physical activity, supplements, and general nutrition.

The Importance of Gluten-Free Whole Grains

Studies have shown that individuals on a gluten-free diet may not be getting enough dietary vitamins, minerals, and fiber. Gluten-free packaged foods are not typically fortified with vitamins and minerals the same way wheat-based products are.

An easy and delicious way to increase the nutrient value of the gluten-free diet is by incorporating naturally gluten-free grains. While you may never have heard of these grains, they're delicious, easy to prepare, and very nutritious. They have the vitamins and minerals often found lacking in the gluten-free diet.

Try incorporating these grains into your meals:

>> Amaranth

>> Buckwheat

>> Millet

>> Oats (gluten-free)

>> Quinoa

>> Rice (flour, brown rice, white rice, wild rice, rice bran)

>> Sorghum

>> Teff

To make life easy, Table A-1 explains how to prepare your new staples.

TABLE A-1   **Grain Preparation Table**

Grain	Amount of Liquid	Amount of Grain	Cooking Time*	Uses
Amaranth	1 cup	1 cup	Simmer 7 minutes, let stand 5 to 10 minutes	Hot cereal
Buckwheat	2 cups	1 cup	Simmer 15 minutes	Hot cereal, side dish, casserole
Millet	1½ cups	1 cup	Simmer 15 minutes and then let stand covered 10 minutes	Hot cereal, side dish
Oats	1 cup	½ cup	Simmer 15 minutes	Hot cereal, binder for meatloaf
Quinoa	2 cups	1 cup	Simmer 10 to 15 minutes	Side dish, cold salad
Teff	2 cups	½ cup	Simmer 15 to 20 minutes	Hot cereal
Wild rice	1 cup	1 cup	Simmer 30 minutes	Side dish, stuffing

Gluten-free broth or soup may be used as a substitution for the water to add flavor to the grain.

Physical Activity and Exercise

Being healthy isn't just about a good, balanced gluten-free diet; it's also about being active! Physical activity has been shown to have a variety of positive effects on your overall health:

>> Improves cardiovascular and respiratory health

>> Decreases risk of developing 13 different cancers

>> Decreases symptoms of anxiety and depression

>> Decreases inflammation, insulin needs, and resting blood pressure

>> Decreases morbidity and mortality

Physical activity recommendations for individuals with celiac disease are the same as those for the general population, unless otherwise specified by a physician.

According to the 2018 Physical Activity Guidelines for Americans published by the United States Department of Health and Human Services, adults should move more and sit less. For substantial benefits, physical activity beyond the daily routine is recommended. Table A-2 outlines time goals for various intensities of exercise.

TABLE A-2

Exercise Recommendations for Adults (ages 18 to 64)

Type/Intensity	Time per Week
Moderate physical activity	150 to 300 minutes
Vigorous physical activity	75 to 150 minutes
A combination of moderate and vigorous physical activity	Proportional equivalent time recommended for each category

Within the total time recommended in Table A-2, adults should perform muscle-strengthening activities at least two days per week.

For more information, check out the physical activity guidelines for Americans from the Department of Health and Human Services and the Centers for Disease Control and Prevention at https://odphp.health.gov/sites/default/files/2019-09/Physical_Activity_Guidelines_2nd_edition.pdf.

General Nutrition, Vitamins, and Minerals

Chapter 10 focuses on the nutritional needs your diet needs to meet. Here are some sites that provide helpful information on healthy eating.

The Center for Nutrition Policy of the United States Department of Agriculture

www.myplate.gov

This branch of government has created MyPlate.gov to provide "steps to a healthier you." On this site you'll find lots of information on healthy eating and, in a clear sign of this digital era, podcasts to download.

The National Institutes of Health Office of Dietary Supplements

https://ods.od.nih.gov

This site provides detailed information on the use of dietary supplements.

Health Canada

https://food-guide.canada.ca/en

Health Canada's highly respected Canada's Food Guide is available at this site.

The National Dairy Council

www.usdairy.com

The National Dairy Council site has, as you might expect, information on dairy nutrition. Here you will find information on vitamin D and calcium, and there are also helpful materials on lactose intolerance.

Gluten-Free Medications

We reviewed medications in Chapter 10. Here are some sites to find more information:

>> **Gluten-Free Drugs** (www.glutenfreedrugs.com)

>> **American Society of Health-System Pharmacists** (www.ashp.org)

Appendix **B**

Resources for Other Nutritional Considerations

As we discuss in Chapter 11, it's not uncommon to have additional dietary restrictions beyond the gluten-free diet. In this appendix, we offer several sites that will help you navigate any of these additional dietary concerns.

Lactose Intolerance

National Institutes of Health

www.nih.gov

The Mayo Clinic

www.mayoclinic.org

Cleveland Clinic Health Library

https://my.clevelandclinic.org/health

The Mayo Clinic Nutrition and Healthy Eating

www.mayoclinic.org/healthy-lifestyle/nutrition-and-healthy-eating/
in-depth/vegetarian-diet/art-20046446

National Health Services

www.nhs.uk/live-well/eat-well/how-to-eat-a-balanced-diet/the-
vegetarian-diet/USDA Nutrition.gov Eating Vegetarian

www.nutrition.gov/topics/basic-nutrition/eating-vegetarian

Food Allergies

The Food Allergy & Anaphylaxis Connection Team

www.foodallergyawareness.org

Food Allergy Research and Education (FARE)

www.foodallergy.org

Other Gastrointestinal Conditions

As we discuss in Chapter 12, if you have celiac disease and you continue to have gastrointestinal (GI) symptoms despite following a gluten-free diet, it could be that you have some other, coexisting GI condition. Here are some websites where you can find more information on some of these conditions.

Inflammatory bowel disease

The Crohn's & Colitis Foundation

www.crohnscolitisfoundation.org

Functional gastrointestinal disorders

Also known as disorders of gut-brain interaction (DGBIs), which include irritable bowel syndrome and functional dyspepsia.

International Foundation for Gastrointestinal Disorders

https://iffgd.org

National Institute of Health, "Management of Functional Gastrointestinal Disorders"

https://pmc.ncbi.nlm.nih.gov/articles/PMC7850201/Rome Foundation

https://theromefoundation.org

Monash University

www.monashfodmap.com

Fructose Intolerance

Fructose is the sugar naturally found in many fruits and vegetables. Some individuals can't tolerate it, as some people can't tolerate lactose.

Cleveland Clinic, "What Is Fructose Intolerance?"

https://health.clevelandclinic.org/what-is-fructose-intolerance

Appendix C

Resources to Help Navigate the Gluten-Free Diet

The Internet and social media can be a source for great up-to-date information or a nightmare of gluten-free horror stories. In this appendix, we provide some recommendations for resources, but please always take what you read online with a very practical view or a grain of salt!

TIP

Some notes before we get to our list:

>> If you're looking for university-based celiac disease centers, celiac disease support groups, or celiac disease foundations, you can find these listed in Appendix D.

>> If you're wondering whether you should trust a site that you come across as you surf the web and it isn't listed in this appendix, have a look at Chapter 1, where we discuss helpful ways to determine the likely worth of an online resource.

>> Most important, always first speak to your healthcare providers before you make any change to your celiac disease (or other health) management based on what you've read online.

One other thing before we move on: Some of the sites listed here are commercial and have products, such as gluten-free cookbooks, for sale. These cookbooks can be very helpful, which is why we mention the sites in the first place. For the record, though, we want to note that we have no affiliation — in particular, no financial interest — whatsoever with any of these sites.

Dining Out or Ordering In

When dining out or ordering in, always be sure to let the restaurant know your meal needs to be gluten-free. There are now smartphone apps (available at the iPhone's App Store or Android's `play.google.com`) with lists of restaurants with gluten-free options. Here are some examples:

» Find Me Gluten Free

» Atly

» Gluten Free Global

» The Celiac App

» Allergy Eats

Traveling Gluten-Free

Having celiac disease and following a gluten-free diet doesn't have to prevent you from traveling the world. It may take a bit more research before you go, but we encourage you to spread your wings and explore! Here are some resources to make your journeys easier:

» **Schar Gluten Free** (`www.schaer.com/en-us/lifestyle/travel`) offers country-by-country tips.

» **Celiac Travel** (`www.celiactravel.com`) is a site devoted to, as you might have guessed from its name, traveling if you have celiac disease.

» **Celiac Disease Foundation** (`https://celiac.org/2023/06/28/traveling-gluten-free`) offers practical suggestions for traveling while following a gluten-free diet.

» **Triumph Dining** (`https://tinyurl.com/3jbvz9py`) sells a gluten-free restaurant guide and a gluten-free grocery guide.

» **Gluten-Free Globe Trotter** (`https://glutenfreeglobetrotter.com`) has all the inside information on traveling the globe as well as the United States.

» **Gluten-Free Allergy-Free Passport** (`https://glutenfreepassport.com`) offers wide-ranging products to assist the person living with celiac disease as they trek around the globe.

Appendix **D**

Organizations for People with Celiac Disease

I n recent years, there has been an explosion in the number of societies, centers, foundations, and support groups for and about celiac disease. You'll find many of them listed in this appendix. We tried to be comprehensive, but the list grows daily!

Celiac Disease Societies and Support Groups

As we discuss in Chapter 1, if you have celiac disease, you may find belonging to a support group helpful. In today's connected world, some groups meet in person and others online. Find a group that has the best options for you.

The organizations we discuss in this appendix include some with local chapters; you can find them listed on the main websites that we provide.

The Canadian Celiac Association (CCA)

www.celiac.ca

The Canadian Celiac Association (CCA) is the longest running celiac disease support organization in North America. It was founded in 1972 by two women, both of whom had family members with celiac disease.

National Celiac Association (NCA)

https://nationalceliac.org

NCA is a patient organization focused on education through meetings (online and in person), webinars, and advocacy.

The Gluten Intolerance Group of North America (GIG)

https://gluten.org

The Gluten Intolerance Group of North America is a large, national, non-profit organization founded in 1974 and based in Washington state. Its mission is to "provide support to persons with gluten intolerances, including celiac disease, dermatitis herpetiformis, and other gluten sensitivities, in order to live healthy lives."

Foundations and Organizations

Over the past few years, a number of foundations and organizations have been created to provide a broad and unified voice for people living with celiac disease.

The Celiac Disease Foundation

https://celiac.org

The Celiac Disease Foundation is a national non-profit group established in 1990 that's "dedicated to providing services and support regarding celiac disease and dermatitis herpetiformis through programs of awareness, education advocacy and research."

Beyond Celiac

www.beyondceliac.org

Beyond Celiac is non-profit foundation created in 2003 with this mission statement: "Beyond Celiac unites with patients and partners to drive diagnosis, advance research and accelerate the discovery of new treatments and a cure."

Societies for the Study of Celiac Disease

These groups provide information, educational grants, webinars, and conferences for both the healthcare professional and the patient.

Society for the Study of Celiac Disease

https://theceliacsociety.org

The SSCD has a wealth of educational activities for members and maintains a Unit Recognition Program for centers that have met the criteria for excellence in celiac disease specialization.

International Society for the Study of Celiac Disease

www.isscd-global.org/home

The mission of the ISSCD is "to promote scientific knowledge regarding the field of celiac disease and gluten-mediated human disease." ISSCD sponsors research and educational events around the world and hosts a biennial international symposium dedicated to celiac disease research.

Celiac Disease Centers

The following university-based centers have a longstanding involvement in celiac disease clinical care, research, and education:

>> Celiac Disease Center at Columbia University, https://celiacdisease center.columbia.edu

>> Celiac Disease Unit at McMaster University, `https://farncombe.mcmaster.ca`

>> Celiac Research Program at Harvard Medical School, `https://hms.harvard.edu/departments/hms-celiac-research-program`

>> Cleveland Clinic Celiac Disease Program, `https://my.clevelandclinic.org/departments/digestive/depts/celiac-disease`

>> Colorado Children's Hospital, `www.childrenscolorado.org/doctors-and-departments/departments/digestive-health/programs/center-celiac-disease`

>> The University of Chicago Celiac Disease Center, `www.uchicagomedicine.org/conditions-services/gastroenterology/celiac-disease`

>> Vanderbilt Celiac Center Clinic, `www.vanderbilthealth.com/clinic/celiac-disease-clinic`

Index

calcium channel blockers, 157

calories, 238–240

Canadian Celiac Association (CCA), 330

cancer, 163–164
  prevention, 171–172
  and refractory celiac disease, 225
  related to celiac disease, 38, 166–170
  risk factors, 163–166, 171
  screening, 171
  and weight loss, 32

candidiasis, 153

canned food, 182, 183

capsule endoscopy (CE), 64–65, 168, 171, 237

carbohydrate counting, 147

carbohydrates, 26, 147, 149, 198

caries, 153

carotenoids, 209

case finding, 111

CCA. *See* Canadian Celiac Association

CE. *See* capsule endoscopy

celiac disease, 8, 23. *See also specific types*
  causes of, 9, 84–91, 90–91
  clinical presentation, changes in, 280
  complications of, 10, 45, 106
  discovering at-risk population, 280
  discovery of, 10
  effects of, 10
  and food allergy/intolerance, 96–97, 178
  and gluten sensitivity, 97–98
  myths about, 307–315
  outgrowing, 291
  prevention of, 276, 280–281, 289
  types of, 68
  up-to-date information about, 298–299

Celiac Disease Foundation, 330

Center for Nutrition Policy, 322

central nervous system, 144

chat groups, 16

chemotherapy, 169

chewing food, difficulty in, 153

children, 276
  ADHD in, 146
  autism spectrum disorder in, 146
  calcium deficiency in, 121
  and celiac disease prevention, 289
  classical celiac disease in, 69
  developmental delay, 143
  diabetes in, 148
  diagnosis of celiac disease in, 256–261
  failure to thrive, 33, 69, 258
  gluten-free diet for, 180, 262–267
  growth of, 233
  involvement in shopping and cooking, 265
  non-classical celiac disease in, 70
  play materials with gluten, 195
  recommended calcium intake for, 201–202
  rickets in, 130–131
  screening of, 260–261, 290
  visits to friends, 264, 300
  vitamin A deficiency in, 117

chromosome defects, 39

chromosome disorders, 159–160

citrus juice, 124

classical celiac disease, 241, 282
  in children, 256
  diagnosis of, 69
  and nutritional deficiencies, 199
  symptoms of, 22, 24, 25, 30, 68, 69

coated iron supplements, 123

coffee, 28, 201

colitis, 64, 219

collagenous colitis, 219

college students, gluten-free diet for, 266–267

colon, 104

colon cancer, 170

colonoscopy, 53, 64, 126, 171

communion wafer, 195

complete protein, 210

confocal microscopy, 272

connective tissue disorders, 152–155

conspiracy thinking, 16

constipation, 23, 124, 233, 241–244, 257

cooking, 302. *See also* food shopping

  and children with celiac disease, 263

  gluten-free food, 184–186

  myths about, 313–314

  in support groups, 19

cornea, ulceration of, 154

cornstarch, 183, 184

corticosteroid-containing creams, 140

corticosteroids, 141, 151, 225

cortisol, 152

cramps, abdominal, 27, 315

cross-contact, 188, 192–193

croutons, 184

crypt hyperplasia, 105

crypts, 105

CT enterography, 168

CT scan, 168

cutting boards, 193

cytokines, 88, 275

D

dairy products, 202, 206, 208

dapsone, 140

deamidated gliadin peptide (DGP), 47, 48

deamidation, 88

defecation, 104

dehydration, 44, 52

denial, after diagnosis, 12–13

dental cavities, 153

dental problems, 38, 131, 132–133, 153, 170

depression, 32, 35, 36, 142–143

dermatitis herpetiformis (DH), 34, 44, 137–140, 141, 311

  in children, 258, 259

  diagnosis of, 138–139

  symptoms of, 137–138

  treatment of, 139–140

developmental delay, 143, 259

DEXA scan. *See* bone mineral density (BMD) test

DGP. *See* deamidated gliadin peptide

DH. *See* dermatitis herpetiformis

diabetes, 37, 104, 147–148

  and blood glucose level, 149

  and celiac screening, 148

  in children, 260

  medications, and endoscopy procedure, 54

  non-classical celiac disease, 75–76

  treatment, 147–148

  and weight loss, 32

diagnosis, 9–10, 41, 287–289. *See also specific diagnostic tests*

  accuracy of, 62–66

  Addison's disease, 152

  blood tests, 44–52

  celiac disease, in children, 256–261

  classical celiac disease, 69

  complications, and gluten-free diet, 60–62

  dermatitis herpetiformis, 138–139

  emotional response to, 12–14, 142

  enteropathy-associated T cell lymphoma, 168–169

  folate deficiency, 118

  future research, 281

  gastroparesis, 220–221

  and gluten sensitivity, 99

  hyperthyroidism, 150

  hypothyroidism, 151

  importance of symptoms, 42–43

  improvements in, 272

  iron-deficiency anemia, 125–127

  lactose intolerance, 207–208

  liver enzyme levels, 157–158

  misdiagnosis, 13, 27, 41

  osteoporosis, 73–74, 129

  pancreatic insufficiency, 219

  potential celiac disease, 78

  refractory celiac disease, 224

gluten-free diet, response to, 212
  antibody tests, 213
  blood tests, 213–214
  intestinal biopsy, 214–215
  nonresponsive celiac disease, 215–223
  symptoms, 212–213
glutenin, 95, 186
gluten-sensitive enteropathy. *See* celiac disease
gnocchi, 188
grains, 92
  gluten-free, 319–320
  myths about, 311
  sources of gluten, 92, 95–96, 176
  vegetarian diet, 210
grand mal seizures, 146
granular IgA antibodies, 138
Graves' disease, 149–150
grilling surfaces, 193
gum disease, 153
gynecological problems, 38

H

H2 blockers, 29
handwashing, 195
Hashimoto's thyroiditis, 150–151
headache, 35, 144
Health Canada, 322
health insurance, 182, 237
healthcare providers, visit to, 230–231
healthy habits, 298
heart rate, 44
heartburn, 28–30
height, examination of, 43–44
hemoglobin, 52, 213
histamines, 97
HLA. *See* human leukocyte associated gene
hordein, 95, 176
hormones
  and digestion process, 104
  endocrine disorders, 147–153
  H2 blockers, 29

hormonal problems, 37
  and infertility, 252–253
hospitalization, 248–249
human leukocyte associated (HLA) gene, 85–86, 271
  HLA DQ2/DQ8 genes, 85–86, 112, 271, 275
  HLA DQ2/DQ8 test, 50–51, 59, 61, 64, 112, 261
  role in disease process, 85
humidifier, 154
hygiene hypothesis, 91
hyperthyroidism, 32, 36, 37, 149–150
hypocalcemia, 143
hypoglycemia, 149
hyposplenism, 134
hypothyroidism, 36, 37, 150–151

I

IBS. *See* irritable bowel syndrome
IELs. *See* intra-epithelial lymphocytes
IgA deficiency, 38, 47–48, 69, 161, 213
IL-15. *See* interleukin 15
ileoscopy, 64
ileum, 64, 102, 103, 118, 145
immediate hypersensitivity reaction, 97
immune response, 84, 87–88, 271
  and dermatitis herpetiformis, 139
  and food allergies/intolerance, 97
  to gluten, changing, 275–276
  and small intestine, 105
  triggers, 89
immune system, 86, 309
  and cancer risk, 165
  and celiac disease, 84
  components of, 86–87
  function of, 86
  and neurological problems, 143
  role in disease process, 87–88
  and vitamin deficiencies, 117, 119
immune-modulating creams, 140

immunoglobulins, 45–50, 69, 161

immunology, 279

indigestion, 30

infants, 206. *See also* children
  gluten exposure of, 91
  introduction of gluten to, 256
  and pregnancy complications, 254
  recommended calcium intake for, 201

infections, 91, 134, 154, 215

infertility, 74–75, 133, 252, 255

inflammation, 142, 215
  and cancer risk, 166, 171
  connective tissue disorder, 152–155
  in intestinal biopsy results, 58
  skin rashes, 34–35, 136–140, 155, 258, 259
  and vitamin B deficiency, 117, 118

inflammatory bowel disease, 222, 324

injection, iron, 124

insoluble fiber, 242–243

insulin, 104, 147, 149

interleukin 15 (IL-15), 274, 283

International Society for the Study of Celiac
    Disease (ISSCD), 331

intestinal biopsy. *See* biopsy, intestinal

intestinal cancer, 32

intestinal permeability, 89

intra-epithelial lymphocytes (IELs), 105,
    167, 215, 220

intrauterine growth restriction, 254

iron, sources of, 122–123

iron deficiency, 123, 214, 293
  dietary strategies for, 200–201
  and pregnancy preparation, 255
  treatment, 123–124

iron-deficiency anemia, 36, 72, 125, 234
  diagnosis of, 125–127
  in elderly people, 126–127
  treatment, 127

irritable bowel syndrome (IBS), 24, 27, 61,
    71, 221, 222

ISSCD. *See* International Society for the Study of
    Celiac Disease

J

JAK inhibitors, 283

jaundice, 158, 170

jejunum, 57, 102, 103, 105, 123

joints, 152–157

K

knock knees, 131

L

lactase, 206, 207, 208

lactose, 206

lactose intolerance, 11, 202, 205–206
  diagnosis of, 207–208
  and lactase levels, 207
  population affected by, 206
  and response to gluten-free diet, 217–218
  symptoms of, 206–207
  treatment, 208
  websites related to, 323–324

larazotide, 274

large intestine, 100
  biopsy, 220
  cancer, 170
  role in digestion process, 104

Latiglutenase, 274

laxatives, 243–244

leakiness, 89

legs, physical examination of, 44

lipstick, 311–312

liver, 100
  cancer, 170
  disease, 38
  disorders, 157–159
  role in digestion process, 102, 104
  tests, 52, 158
  transplant, 158

local support groups, 18–19

lower esophageal sphincter, 28

low-impact fracture, 73, 74

lupus. *See* systemic lupus erythematosis (SLE)

lymphocytes, 105

lymphocytic colitis, 219

lymphoma, 166–169

M

macrophages, 87

magnesium, 130, 146

malabsorption, 24, 106, 115, 199, 203, 236, 238, 258, 308

  and blood glucose level, 75

  and BMI, 44

  and cancer risk, 165

  and classical celiac disease, 69

  and diabetes, 149

  effects of, 25

  and epilepsy, 146

  and infertility, 252–253

  mineral deficiency, 121–125

  and neurological problems, 143

  and non-classical celiac disease, 73–74

  nutritional tests, 52

  and osteomalacia, 131–132

  and osteoporosis, 73–74

  and pancreatic insufficiency, 219

  and peripheral neuropathy, 145

  rickets, 130–131

  and vitamin deficiency, 116–121

  and weight loss, 31, 32

malnutrition, 198–205, 259

malt vinegar, 312

malt-based products, 183

MASH. *See* metabolic dysfunction-associated steatohepatitis

mast cells, 87, 97

matzah/matzoh, 188, 195

meal plan, 186, 266

meat, 184, 185, 187

medical history, 42–43, 246

medications, 246

  causing oral dryness, 154

  dermatitis herpetiformis, 139–140

  and endoscopy procedure, 54

  for fibromyalgia, 157

  for gastroesophageal reflux, 29–30

  gluten-free, 322

  glutens hidden in, 194

  and microscopic colitis, 220

  for migraine headache, 144

  for osteoporosis, 130

  for psoriasis, 141

  for Raynaud's phenomenon, 157

  refractory celiac disease, 225

megaloblastic anemia, 128

menstrual periods, 126, 252

metabolic dysfunction-associated steatohepatitis (MASH), 158

microscopic colitis, 219–220

microvilli, 103–104, 106

migraine headache, 35, 144

mineral deficiency, 121–125

mineralocorticoid deficiency, 151

minerals, 106, 198. *See also specific minerals*

miscarriage, 117, 133, 253, 254, 255

misinformation, 277–278

modified food starch, 183

monitoring, of celiac disease, 229–237

  frequency of visits to healthcare providers, 230–231

  healthcare professional responsible for, 231–232

  improvements, 272–273

  and rules, 230

  topics of discussion, 232–237

mood disorders, 35, 156

mouth

  ailments, 38, 123, 133, 153

  and digestion process, 101

  guard, 55

  physical examination of, 44

mucosa, 58

mucosal immune system, 86

mucosal surfaces, 86

Murray, Joseph, 280

musculoskeletal problems, 37, 152–157

N

National Celiac Association (NCA), 19, 330
National Dairy Council, 322
National Institutes of Health, 322, 323
natural broths, 188
nausea, 315
NCA. *See* National Celiac Association
nerve damage, 118, 120, 144–145
neurological disorders, 35, 143–146. *See also*
    specific disorders
neutrophils, 87
new information, making sense of, 278–279
night blindness, 117
night sweats, 159
non-celiac gluten sensitivity. *See* gluten, sensitivity
non-classical celiac disease, 68, 70–71, 280, 282
    in children, 257
    and nutritional deficiencies, 199
    symptoms of, 22, 25, 30, 68, 71–76
non-Hodgkin lymphoma, 164, 167
nonresponsive celiac disease, 215
    conditions coexisting with celiac
        disease, 221–222
    conditions complicating celiac disease, 217–221
    continued exposure to gluten, 216–217
    enteropathy-associated T cell lymphoma, 226
    overall approach to, 223
    refractory celiac disease, 224–225
    wrong diagnosis, 222
non-tropical sprue. *See* celiac disease
non-ulcer dyspepsia, 221
numbness, 35, 144
nutrition, 197, 321–325. *See also specific entries*
    deficiencies, 198, 199, 200
    and gluten-free diet, 198–205
    issues, mangement of, 237–244
    tests, 52

O

oats, 95, 192, 278, 295
obstetrical problems, 38

occult GI blood loss, 126–127
Office of Dietary Supplements, National Institutes
    of Health, 322
ongoing care, celiac disease
    advocacy, 247–249
    doctor visits, 245–246
    gaining expertise on celiac disease, 247
    monitoring, 229–237
    nutrition issues, 237–244
    rules for management, 229–230
online advertising, 15
online support groups, 16–18
oral cavity, cancer of, 170
oral health, 132–133
oral hygiene, 154, 155
organizations, celiac disease, 277–278, 329–332
osmotic laxatives, 243
osteomalacia, 131–132
osteoporosis, 33, 37, 129, 234
    and calcium deficiency, 121
    and non-classical celiac disease, 73–74
    versus osteomalacia, 131–132
    and vitamin D deficiency, 119
overeating, and reflux, 28
ovulation, 252, 253

P

pancreas, 100, 149
    cancer, 170
    role in digestion process, 102, 104
pancreatic enzyme supplements, 219
pancreatic insufficiency, 32, 219
papier-mâché, 195
partial villous atrophy, 105
pasta, 184, 185
pathogenesis, 279, 280
PBC. *See* primary biliary cholangitis
PEG. *See* polyethylene glycol
peptic duodenitis, 63
peripheral nervous system, 144
peripheral neuropathy, 35, 144–145

peristalsis, 64–65

pernicious anemia, 128

PET scan, 168

pharmacists, 194

phosphates, 123

physical activity, 320–321

physical examination, 42, 47–48, 138, 168, 259

phytates, 201, 210

pizza, 185

play dough, 195

pneumococcus, 134

policy, public, 276–277

polyethylene glycol (PEG), 243

positive thinking, 14

potassium competitive acid blockers, 29

potential celiac disease, 68, 78–79, 113, 281, 310

  diagnosis of, 78

  and silent celiac disease, difference between, 78

  symptoms of, 68

pregnancy

  complications of, 133, 253–255

  and folate deficiency, 117

  and heartburn, 28

  preparation for, 255

premature delivery, 254

preschool children, gluten-free diet for, 263–264

pre-term delivery, 254

primary biliary cholangitis (PBC), 158

primary healthcare provider, 231

primary sclerosing cholangitis (PSC), 159

processed food, 182, 183, 192, 204

prolamins, 92

proteins, 198, 210

proton pump inhibitors, 29

PSC. See primary sclerosing cholangitis

psoriasis, 35, 141

psyllium, 242

public awareness, 276–279, 283

push enteroscope, 65

pylorus, 56

Q

quinoa, 210

R

radiation therapy, 169

rashes, 34–35, 136–140, 155, 258, 259

Raynaud's phenomenon, 37, 157

RCD. See refractory celiac disease

rectal examination, 44

rectum, 100, 104

reflux. See gastroesophageal reflux

refractory celiac disease (RCD), 224–225, 244, 282–283

relative risk, 164, 165

respiratory system, 154

restaurant dining, 179–180, 187–188, 267, 299, 301, 302, 328

rheumatologic disorders, 37, 152–157

rickets, 37, 69, 119, 121, 130–131, 258

roughage, 242–243

rye, 95

S

sadness, after diagnosis, 13, 142

salad, 184, 185

saliva, 101, 133, 153

saliva tests, 59

saturated fats, 204–205

scientific knowledge, updating, 298–299

scientific research, 15, 16, 270

  areas of further investigation, 279–283

  decreasing gluten uptake, 274

  diagnostic improvements, 272

  digestive enzyme supplements, 273–274

  genetic susceptibility, 270, 271

  and misinformation, 278

  monitoring improvements, 272–273

  silent celiac disease, 79

screening, 107, 108, 257

  asymptomatic individuals, 113

  cancer, 171

primary biliary cholangitis, 158
primary sclerosing cholangitis, 159
psoriasis, 141
Raynaud's phenomenon, 157
reflux, 28–30
refractory celiac disease, 225
reputable websites, 15–16
and screening, 111
silent celiac disease, 76–77, 113
Sjogren's syndrome, 154–155
small intestine adenocarcinoma, 169
triglyceride, 102
triptans, 144
triticale, 95
TTG. *See* tissue transglutaminase
Turner syndrome, 160
type 1 diabetes, 37, 75–76, 147–148, 260
type 2 diabetes, 147

U

ultrasound, 171
United States Department of Agriculture, 322
universal screening, 109
university-based celiac disease centers, 331–332
unsaturated fats, 204
upright toasters, 314
utensils, cooking, 193, 313–314

V

vaginal dryness, 150
vaginal lubricants, 155
vegans, 127, 209–210
vegetarians, 127, 209–210
verifiable facts, in websites, 16
villi, 58, 103–104, 105, 106
villous atrophy, 214, 215
vinegar, 312
vitamin A, 116–117
vitamin B_9, 72, 125
anemia, 128
deficiency, 117–118, 128
sources of, 117

vitamin B_{12}, 125
anemia, 72, 128
deficiency, 118, 128, 145
sources of, 118
and vegetarian diet, 210
vitamin C, 124, 201
vitamin D, 33, 130, 131, 132, 141
and calcium deficiency, 122
deficiency, 119, 213–214, 234, 258
and osteoporosis, 73
sources of, 119
vitamin E, 120
vitamin K, 120–121
vitamins, 198. *See also specific vitamins*
deficiencies, 116–121
dietitian consult, 116
effects of celiac disease, 106
supplements, 116, 118
vitiligo, 35, 140–141

W

water-soluble vitamins, 198
websites
benefits of, 247
BMI calculator, 44, 238
FGID, 222
food allergy, 324
fructose intolerance, 325
gastrointestinal conditions, 324–325
gluten-free medications, 322
lactose intolerance, 323–324
medications with gluten, 194
navigating gluten-free diet, 327–329
objective information in, 15
physical activity guidelines, 321
related to nutrition, 321–325
reliability of sources, 15–16, 277
support groups, 16–18
tax deductions for gluten-free diet, 181
travel, 328

About the Authors

Benjamin Lebwohl, MD, MS, is Professor of Medicine and Epidemiology at Columbia University Irving Center, where he practices as a gastroenterologist and serves as Director of Clinical Research at the Celiac Disease Center. He is the past president of the Society for the Study of Celiac Disease and collaborates with investigators in the United States and abroad in epidemiology, patterns of care, natural history, and therapeutics. Ben has coauthored more than 350 peer-reviewed publications, including national guidelines for the diagnosis and management of celiac disease. His research has been supported by the National Institutes of Health, the American Gastroenterological Association, the Celiac Disease Foundation, and the American Scandinavian Foundation. Dr. Lebwohl served on the Gastrointestinal Drugs Advisory Committee of the United States Food and Drug Administration (2017–2025), including a term as chairperson. He is heavily involved in medical education and lectures regularly to trainees on topics including celiac disease, evidence-based medicine, clinical decision-making, pseudoscience, diarrhea, the Beethoven string quartets, and colorectal cancer screening.

Anne Roland Lee, EdD, RDN, LD, is an Assistant Professor of Nutritional Medicine in the Department of Medicine and the Institute for Human Nutrition at Columbia University. She is the lead dietitian for the Celiac Disease Center and its nutrition research. Anne is involved in patient care and research. Her research and published work focus on quality-of-life issues, dietary adherence, concerns of the nutritional quality of the gluten-free diet, and eating patterns and behaviors. Anne's research on eating behaviors has provided insight into the impact of the rigidity of the gluten-free diet on eating patterns and behaviors and has created a paradigm shift in the education and counseling of individuals with celiac disease. Currently, she is leading an international group to define standards for nutritional assessment, education, and adherence of individuals with celiac disease.

Dedication

Ben: This book is dedicated to my immediate family: my children, Lily, Jakey, and Miri; my parents, Oscar and Vida; my brothers, Martin, Zachary, and Isaac; and most of all, my wife, Rachel. They have provided a loving home and foundation from which all else springs, including a fulfilling professional life of medicine and discovery.

Anne: This book is dedicated to my family and colleagues, and our patients who have provided their support, direction, and inspiration for both this book and my professional path. I also want to give a special acknowledgment to my three children and their children, who are truly the wind beneath my wings.

Authors' Acknowledgments

Both: First, a huge acknowledgment to Drs. Ian Blumer and Sheila Crowe, the authors of the first edition of this book. The current edition builds on their work. Much of their writing is retained, and we are grateful for their permission to update their text. We would not be in the position to write this book if it were not for our mentor, Peter Green, MD. Peter's curiosity, enthusiasm, and generosity have been the driving force for The Celiac Disease Center at Columbia University, which has been at the forefront of patient care, research, education, and advocacy. Our colleagues at the center — including physicians, research coordinators, and staff — work daily to advance our mission to improve the lives of people living with this condition.

Ben: I am particularly grateful to Anne Lee. Anne's expertise is unparalleled, and I'm lucky to have the opportunity to be her partner in authoring this book and in taking care of patients at our center.

Anne: I cannot express enough gratitude to Ben. Without his intellect, guidance, support, and compassion, this book would not be possible.

Publisher's Acknowledgments

Acquisitions Editor: Elizabeth Stilwell

Project Manager: Charlotte Kughen

Copy Editor: Charlotte Kughen

Managing Editor: Ajith Kumar

Production Editor: Magesh Elangovan

Cover Images: © illustrart/Getty Images, © 9dream studio/Shutterstock

12 301

SAVING FOR DEVELOPMENT